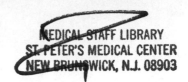

CLUSTER HEADACHE SYNDROME

Volume 23 in the Series

Major Problems in Neurology
LORD WALTON OF DETCHANT, TD, MD, DSc, FRCP
PROFESSOR CP WARLOW, BA, MB, BChir, MD, FRCP
Consulting Editors

OTHER MONOGRAPHS IN THE SERIES

CLUSTER HEADACHE SYNDROME

OTTAR SJAASTAD
Professor of Medicine
Regionsykehuset i Trondheim
Neurologisk avdeling
7006 Trondheim
Norway

W. B. Saunders Company Ltd   London   ·   Philadelphia
Toronto   ·   Sydney   ·   Tokyo

This book is printed on acid free paper.

W. B. Saunders Company Ltd   24–28 Oval Road
London NW1 7DX, England

The Curtis Center
Independence Square West
Philadelphia, PA 19106–3399, USA

55 Horner Avenue
Toronto, Ontario M8Z 4X6, Canada

Harcourt Brace Jovanovich Group
(Australia) Pty Ltd
30–52 Smidmore Street
Marrickville, NSW 2204, Australia

Harcourt Brace Jovanovich Japan Inc.
Ichibancho Central Building, 22–1 Ichibancho
Chiyoda-ku, Tokyo 102, Japan

Typeset by Paston Press, Loddon, Norfolk
Printed in Great Britain by The University Press, Cambridge

A catalogue record for this book is available from the British Library

ISBN 0–7020–1554–7

To John R. Graham and the memory of Bayard T. Horton, two great men and teachers in this field. To all my previous, present, and future collaborators in headache research, and last, but not least, to Ellen.

Contents

Foreword

Headache is *the* most common neurological symptom both in general practice and in specialist neurological practice. The vast majority of patients have no physical signs and the diagnosis, and hence prognosis and treatment, depends almost entirely on the history. Amongst the morass of migraine and tension headaches lie not just a few serious conditions such as intracranial tumours and giant cell arteritis, but some specific syndromes which although not threatening to life can be extraordinarily debilitating if they are not treated correctly. Cluster headache and the related syndromes fall into this last category. Ottar Sjaastad has contributed to our knowledge of cluster headache for more than twenty years and has made particular contributions to our understanding of chronic paroxysmal hemicrania. In this monograph he has packed all his experience between two hard covers and provides a source of reference for all neurologists, since we all have to deal with headache every day of our professional lives. Not only are the syndromes described, but so are the differential diagnosis, pathophysiology and aetiology and there are detailed accounts of what treatments work and what do not. I am sure that I for one will be turning to this book when my next cluster headache patient does not do as well as anticipated, or when I am beginning to wonder whether I have got the diagnosis right.

C. P. WARLOW

Preface

Cluster headache is not an 'old' headache. The number of articles dealing with this headache until the late 1950s was limited. Since then, the number of articles on cluster headache has increased exponentially. Not all these articles contain brand-new information. It may, nevertheless, be difficult for the newcomer and the old-timer alike to gather all the information available.

This book represents an endeavour to give a more or less complete review of cluster headache syndrome, to cover the relevant hypotheses and investigations, and to give an overview of the pathogenesis of the syndrome. There are still minor items left untouched. This is due partly to space considerations and partly due to the fact that the available evidence on these items is insufficient at the present time.

There are many ways to kill a cat—there are admittedly also many ways to write a book. The frame of the present book is one of first dealing with the clinical aspects of the syndrome—clinical picture, differential diagnosis, and therapy—in a fairly complete way. Current theories on pathogenesis, and a synthesis of these, are one of the main topics covered. In order to cover all the facets of these theories in a comprehensive way, actual studies carried out on cluster headache had to be dealt with, some of them in some detail. If the theories had been included in the pathogenesis section proper, this section would have been so large as to be difficult to use. The various tests, therefore, constitute a separate section which precedes the pathogenesis chapter. In the pathogenesis chapter, reference is made to various parts of the test section for detailed information.

The present book is in many ways a personal book. The various items could have been dealt with in a (much) briefer manner. My intention has been to show the background of the various hypotheses as well as to show the results obtained in some detail. In these respects, an attempt has been made to dig a little deeper into the problems as far as my own fields of research are concerned; through exemplification, I hope to show the difficulties encountered in trying to explore the pathogenesis of the syndrome. It may be as important to show the weaknesses and limitations of the approaches and techniques used, as to show their virtues. We probably are more familiar with the imperfections and shortcomings of our own work than with those in fields more distant to us. And we are supposedly more familiar with some of the intricacies of and the difficulties encountered in investigative approaches in our own fields than in fields in which we are not well versed. Pointing out such shortcomings may—hopefully—serve as inspiration, incitation, and guide-lines for a renewed push to move the border of insight in the desired direction. A further reason for detailing some of my own work is to emphasize the thread that runs through the line of reasoning used.

The descriptions and lines of arguments detailed in the section on cluster headache proper may seemingly slavishly have been repeated in the section on chronic paroxysmal hemicrania. However, in my opinion, one cannot take it for granted that features typical of, or reasonings having a bearing on, cluster headache and its pathogenesis have a bearing on chronic paroxysmal hemicrania.

It is my hope that this book will prove useful to the students and trained migrainologists (cephaliatrists) alike.

OTTAR SJAASTAD
Trondheim, August 1990

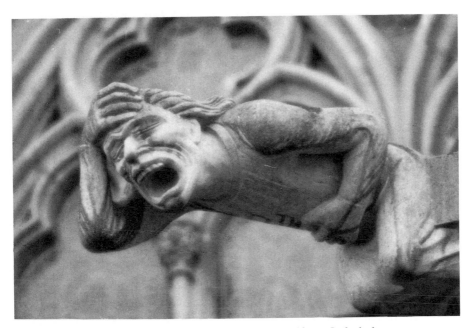

The headache sufferer: sculpture on the north wall of the Nidaros Cathedral, Trondheim, Norway.

1

Cluster Headache as Such

TERMINOLOGY

In their first publication concerning cluster headache, Horton *et al.* (1939) used the term 'erythromelalgia of the head'. Horton (1941, 1944) then proposed the term 'histaminic cephalgia', and he stated (1941) that he would use this term thereafter. Nevertheless, in some later communications he used the term 'histaminic cephalalgia' (1956b). The term 'histaminic cephalgia' (or 'cephalgia') has, however, gradually vanished from the headache literature, mainly because of a growing belief that the theory of a causal relationship between histamine and this type of headache was not well founded (e.g. Sjaastad, 1975a). This term is now mainly of historic interest.

Many investigators have used the term 'Horton's headache' for this type of headache (e.g. Lovshin, 1961; Ekbom and Kugelberg, 1968; Hasan *et al.*, 1976; Sjaastad *et al.*, 1976; Sjaastad, 1978). As far as our group is concerned, this has been done as a tribute to Bayard T. Horton's fundamental work in this field. 'Horton's headache' may be used in the future as a synonym for 'cluster headache'.

The term 'cluster headache' was coined by Kunkle and co-workers (1952, 1954). This term illustrates a typical trait of this pain syndrome, i.e. the occurrence of attacks within a relatively limited time-span. This catchy term has become popular and, at present, is the term usually used. It is also in all probability going to be the term most used in the future, at least until the aetiology and pathogenesis of this headache are disentangled.

Direct translations of this term into other languages have been made, e.g. in Italian it is *cefalea a grappolo* (Nappi and Savoldi, 1983), or approximations having similar connotations have been made: in French, *mal de tête en salves* (Bousser and Baron, 1979); and in Spanish, *la cefalea acuminada* (Guerra, 1981), *cefalea en grupo, cefalea en acúmulos,* or *cefalea en racimos* (Espadaler, 1986). In Portuguese, many terms have been formed, e.g.: *cefaléia em cachos* (da Silva, 1974; Raffaelli, 1986); *cefaléia agrupada* (da Silva, 1974); *cefaléia aglomerada* and *cefaléia acuminada* have also been employed. The presently preferred term, however, seems to be *Cefaléia em salvas* (Raffaelli, 1979; 1984; da Silva, 1983). In German, a 'mixed' term has been innovated: *'Cluster' Kopfschmerz* (Heyck, 1976). In Chinese, the term is *Chong Ji Xing Tou Tong*, which literally means 'a headache that occurs in clusters'.

HEADACHES DESCRIBED UNDER OTHER HEADINGS

HEADACHES PROBABLY IDENTICAL WITH, OR CLOSELY RELATED TO CLUSTER HEADACHE

1. Hemicrania angioparalytica or neuroparalytica (Eulenburg, 1878).
2. Ciliary neuralgia (Harris, 1926).
3. Migrainous neuralgia (Harris, 1936).
4. Erythromelalgia of the head (Horton *et al.*, 1939).
5. Histaminic cephalgia (Horton, 1941).
6. Histaminic cephalalgia (e.g. *Ad Hoc* Committee on Classification of Headache, 1962).
7. Horton's headache (various later investigators).
8. Greater superficial petrosal neuralgia (Gardner *et al.*, 1947).
9. A particular variety of headache (Symonds, 1956).
10. The periodic migrainous neuralgia of Wilfred Harris (Bickerstaff, 1959).

SYNDROMES PARTLY IDENTIFIED WITH CLUSTER HEADACHE, BUT PROBABLY DIFFERING FROM IT

1. Romberg's description (1840).
2. Möllendorff's Hemikranie (1867).
3. Sluder's sphenopalatine neuralgia (Sluder, 1908, 1910).
4. Erythroprosopalgie (or erythroprosopalgia) (Bing, 1913, 1930).
5. Vail's vidian neuralgia (1932).
6. Syndrome de vasodilatation hémicéphalique d'origine sympathique (Vallery-Radot and Blamoutier, 1925).
7. Atypical (facial) neuralgia (e.g. Fay, 1927, 1932; Glaser, 1928, 1940).
8. Autonomic faciocephalalgia (Brickner and Riley, 1935).

CLASSIFICATIONS AND DEFINITIONS

Various classifications and definitions have been attempted (see Table 1.1). According to the *Ad Hoc Committee on Classification of Headache* (1962), cluster headache is clearly viewed as a vascular headache and as a subgroup of 'headaches of the migraine type' in line with 'classic' and 'common' migraine. Cluster headache was described as follows by the committee: 'Vascular

Table 1.1   Various classification systems of cluster headache

Source	
Vascular headaches of the migraine type	
Ad hoc Committee on Classification of Headache (1962)	(A) 'Classic' migraine (B) 'Common' migraine (C) 'Cluster' headache (D) 'Hemiplegic' migraine and 'Ophthalmoplegic' migraine (E) 'Lower half' headache
Migraine	
World Federation of Neurology's Research Group on Migraine and Headache (1970)	(A) Conditions generally accepted as falling within the above definition: (1) classical migraine; (2) non-classical migraine (B) Conditions which may fall within the category of migraine: (1) cluster headaches; (2) facial 'migraine'; (3) ophthalmoplegic 'migraine'; (4) 'hemiplegic migraine'
Cluster headache	
Kudrow (1980)	(A) Episodic (periodic) (B) Chronic: (1) primary; (2) secondary; (3) chronic paroxysmal hemicrania (C) Atypical variant: (1) cluster-migraine; (2) cluster-vertigo
Cluster headache syndrome	
Sjaastad (1986a)	(A) Cluster headache: (1) episodic form; (2) chronic form (a) primary, (b) secondary (B) Chronic paroxysmal hemicrania: (1) pre-chronic form; (2) chronic form
Headache Classification Committee of the International Headache Society (1988)	Cluster headache and chronic paroxysmal hemicrania

headache, predominantly unilateral on the same side, usually associated with flushing, sweating, rhinorrhea and increased lacrimation, brief in duration and usually occurring in closely packed groups separated by long remissions. Identical or closely allied are erythroprosopalgia (Bing), ciliary or migrainous neuralgia (Harris), erythromelalgia of the head or histaminic cephalalgia (Horton), and petrosal neuralgia (Gardner *et al*.)'.

In 1969, the *World Federation of Neurology's Research Group on Migraine and Headache* (1970) redefined and reclassified migraine (Table 1.1). Cluster headache was then, together with 'facial migraine', 'ophthalmoplegic migraine' and 'hemiplegic migraine', placed under the heading 'conditions which may fall within the category of migraine'. Cluster headache was thus still not classified as a separate entity; it was still in the migraine group, though with a question mark. It was defined as follows:

> Unilateral intense pain involving the eye and head on one side usually associated with flushing, nasal congestion and lacrimation, attacks recurring one or more times daily and lasting for twenty to one hundred and twenty minutes. Such bouts commonly continue for weeks or months and are separated by remissions of months or years.

Ekbom (1970) proposed the addition of some criteria: 'pain being strictly unilateral', but 'During another period, the pain might occur exclusively on the contralateral side, attacks might be associated with one or more of the following signs: conjunctival injection, lacrimation, nasal congestion, rhinorrhea, sweating, partial Horner's syndrome'. 'The patients must have had at least two typical headache periods'. 'Absence of neurological signs (with the exception of a partial Horner's syndrome) which might explain the headache'.

In *Kudrow's classification* (Kudrow, 1980), cluster headache was for the first time separated entirely from migraine (Table 1.1). In my opinion, 'cluster migraine' probably does not deserve a place in the classification system. As far as is known at present, this headache is basically a migraine or migraine-like headache, but with accumulated attacks. Until proven otherwise, it should accordingly be categorized under 'migraine', and a more appropriate term would probably be 'cyclical migraine'.

'Cluster vertigo' (Gilbert, 1965, 1970) was described more than 20 years ago. To the best of my knowledge, only one possible similar case has been described since the original one (Sutherland and Eadie, 1972). Moreover, none of the members at the International Cluster Headache Research Group meeting in 1980 had seen a single case, even though its members had seen a total of more than 2000 cluster headache patients. Until corroborated by further evidence, cluster vertigo should, therefore, not be included in the classification system.

There are arguments in favour of placing the cluster-tic syndrome (Green and Apfelbaum, 1978; Solomon *et al*., 1985) on the list. For the time being, however, it should be placed on the waiting list, as it remains to be clarified whether we are in fact faced with the fortuitous co-existence of two separate and relatively rare headaches (see later).

In the classification of 'cluster headache syndrome' which I have proposed (Sjaastad 1986a,b,c), cluster headache is separated from migraine. Chronic paroxysmal hemicrania is not classified as a *subgroup* of cluster headache but is placed at the same level as cluster headache (Table 1.1). Neither the prevalence of the two disorders nor the fact that one disorder was discovered before the other should be decisive for the classification of the specific disorders or for a possible sub- or super-ordination of a disorder.

In the *classification/description system of the International Association for the Study of Pain (IASP)* (Merskey *et al.*, 1986), the 'pre-chronic form' of chronic paroxysmal hemicrania was not distinguished as a separate group. Otherwise, there is conformity between this and the latter two classifications. The IASP description of the episodic form of cluster headache is as follows (with the courtesy of the chairman of the committee, Prof. H. Merskey, London, Ontario).

Definition: unilateral pain principally in the ocular, frontal and temporal areas recurring in separate bouts with daily attacks for several months, usually with rhinorrhoea or lacrimation.

Site: ocular, frontal, temporal areas; considerably less frequently in infraorbital areas, ipsilateral upper teeth, back of the head, entire hemicranium, neck or shoulder. Unilateral pain is characteristic. The side may change even within a cluster period, but a change of side is rare.

System: uncertain. Possibly vascular or autonomic nervous system.

Main features: (i) Occurrence—approximately 4 per 10 000 population. 85–90% male. Most frequently headaches start between 18 and 40.
        (ii) Pain—constant stabbing, burning or throbbing.
     (iii) Attacks—grouped in bouts of several weeks to months duration with more or less attack-free intervals of some months duration in between. Bouts most often last 4–8 weeks. Range 1 week to 12 months. Usually one cluster period per 6–18 months. Usually 1–3 attacks lasting 0.5–2 h each per 24 h in the cluster, frequently at night. Maximum 8 attacks per 24 h. Attacks may skip a day or two or more during the cluster. At maximum, the intensity is excruciating. Abortive or mild attacks may nevertheless occur. Patients characteristically pace the floor, bang their head against the walls, etc., during attacks and are usually unable to lie down.

Associated symptoms: usually no nausea but some may occur, probably with the more severe attacks or at the peak of attacks. Vomiting is still less frequent than nausea. Ipsilateral ptosis/ miosis are associated with some attacks; occasionally they persist after attacks and sometimes permanently. Ipsilateral conjunctival injection and lacrimation occur in most patients. Ipsilateral nasal stuffiness and/or rhinorrhoea occur in most patients. Hyperacusis and photophobia occur in many patients. A reduction in heart rate is a feature in some patients, especially during severe attacks.

Signs: ptosis/miosis, tearing, rhinorrhoea and blocked nose, and changes in heart rate.

Relief: from ergot preparations, oxygen, prednisone, methysergide, etc.

Pathology: unknown.

Differential diagnosis: sinusitis, chronic paroxysmal hemicrania, chronic cluster headache, cluster-tic syndrome and migraine.

According to the *Headache Classification Committee of the International Headache Society* (IHS) (1988), the 'cluster headache and chronic paroxysmal hemicrania' group should be divided into three subgroups: cluster headache, chronic paroxysmal hemicrania and cluster headache-like disorder not fulfilling the above criteria. In this classification, under ordinary cluster headache, a new group, 'cluster headache periodicity undetermined', is added to the 'episodic' and 'chronic' cluster headache groups. The 'primary' and 'secondary' chronic cluster headache subgroups are termed 'chronic cluster headache unremitting from onset' and 'chronic cluster headache evolved from episodic', respectively.

The classification systems of IASP (Merskey *et al.*, 1986) and IHS (1988) are used in this book. In older studies, the *Ad Hoc* Committee classification (1962) has been used.

CLUSTER HEADACHE AND SIMILAR HEADACHES: EARLY DESCRIPTIONS

In the decades prior to the authoritative description by Horton and co-workers in 1939 there were several communications probably pertaining to the disorder later termed 'cluster headache'. These early descriptions are detailed in the following (Tables 1.2 and 1.3). In several of these reports, there were, unfortunately, small or large shortcomings in the description of the headache. Sometimes, various types of headache were mixed, and the accompanying phenomena may have been of greater interest to the investigators than the pain. At times, therefore, it is next to impossible to make head or tail of the reported condition. Modern diagnostic procedures could probably have determined with reasonable certainty whether these early cases belonged to the cluster headache syndrome. However, even on the basis of the purely clinical—and inadequate—descriptions available, it is possible to make assumptions as to the nature of the headache described. Some of the most unlikely candidates, such as Sluder's neuralgia, are dealt with here in connection with differential diagnosis.

ROMBERG'S DESCRIPTION

Opinions are divided as to the nature of the disorder described by Romberg (1840). Heyck (1976, 1981) believes that the 'ciliary neuralgia' referred to by Romberg may generally be classified as iridocyclitis, whereas Lance (1982) apparently believes that Romberg described cluster headache. Since opinions are so markedly divided, a translation of the pertinent sections in Romberg's report are reproduced below. Romberg wrote partly about the causes of this neuralgia and partly about its treatment; these sections are *not* included here.

Ciliary neuralgia.
    Pain in the eye, initiated and enhanced by the influence of light and by using the eyes, is the constant characteristic. To a higher degree, there is a sensitivity to light, for which reason one also has termed this disease *photophobia*. The patient avoids sun- and candle-light, the influence of which will make the eyeball painful and the eyelids will immediately close forcefully. The pupil is contracted. The pain not infrequently extends over the forehead and head. The eye usually weeps and becomes red.

    Any (forceful) use of the eyesight, in particular for near vision, leads to a painful feeling of fatigue in the eye, which frequently increases to a stronger pain, which causes objects to appear unsharp, eventually to disappear totally. With continued forceful use, tearing will

Table 1.2 A summary comparison of the first possible descriptions of cluster headache (see also Table 1.3)

Authors	Unilaterality	Persistent unilaterality	Maximum pain in ocular area	Other painful areas	Special features
Romberg (1840)	+	?	Probably	Forehead/head	Frequent blinking. Unsharp vision, even amaurosis
Möllendorff (1867)	+	No. Sideshift, even during same day	Possibly (starts above arcus superciliaris)	Temporoparietal area	Tinnitus. Hereditary forms. 'Rotating star' in the visual field before onset of pain. Unilateral obscuration of visual field. Stops at climacterium. Connected with menstrual period
Eulenburg (1878)	+	–	–	'Hemicrania'	Long free intervals. Hot ear, symptomatic side
Bing (e.g. 1945)	–(+)	?	Face	–?	Increased temporal artery pulsation
Vallery-Radot and Blamoutier (1925)	+ As well as global headache	+	Eye, nape of neck	Vertex, temporal area, neck	Rather continuous headaches. Transitory erythema face (symptomatic > non-symptomatic), neck, chest
Brickner and Riley (1935)	+	Generally +	Face and head	Ear region	Association with menstruation
Harris (1936)	+ 'usually strictly unilateral'	Probably +	'in, behind or around the eyeball' ('ciliary neuralgia')	Temple, side of the forehead, often both jaws, sometimes extending to the back of head	'injected the Gasserian ganglion with alcohol'. 'with apparently lasting cure'. Also injected infra- and supra-orbital nerves. 'Usually—highly strung individuals with a nervous heredity'
Horton et al. (1939)	+	+	+	Temple, neck, face	No familial characteristics. Clock-like regularity of attacks. Scotoma not present

(continued)

Table 1.2 *Continued.*

Authors	No. of attacks per day	Duration of attack	Nocturnal attacks	Pacing during attack	Excruciating severity	Hyper-sensitivity to touch	Character of pain
Romberg (1840)	?	?	?	?	+(?) Influenced by sunlight	?	Pressing
Möllendorff (1867)	?	12–15 h	–?	Improved by lying down	Severe (?), not excruciating	+	Pulsatile
Eulenburg (1878)	<1	Generally some hours to ½ day	?	?	Moderate	?	Piercing
Bing (e.g. 1945)	?	Few minutes to some hours	?	?	+ (1952)	+	'Burning', 'piercing'
Vallery-Radot and Blamoutier (1925)	?	Partly *continuous* pain	?	?	Probably 'severe' at maximum (?)	?	?
Brickner and Riley (1935)	≤1	Around 24 h. 'Several hours' to 3–4 days (or 'almost constant')	(±)	Bedrest specifically mentioned in the worst-affected case	Probably moderate pain (2 of 3 patients); severe in one	?	'Pressing', 'sharp'
Harris (1936)	≥3 (up to 6)	10–30 min to 5–6 h (30 h)	+	?	+	?	?
Horton *et al.* (1939)	2–20 per week	15 min to several hours	+	+	+	?	Burning, boring

(continued)

Table 1.2 *Continued.*

Authors	Lacrimation	Miosis	Ptosis	Sweating	Con-junctival injection	Facial flushing	Oedema	Temporary vessel dilatation	Rhinorrhoea/ nasal stuffiness	Autonomic features present
Romberg (1840)	+	+	+	?	+	+ – ?	?	?	?	+
Möllendorff (1867)	?	+ Bilateral	?	Reduced (or visible ipsilaterally)	+	?	?	?	Greenish secretion in one case	+
Eulenburg (1878)	+	+	±	+ (Partially unilateral)	+	+	?	+	?	+
Bing (e.g. 1945)	? (1952: 'occasionally')	±	±	–	?(++)	+ (+ Ocular area)	+ (Swelling)	?	++ –/	+
Vallery-Radot and Blamoutier (1925)	++	?	?	Generalized sweating (symptomatic side > non-symptomatic side)	++	++	*'Congestion de la face'*	?	++/?	+
Brickner and Riley (1935)	+(–)	?	?	+ No relationship to headache (–)	?	+	+	?	–	+
Harris (1936)	+	?	?	?	+	?	?	?	?	+
Horton et al. (1939)	+	?	?	?	+	+	+ Engorgement of the soft tissues of the eye	+	+/+	+

(continued)

Table 1.2 *Continued.*

Authors	Cluster phenomenon	Intolerance to alcohol	Male preponderance	Blepharo-spasm	Photo-phobia	Bradycardia	Nausea/vomiting
Romberg (1840)	?	?	?	++	++[a]	?	?
Möllendorff (1867)	?	?	Mentions females in particular	?	+	+	+/+
Eulenburg (1878)	−	?	Females:males = 6:1	−	−	+	+
Bing (e.g. 1945)	?	?	−	−	−	?	?
Vallery-Radot and Blamoutier (1925)	2 periods: >5 and 1 y long; 16 y between them	?	− Solitary case (female)	+	+	Tachycardia	?(−?)
Brickner and Riley (1935)	?	?	Only females (*n* = 3)	?	?	?	−/++ −/− +/+ (*n* = 3)
Harris (1936)	'6 to 8 weeks yearly'	?	?	?	?	?	+/'rare'
Horton *et al.* (1939)	Mentions: 'remissions and exacerbations'	+	?	?	?	?	Occasionally +/−

?, Information not given; −, phenomenon not present; +, phenomenon present.
[a]The photophobia (and blepharospasm) are emphasized more than the pain. He states that 'this disease has also been termed "photophobia"'. He also mentions that this condition can lead to blindness.

Table 1.3 Presence of crucial cluster headache features in the first possible descriptions of cluster headache

Authors	Male preponderance	Cluster phenomenon	Autonomic features	Excrutiating severity	Persistent unilaterality
Romberg (1840)	?	?	+	+(?)	+(?)
Möllendorff (1867)	− (Females!)	?	+	+?	−
Eulenburg (1878)	−	−	+	−(+)	−
Bing (e.g. 1945)	−	?	+	+	∓
Vallery-Radot and Blamoutier (1925)	−	+?	+	−	+?
Brickner and Riley (1935)	−	?	+	−	+(−)
Harris (1936)	?	+	+	+	+(?)
Horton *et al.* (1939)	?	+	+	+	+

start in the eye and the upper eyelid will be heavy and will close; finally, a pressing headache in the forehead will be added. Such patients cannot at all open the eyelids so completely as those of a healthy eye can be opened, for which reason the eye appears smaller than the healthy one. In many cases, I have, furthermore, observed frequent blinking. All such cases improve upon rest.

Among the other symptoms of ciliary neuralgia are also the tearing and the injection, which could be viewed as being of trophic nature. Some ophthalmologists have also observed a neuralgia of the lacrimal gland, which manifests itself through piercing pains in the area of the lacrimal gland, through photophobia and irritability of the eye, and through a periodic tearing. . . . The ciliary neuralgia is often associated with hemicrania and hysteria.

A cure is generally difficult to obtain, in particular with regard to the sensitive and irritable eye. The longer the duration, and the more difficult the determination and the removal of the causes, the lower the expectations. Even amaurosis has occasionally been observed.

A summary of the main findings are given in Tables 1.2 and 1.3. Evidently, several main factors of cluster headache are lacking in Romberg's description: unilaterality and autonomic phenomena are mentioned, but the cluster phenomenon and the male preponderance are not (see Tables 1.2 and 1.3). On the other hand, miosis/ptosis are mentioned, as is photophobia. However, photophobia and blepharospasm appear to be out of proportion to what is usually found in cluster headache. The headache is described as being *in* the eye, which is not usual in cluster headache (where it is typically *behind* and *around* the eye), and it is partly described as a *consequence* of the ocular irritability. The visual acuity is described as partly reduced. This picture is clearly at variance with cluster headache. It may be that cases of cluster headache are hidden in this global description, but the main part of the description deals more with an ocular disorder. There appears to be positive evidence in favour of iridocyclitis, i.e. marked photophobia, blepharospasm, miosis and even amaurosis being constituents of this picture.

MÖLLENDORFF'S DESCRIPTION

Möllendorff's description (1867) has been considered by several migrainologists to pertain to cluster headache. I do not share this view. Möllendorff did not describe particular cases but only 'hemicrania' in general and classic migraine attacks with the initial occurrence of 'a rotating star'. Other typical migraine traits were also described: the headache alternated between sides, the attacks were rather long-lasting, and nausea and vomiting were present in severe attacks. The pain was described as throbbing and increased on bending forwards. Females were frequently affected in connection with their menstrual periods. Nevertheless, he observed typical traits of cluster headache in his patients, such as hypersensitivity when touching the hair, bradycardia (Tables 1.2 and 1.3), and ipsilateral rhinorrhoea (although the patients apparently at times had a greenish exudate). Typical characteristics of cluster headache attack, such as the brevity and excruciating severity of attacks and other accompanying phenomena, like lacrimation and conjunctival injection, to specify but a few important parameters, were not mentioned. The cluster phenomenon was not mentioned. So, all in all, what Möllendorff described does not seem to be cluster headache, although it is possible that there may have been some cases of cluster headache among those he described. If so, the typical cluster features were overshadowed, and possible cases were not recognized for what they were. Möllendorff was, therefore, probably not the first to describe a homogeneous picture of cluster headache. Heyck (1981) is of the same opinion.

EULENBURG'S DESCRIPTION

Eulenburg (1878, 1883) described 'hemicrania angioparalytica' and 'hemicrania neuroparalytica' and in this manner tried to separate his cases from the usual type of migraine—the 'pale' or 'angiospastic migraine'. Eulenburg described a severe, mostly *unilateral* headache, the attack being associated with ipsilateral lacrimation and conjunctival injection. A transitory Horner's syndrome on the symptomatic side was also observed. Ipsilateral reddening in the frontotemporal area and temporal artery swelling were also noted, as was occasional forehead/facial sweating. The attacks lasted from several hours to 'half a day'. Some of the clinical features of cluster headache are lacking in his description, such as rhinorrhoea and the male preponderance (the female: male ratio was 6:1!). The attacks were rather long-lasting and did not appear in clusters. This is, however, in other ways a passable description of cluster headache (see Tables 1.2 and 1.3). Even ptosis and miosis were observed, aspects of cluster headache that were overlooked in later descriptions (Harris, 1936; Horton *et al.*, 1939).

There is probably no earlier report outlining cluster headache this well. Heyck (1975) is of the same opinion. This description would, however, not suffice as a guideline for others to make the diagnosis of cluster headache on their own. The test of time seems to have shown that Eulenburg's description did not lead to a flow of communications concerning this specific item.

BING'S ERYTHROPROSOPALGIA

As early as 1913, Bing (1930, 1945, 1952) described erythroprosopalgia, first one case (1913) and later a total of three cases (1945, 1952). In all contexts Bing stressed the localization of the pain as facial (*Smerzen in der einen, seltener in beiden Gesichtshälften* (Bing (1952); 'prosopalgie'). Horton *et al.* (1939) emphasized the eye and the head. The disorder started in the fourth or fifth decade and was characterized by 'spectacle'-like distribution of oedema, flushing with burning pain, conjunctival injection and, in one case, nasal secretion. Infraorbital trigeminal branches were extremely tender to pressure, and attacks could even occasionally be elicited from these points. Finger oedema of Quincke's type was even observed during attacks. Haemoglobin levels were increased, as in erythromelalgia. This account forms the basis of the assumption that Bing provided the first description of cluster headache. In German-speaking countries (e.g. Heyck, 1975, 1976), the term *Bing–Horton syndrom* (or *Kopfschmerz*) has sometimes been used. Bing, however, clearly stressed the facial flushing and oedema, features that are not usually very prominent in cluster headache, whereas lacrimation, duration, frequency, nocturnal appearance, unilaterality and, above all, the severity of the pain are not emphasized or even mentioned in his original paper. However, he did specify some of these characteristic traits later (Bing, 1952). The precipitation of attacks due to pressure exerted towards the trigeminal branches substantiates the difference between this headache and cluster headache (see Tables 1.2 and 1.3).

There certainly are cases involving a combination of unilateral headache/facial pain and autonomic phenomena such as flushing and conjunctival injection, but without the typical cluster headache features such as the cluster phenomenon. These pain conditions are poorly understood and have by no means been classified properly. Some of them may belong to the 'cervicogenic headache' group (see later), whilst others may not.

In his later publications, but not in the first one, Bing (1945, 1952) also emphasized the unilaterality of the pain (see also, e.g. Heyck, 1975). He even mentioned Horner's syndrome as an integral part of the picture. In his last treatise, Bing (1952) claimed that he had originally described cluster headache. Heyck, in his earlier publications (1975, 1976), felt that Bing (1913) really had described cluster headache; in later years, however, he was inclined to believe that this was not the case (personal communication from Heyck, H., 1980).

It is my considered opinion that Bing's first case is definitely at variance with cluster headache (and this also goes for his later cases). The term 'Bing–Horton headache', as partly used in German-speaking countries, is probably wrong and should be abandoned. The headache that Bing described may be similar to the one described later by Vallery-Radot and Blamoutier (1925).

VALLERY-RADOT AND BLAMOUTIER'S CASE: 'SYNDROME DE
VASODILATATION HÉMICÉPHALIQUE D'ORIGINE SYMPATHIQUE
(HÉMICRANIE, HÉMIHYDRORRHÉE NASALE, HÉMILARMOIEMENT)'
(1925, 1951)

Vallery-Radot and Blamoutier (Vallery-Radot and Blamoutier, 1925; Vallery-
Radot *et al.*, 1951) described under this heading the case of a 35-year-old
woman. This account has been accepted by many authors as an early description of cluster headache (e.g. Bickerstaff, 1968; Sutherland and Eadie, 1972;
Heyck, 1981). I do not agree with these interpretations. First of all, the patient
was a woman; this, of course, does not exclude the possibility of cluster
headache but certainly raises the index of suspicion. She had hemicrania, with
a maximum around the eye and the nape of the neck, although she also
apparently had a basic, global headache (*'elle souffrait de toutes les regions de la
tête'*). The patient had long-lasting attacks, although the headache was not
quite chronic (*'s'etait une douleur permanente. . . .'* *'. . . la cephalée durait toute la
matinée, puis s'atténuait et même disparaissait souvent dans la journée'*). There may
have been a more or less permanent background headache. Profuse lacrimation and rhinorrhoea on the side of hemicrania were so disturbing that she
always had to carry a handkerchief ready for use. She had an intense,
conjunctival injection and congestion of the face on the most painful side, and
large areas of rapidly appearing and vanishing redness on the neck and chest
(see Tables 1.2 and 1.3).

It is also remarkable that atropine and pilocarpine had little influence on the
lacrimation and nasal secretion (which they clearly have in the cluster headache syndrome (Sjaastad, unpublished data; Saunte, 1984b)). The pain level is
described as *'des maux de tête tenaces'*. There is no mention of clustering of the
paroxysms. There were probably no nocturnal attacks. The emphasis was
clearly on the hemilacrimation, hemirhinorrhoea and the erythema (*'vasodilatation hémicéphalique'*) and seemingly not so much on the severity of the pain.
The finding that attacks could be triggered by pressure against cranial nerves
and the supraorbital nerve on the most painful side is clearly at variance with
the regular picture of cluster headache.

Later, Vallery-Radot and co-workers (1951) returned to their original case
and claimed that their clinical picture (Valery-Radot and Blamoutier, 1925) was
similar or identical to that of Horton *et al.* (1939). However, even their later
communication gives rise to some strong reservations with regard to a diagnosis of cluster headache. There is distinct, facial erythema in the *'syndrome de
vasodilatation hémicéphalique'*, even with *'placards érythémateux'*. The degree of
pain is still not stressed, the duration of the attacks is not given, and the
presence of possible nocturnal attacks is not mentioned.

On the other hand, Vallery-Radot and co-workers dismissed the possibility
of a similarity between their *syndrome hémicéphalique* and the syndrome described by Gardner *et al.* (1947), as a neuralgia stemming from the greater
superficial petrosal nerve. One reason for this is apparently the lack of

cutaneous vasodilatation in the cases described by Gardner, which was a characteristic feature of the *syndrome hémicéphalique*. It is noteworthy that Gardner's 'greater superficial petrosal neuralgia' is considered by most clinicians in this field to be identical with cluster headache (see e.g. Sutherland and Eadie, 1972; Kudrow, 1980). It should be mentioned in this connection that the status of the erythema/flush in cluster headache symptomatology is a little dubious (Ekbom and Kudrow, 1979). Many experienced headache specialists seem to have observed erythema during the attack (e.g. Heyck, 1976) (see 'Oedema', page 66), but it is under no circumstances a major feature of the attack. In Vallery-Radot and Blamoutier's case, cutaneous vasodilatation was pronounced. Furthermore, in their case, subcutaneous injections of adrenaline ameliorated the symptoms.

Vallery-Radot and Blamoutier seem to have described a cluster headache-like picture, but a picture nevertheless at variance with cluster headache (and, in my opinion, very clearly at variance with it). There seem, however, to be some similar traits between the picture they described and Bing's (1913) erythroprosopalgia.

AUTONOMIC FACIOCEPHALALGIA

Several authors have contended that the headache described by Brickner and Riley (1935) is identical to that later described by Horton (e.g. Bickerstaff, 1968; Heyck, 1981). This point of view is difficult to accept;. Brickner and Riley described three female patients; the headache in one of them had started by the age of 12 years, and the attacks were long-lasting (that is >24 h). One of the patients awoke nightly from pain, and the pain attacks were accentuated during menstruation. There was occasional, attack-related, profuse vomiting and vertigo and reduced visual acuity, whereas rhinorrhoea was absent (see Tables 1.2 and 1.3). In one of the cases, the limbs on the headache side felt heavy and weak during the most severe attacks. Together these traits are strong evidence against the presence of cluster headache.

The authors themselves felt that these patients represented a special group of headaches, different from migraine and 'atypical facial neuralgia'. These cases may well be special. They bear a clear resemblance to the case described by Vallery-Radot and Blamoutier (1925), an idea that also struck the authors.

HARRIS' CILIARY (MIGRAINOUS) NEURALGIA

Many of the cases in the reports by Harris (1926, 1936) probably had cluster headache and, with a few exceptions, his descriptions are better than that of Eulenburg (1878). He states that he prefers the term ciliary neuralgia 'when the eyeball itself is prominently affected', without specifically indicating that the pathology of the condition is associated with the ciliary ganglion or ciliary body. Harris even briefly described the cluster phenomenon *per se* (headaches 'for periods of six to eight weeks yearly') and was probably the first to do so. He described the excruciating severity, the usual absence of migraine features ('visual spectra and transient hemianopia are never met with'), the unilaterality, the frequency, and the relative brevity of attack (that is, 'ten minutes to half an hour' or somewhat longer) and stresses the localization in the ocular area. It is striking, however, that, although he had seen 23 cases (Harris, 1936), he did not observe (or, to put it more correctly, did not describe) the male preponderance. Nor did he notice signs indicating a possible Horner's syndrome (see Tables 1.2 and 1.3). The other autonomic symptoms and signs are also inadequately described.

In spite of the relative clarity of his description, *some* inaccuracy seems to have sneaked into his material: he thus describes occasional attacks lasting 24–30 h, 'one or more every week'. One patient in this category even proves to be a girl of 12 years. He also claims that the onset may have been in 'infancy' in this very patient, and her attacks were accompanied by nausea and vomiting, 'a point which is strongly suggestive of the association of the pain with migraine'.

There are thus 'contaminations' in his case material. Nevertheless, the features of cluster headache emerge, and his contribution is indisputable. Unfortunately, not even this contribution led to a general recognition of the disorder.

HORTON AND CO-WORKERS' 'ERYTHROMELALGIA OF THE HEAD' OR 'HISTAMINIC CEPHALGIA'

Even though several traits of cluster headache had in all probability been described by Eulenburg (1878) and Harris (1926, 1936), Horton's (Horton *et al.*, 1939; Horton, 1941) contribution was of crucial importance. The previous descriptions had not led to a general awareness and acceptance of this headache, and Horton and co-workers were apparently unaware of the earlier descriptions. Horton (Figure 1.1) focused attention on this headache. Through the work of Horton and co-workers this headache became part of the general knowledge not only of specialists, but also of general practitioners. Their succinct, almost definitive description, and the clarity and the completeness of it (see e.g. Lovshin, 1961), made this process a rather easy one. There does not seem to be any sizeable contamination of other types of headache in their description.

Horton and co-workers described almost all the most important clinical features of this headache (see Tables 1.2 and 1.3). Their description is, therefore, better than any of the prior ones. However, they missed three features, two of them significant: (1) Horner's syndrome or a 'Horner-like syndrome'; this is a minor flaw, this syndrome being insignificant or even absent in many cases; (2) photophobia; and (3) the fluctuating course of the disease, i.e. the tendency to clustering. Although Horton and co-workers were aware that 'remissions and exacerbations in many cases occurred spontaneously', they apparently did not recognize the full implications of these fluctuations. The latter flaw was a rather tragic one, because this in all probability was what led to

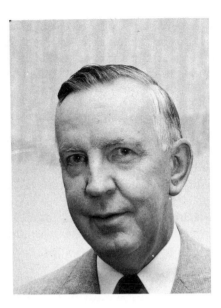

Figure 1.1   Bayard Taylor Horton, 1895–1980.

the misinterpretations regarding the therapeutic efforts with 'histamine desensitization' (see later). In their first publications, Horton and co-workers did not mention the male preponderance of the syndrome.

We all make blunders—*errare humanum est*. This having been said, it should be stated that Horton's contribution to this field is an impressive and decisive one.

COMMENTS CONCERNING PRIORITY

Who, then, is going to be given the honour of having been the first to describe cluster headache? The *standard* should be discussed before making any decisions. Is it the completeness of the description that matters—or only the 'firstness'—or both? The exactness of the description is of considerable importance; the disorder should be described in such a manner that it can be recognized by other workers in the field. This requires exactness and completeness.

There is no doubt that Horton *et al.* (1939) gave such a complete and exact description that others had little difficulty in recognizing such cases and in establishing the diagnosis on their own (Tables 1.2 and 1.3). Furthermore, it is clear that Bing (1913), Vallery-Radot and Blamoutier (1925), and Brickner and Riley (1935) did *not* describe cluster headache, but other interesting headache types. These authors *may* have described one and the same disorder, or rather similar headaches.

What about the other authors who preceded Horton and co-workers? Romberg (1840) did not describe cluster headache, and Möllendorff (1867) described only some *traits* of cluster headache. The description given by Eulenburg (1878) is a much improved version. There is a clear development in description from that of Möllendorff to that of Eulenburg. The difference between Eulenburg's and Harris' (1936) descriptions is sizeable. Möllendorff and, in particular, Eulenburg are to be commended for their descriptions of cluster headache traits. Unfortunately, since they described 'hemicrania' and not single cases, they missed many essential characteristics. Harris' contribution is a great one—being an almost complete and exact description of this headache based on case histories. But even Harris' description, although containing most of the elements, contains some contamination. There are apparently no reports on cluster headache in the literature between Harris' and Horton's contributions, and the diagnoses *then* were made with reference to the work of Horton and co-workers.

The question of priority can hardly be answered with a single name or a single group. The contribution of Horton and co-workers is, however, of crucial importance because they delivered the most authoritative and concise semiological description; their contribution was seminal in bringing about the general recognition of this headache. Most of the honour for having revealed this entity to the medical world, therefore, belongs to Harris and Horton.

PREVIOUS SERIES

Surveys of cluster headache symptomatology have been given by Horton *et al.* (1939), Horton (1961), Symonds (1956), Friedman and Mikropoulos (1958), Robinson (1958), Bickerstaff (1959), Duvoisin *et al.* (1961), Nieman and Hurwitz (1961), Kunkle *et al.* (1954), Lovshin (1961), Balla and Walton (1964), Hornabrook (1964), Graham (1972, 1975), Graham *et al.* (1970), Ekbom (1970), Lance and Anthony (1971a), Sutherland and Eadie (1972), Kudrow (1980), Pearce (1980), and Manzoni *et al.* (1983b).

The main drawback of many of the clinical studies is that they are retrospective, and that the authors only rarely, if ever, observed attacks themselves. This has to some extent been compensated for by attack provocation (e.g. by histamine or nitroglycerine) in some studies. The crucial point in this connection is, however, whether provoked and spontaneous attacks are identical (see later). In a few studies, spontaneous attacks were observed in the majority of the patients (e.g. Manzoni *et al.* (1983b), in 145 out of 180 patients). This strengthens the description of the attack symptomatology, and for some features of the syndrome the findings of such studies have to be relied upon.

Some workers have compared the findings in a cluster headache population with those in healthy controls, migraine patients and tension headache patients (Manzoni *et al.*, 1983b). Ekbom (1970) has also partly compared the

Table 1.4   Cluster headache: large clinical series[a]

Authors	No. of patients
Horton (1961)	1402
Lovshin (1961)	492
Ekbom (1970)	105
Lance and Anthony (1971a)	60
Sutherland and Eadie (1972)	58
Kudrow (1980)	500 (425)
Pearce (1980)	95
Manzoni *et al.* (1983b)	180
Andersson (1985)	127

[a]In addition, Graham (1975) (>500 cases) and Sjaastad *et al.* (around 280 cases, unpublished data) have described various features on the basis of a large series of patients.

findings in a cluster headache population with those in a migraine control group. The inclusion of a control group would appear particularly important with regard to assessing the non-headache features that accompany cluster headache.

My own experience is based on approximately 280 cases of cluster headache. A total survey of this series has never been published. Some of the clinical data on some of these patients have been dealt with in detail (e.g. Russell, 1981, 1985; Saunte, 1984b). In these studies, only spontaneously occurring attacks in patients not receiving drugs at the time were described. This may be of importance in assessing the symptomatology of cluster headache as such. In a previous review (Sutherland and Eadie, 1972), the second largest series of cluster headache comprised only 58 patients. In recent years, several good-sized series have been collected, on the basis of which several new features of cluster headache have been described (Table 1.4).

PREVALENCE OF CLUSTER HEADACHE

Prevalence studies of cluster headache in adults have only appeared in recent years. The following aspects of the syndrome have been studied:

1. the prevalence of cluster headache in 18-year-old draftees (Ekbom *et al.*, 1978);
2. the relative frequency of migraine and cluster headache in clinical headache materials (Lieder, 1944; Ekbom, 1970; Heyck, 1976; Kudrow, 1980); and
3. the prevalence of cluster headache in a relatively well-defined population (Sutherland and Eadie, 1972; D'Alessandro *et al.*, 1986).

Studies of the first-mentioned type may, in addition, to some extent help elucidate how early in life cluster headache first occurs (see later). In their study of Swedish conscripts, Ekbom *et al.* (1978) initially used a questionnaire. Later, the suspected cluster headache patients were examined by a neurologist. Of a total of 9803 boys enrolled (18 years old), eight cluster headache patients were found, giving a prevalence of 0.09%.

Three of the investigations concerning the prevalence of cluster headache among adults (i.e. Sutherland and Eadie, 1972; Heyck, 1976; D'Alessandro *et al.*, 1986) are described here in detail, and Kudrow's estimations (1980) are commented upon.

Sutherland and Eadie (1972) found 58 cases of cluster headache over a period of 7 years in practices drawing on a population of about 1.3 million people (Brisbane). 'This experience would suggest a minimal prevalence figure of 4.5 cases per 100 000' and 'a true prevalence rate of 5 per 100 000 might be considered a minimum estimate' (Table 1.5). The investigators are thus fully aware that their estimates may be too low. Small countries like Norway would be well suited for such epidemiological surveys. The estimate given by Sutherland and Eadie, i.e. 5:100 000, would mean that in the whole of Norway (population 4.2 million) there are just over 200 cases of cluster headache. In my opinion, this estimate is too low. The background for this statement is as follows.

In collaboration with Dr David Russell in Oslo, I have seen upwards of 280 cases during the past 14 years. In the last 9 years of this period, Norway has been divided into five health regions, two of which constitute our primary catchment areas (total population of slightly more than 2 million, i.e. just under half the population of Norway). Referrals may be made across the borders of these regions when it is considered that the patient will receive better treatment outside their 'home region'. Therefore, although our special interest in headache may be known outside our health-regions, many new (and old!) cases from the other regions will not have been referred. Moreover, in our own health regions we sometimes discover patients who have had cluster headache for years, even decades, but have been mis-diagnosed. Therefore, a figure of just over 200 cases would clearly be a minimum figure for the prevalence of cluster headache in Norway. The number can safely be estimated to be three times as high and probably 8–10 times as high.

Table 1.5 The prevalence of cluster headache as calculated in various surveys on adults

Authors	Estimated prevalence
Sutherland and Eadie (1972)	5:100 000[a]
Heyck (1976)	40:100 000
Kudrow (1980)	240:100 000[b]
D'Alessandro *et al.* (1986)	69:100 000

[a]Considered by the authors to be a 'minimum estimate'.
[b]Males: 400/100 000; females 80/100 000; Kudrow considers that the prevalence may be even as much as 0.9% or 900 per 100 000.

An even better Nordic country on which to make epidemiological studies of this sort would be Iceland, which has a clearly defined area, a fixed population and an inland health service. However, according to Professor G. Gudmundsson, Reykjavik (personal communication), no such survey has been carried out. Heyck (1976) reasoned as follows: approximately 6% of the general population suffer from migraine. Approximately one-third of these patients consult a physician for their headache. The ratio between cluster headache and migraine in his subjects (hospital outpatients) was approximately 2:100 (or, to be exact, 1:39.4). Accordingly, approximately 0.4 per 1000 people in the general population would have cluster headache (Table 1.5). This should indicate that approximately 1700 Norwegians have cluster headache, the corresponding figure for North Americans being >80 000.

The culmination of the age-of-onset curve for cluster headache is around the age of 25–30 years (see later). According to data given by several investigators, only a proportion of those with cluster headache in clinical materials had their first attack at 20 years. Thus, in Sutherland and Eadie's study (1972), only 17% of the patients had already experienced their first attack at that age. This must be taken into account when assessing the data of Ekbom *et al.* Furthermore, Ekbom *et al.* (1978) examined only males, whereas Heyck (1976) gives data for both sexes. Cluster headache is a disease mostly affecting the male sex, around 84% of the cases being males (see Table 1.6). Even when making due allowance

Table 1.6 Sex distribution in episodic cluster headache

Authors	Total No.	No. females	No. males	Males (%)
Kunkle *et al.* (1952)	30	6	24	80
Symonds (1956)	17	3	14	82
Friedman and Mikropoulos (1958)	50	9	41	82
Robinson (1958)	20	2	18	90
Bickerstaff (1959)	30	9	21	70
Horton (1961)	1402	176	1226	87
Duvoisin *et al.* (1961)	32	2	30	93
Lovshin (1961)	492	64	428	87
Nieman and Hurwitz (1961)	50	15	35	70
Balla and Walton (1964)	28	6	22	79
Hornabrook (1964)	21	4	17	81
Lance and Anthony (1971a)	60	8	52	87
Sutherland and Eadie (1972)	58	12	46	79
Ekbom (1974b)	163	20	143	88
Heyck (1976)	48	8	40	83
Kudrow (1980)	425	70	355	84
Pearce (1980)	95	7	88	93
Manzoni *et al.* (1983b)	161	21	140	87
Mean of means				84

If only the series with ≦60 patients are included: mean 88% males.

for these facts, there may seem to be a discrepancy between the figures of Ekbom *et al.* (1978) and Heyck (1976), that is 90:100 000, and 40:100 000, respectively. The data of Ekbom *et al.* could thus indicate that Heyck's estimate is far too low. The prevalence given by Ekbom *et al.* (1978), 0.09% in 18-year-old men, therefore, indicates a rather high total prevalence in adult men, even as high as the estimates given by Kudrow. There may be various explanations for this: first, Heyck's estimations are based on the prevalence of migraine in the general population. Because of the very poor criteria for the migraine diagnosis (particularly the 'common form') and because questionnaires were used in many of the studies (Waters and O'Connor, 1970), the estimation of the prevalence of migraine has been far from accurate enough. Furthermore, the ratio of migraine patients consulting their physician may have been stipulated incorrectly. Heyck's practice was a referral practice, so the percentage of referrals of cluster headache and migraine patients from the patients' primary physician would need to have been approximately the same to justify this method of calculation. Heyck's estimate is based on the assumption that all cluster headache patients consult their physician. All these factors could theoretically heighten the prevalence compared with Heyck's calculations. Caution should, therefore, be exercised in evaluating these figures. It should, for example, be noted that in other surveys the ratio between migraine and cluster headache has been found to be very different from Heyck's ratio (i.e. 50); Ekbom (1970) found a ratio of 25.

With this complex situation, it would in all probability be far better to rely on the diagnostic criteria for cluster headache only and not to make an indirect estimate via the prevalence of migraine.

The prevalence figures given by Kudrow (1980) are so high (that is, upwards of 240 per 100 000; see Table 1.5) that they are not readily acceptable at face value. The following points may be relevant, however, when assessing Kudrow's estimates.

1. The prognosis of early onset cluster headache may differ from that of cluster headache of later onset. Cluster headache may become milder and may even possibly go into spontaneous remission with time. With long-lasting remission, the patients may even have forgotten the previous episode(s). It should in this context be remembered that early-onset migraine has a tendency to remit (Bille, 1981).
2. Conceivably, some patients in this category do not consult physicians, despite their complaints, owing to the relative mildness of their symptoms. The *severity* of cluster headache may show a Gaussian distribution (Sjaastad and Salvesen, 1986).

The last mentioned possibility may be worth considering, since the cases amongst Swedish conscripts were discovered as a consequence of the filling in of questionnaires and *not* as a consequence of consultation (Ekbom *et al.*, 1978).

Kudrow (1980) estimates that as many as 0.5–2 million Americans may conceivably have cluster headache. This would indicate that as many as 10 000–

40 000 Norwegians have cluster headache. We then have a spectrum from Sutherland and Eadie's estimate to Kudrow's, which, applied to the Norwegian population, would give between 200 and 10 000–40 000, a ratio of up to 200. On the basis of this reasoning, Sutherland and Eadie's estimate is clearly too low. Kudrow's estimate seems to be too high, if only patients consulting a physician are taken into consideration. Conceivably, Heyck's estimate is not too far off the real value, although perhaps the estimate of the proportion that consult their physician is wrong. There may be quite a large 'hidden' or undiagnosed cluster headache population. This proportion may be as high as the diagnosed one, or even higher. The higher this fraction, the more marked the influence will be on the given estimate.

Recently, information has been obtained that can fill in some of the gaps in our knowledge. Members of the Bologna group (D'Alessandro *et al.*, 1986) have recently tried to estimate the prevalence of cluster headache in a defined, circumscribed population—that of the Republic of San Marino with a population of 21 792 inhabitants. They accomplished this by going through patient files of the neurological, ophthalmological and otorhinolaryngological services. In addition, a letter was sent to each inhabitant in the Republic. Moreover, a control study of the case collection method was carried out on a random sample of 1314 inhabitants of more than 7 years of age. D'Alessandro *et al.* (1986) arrived at a prevalence of 69 per 100 000 inhabitants (Table 1.5).

We have recently been forced to re-evaluate somewhat our beliefs as to the prevalence of cluster headache (Sjaastad and Salvesen, 1986; Sjaastad *et al.*, 1988c). Cluster headache has, so far, been considered to be an excruciatingly severe headache, a 'suicide headache', probably the worst headache imaginable (together with chronic paroxysmal hemicrania). Nocturnal pain attacks have by many investigators been considered almost a *sine qua non*.

One of the brothers in a pair of apparently monozygotic twins (40 years old) had experienced typical bouts of cluster headache for 7 years, with clear-cut remissions. The typical unilateral, severe attacks (1–2 per day) were accompanied by ipsilateral autonomic phenomena, and the attacks also occurred during the night (Sjaastad and Salvesen, 1986). During one consultation, it was mentioned that the twin brother had also had headaches (since around the age of 28 years), but these were so mild that he never consulted a physician for them, hardly used any drugs for the pain attacks, and was never awakened during the night by them. The twin brother himself said that he had never had to stop his work as a teacher because of headache, and his pupils would not even notice that he was having attacks. The frequency of attacks was up to 2–3 per day. The pain was strictly unilateral, its maximum being localized in the periocular area, and it was associated with autonomic phenomena. The attacks usually lasted 2–3 h, and each bout usually lasted no more than 3–4 days ('mini-bouts') (Sjaastad *et al.*, 1988e), the interval between bouts usually being a couple of weeks.

Cluster headache sometimes occurs in families and also in twins. It is highly likely that the twin also had cluster headache, despite the mildness of the attacks. We would, however, probably not have been inclined or able to make a diagnosis of cluster headache in the latter case if he had consulted us on his own, without the information that the twin brother had clear-cut cluster headache. In retrospect, we have seen other patients with similar mild attacks and with only a slight tendency to clustering (Sjaastad *et al.*, 1988c, 1988e). Because of the mildness of the pain, such patients may never consult a physician.

These observations *may* have a bearing on the true prevalence of cluster headache in the general population. Such cases may constitute the left-hand side of a Gaussian distribution curve based on the severity of cluster headache. Such mild cases may escape the diagnostic 'detection system'. It may, therefore, be that even with the painstaking and vigilant detection system of the Bologna group, some patients in the left-hand part of the Gaussian distribution have been sifted through the diagnostic sieve. At present, the magnitude of this possible shortcoming of the system can only be guessed at. Some of the apparent discrepancy between the findings of Ekbom and co-workers and those of the Bologna group may theoretically be explained in this way. There *may* also be other explanations for this discrepancy, as previously mentioned, such as a more favourable prognosis of cluster headache (or cluster headache-like pictures) arising early in life.

Until proven otherwise, however, we should continue to believe that there exists a proportion of 'mild' cluster headache cases (Sjaastad *et al.*, 1988c) and, therefore, the figures calculated by the Bologna group should, for the time being, be considered as minimum values, as far as the population at large is concerned. With regard to the fraction of cluster headache patients who consult a physician, I am inclined to believe that the results of the Bologna group (D'Alessandro *et al.*, 1986) represent a fairly correct estimate.

There may be differences between races as to the prevalence of cluster headache. It should also be mentioned in this context that Lovshin (1961) has claimed that negroes are more frequently affected than whites. Joubert (1988) has recently described cluster headache in seven African black patients.

FAMILIAL OCCURRENCE OF CLUSTER HEADACHE

Cluster headache seems to be more frequent among family members of cluster headache patients than in the population as a whole. In a review of the literature, Andersson (1985) found an average of 3% of family members with cluster headache (Andersson's personal data: 5%). This contrasts with a prevalence of cluster headache in the general population of 0.07% (d'Allessandro *et al.*, 1986). However, the prevalence of cluster headache in the family of cluster headache patients is vastly different from that of migraine in the family of migraine patients.

ISTICS OF THE PATIENT

ad to be more frequent and extensive in cluster headache
ls. Sadjadpour (1975) questioned 36 patients about their
ound that the patients had 'with a few exceptions, a
/or heavy cigarette (occasionally cigar or pipe) smoking
smoking dated back to the teenage years and had been
(1980) compared cigarette smoking in cluster headache
d found a significantly higher frequency of smoking (i.e.
) and a higher number of cigarettes smoked per day (33
e cluster headache group. An even higher percentage of
er headache patients was found by Manzoni *et al.* (1983b):
ine sufferers.
of importance with regard to the symptoms of cluster
ay *aggravate* the headache. However, smoking cannot be
headache because there are many patients with typical
o do not smoke.

MPTION

h was found to be higher in cluster headache patients than
1980; Manzoni *et al.*, 1983b). This behaviour may possibly
psychological habitus of these patients. Alcohol may be
the remission phase, without any tendency to attack
luster phase, however, most patients are most careful with
ey know that if they do drink then they will have attacks.
s to this rule. It has been said that chronic cluster headache
lar, may lessen the tendency to attacks by consuming
varius, 1971). Several such patients were initially reported
oholics.
ohol may depend on the mode and extent of consumption.
uantities are consumed and at relatively long intervals,
th some regularity. If larger quantities are consumed and
y, attacks may be prevented. Whether there really is any
between the chronic and recurrent forms of cluster head-
ct is not fully known. The temporal pattern of alcohol
ttack development has not been studied in detail.

N

arris (1936) did not mention the male preponderance of
and Horton *et al.* (1939) did not mention a specific sex
ir first report. In a report from 1941, Horton mentions 45

FAMILIAL OCCU[
PATIENTS

The average familial
around 22% (Ander
was 24%. The diagn
further major short
migraine has been m
what is meant by far
siblings/children, or
ever, in a comparison
most of the relatives
history for migraine a

These figures are cl
migraine population;
than the prevalence o
researchers such as G1
between migraine and
Andersson may provi
among mothers of fem
did a father have migi
trend also observed by

CO-EXISTENCE OF C

The occurrence of migra
various studies. It shoul
small, and in many of th
simply 'headache' that w

The occurrence of migi
by Andersson (1985), wh
data: 17%). In view of the
male sex, the figure for mi
to be clearly higher than tl
exceptionally high figure
relatively high. Migraine
female than among male c
1981; Manzoni *et al.*, 1988).
and 3.5% in the two groups
(1985) own studies, migrain
headache in only 11% of su
two headache types appea
patients. The occurrence of
indicate that cluster headac.
migraine is a frequent head

SOME CHARACTER[

SMOKING HABITS

Smoking has been fou
patients than in contr
smoking habits and
history of chronic an
for many years'. Thei
continuous. Kudrow
and control groups an
78% vs. 52%, $p < 0.0$
vs. 21, $p < 0.01$) in th
smokers among clust
84% vs. 42% in migr

Smoking may be
headache in that it n
the cause of cluster
cluster headache wh

ALCOHOL CONSU

Alcohol consumptio
in controls (Kudrow
be ascribed to the
consumed freely ir
provocation. In the
drinking, because t
There are exception
patients, in particu
alcohol (de Fine Ol
to have become alc

The reaction to al
If relatively small
headaches occur w
with some regular
marked difference
ache in this resp
consumption and

SEX DISTRIBUTIO

Oddly enough, H
cluster headache
distribution in th

males and 27 females with the condition. In 1956, Horton stated that about 90% of cluster headache patients were men more than 40 years old (Horton, 1956b). He later observed a male preponderance of 87% (Horton, 1961) (Table 1.6).

There is a clear preponderance of the male sex in all the *large* series (see Table 1.6), the percentage of females ranging from 7% to 30%, with an average of 16.5%. The only exception to this clear male predominance is the series studied by Hardman and Hopkins (1966), in which females and males were equally frequently affected. This series was based on questionnaires, and the deviating result obtained probably attests to the many shortcomings of using such techniques in headache work. This work is not included in Table 1.6. The series of Duvoisin *et al.* (1961) has the highest reported male preponderance (93%) and might have been biased, since the authors were linked with the Air Force. This study should, therefore, probably have been excluded (Table 1.6). However, exclusion of these data would not change appreciably the percentage of males in the total material and so it has been retained.

There are, in other words, about five male cluster headache patients for every female patient. This figure may possibly be even higher: some females given the cluster headache diagnosis have atypical traits and may have one of several similar disorders. One such case has been described by us (Sjaastad *et al.*, 1976, 1988b). Some female patients in older series may have been chronic paroxysmal hemicrania patients. The reason for the male predominance is unknown. The proneness of males to head injuries is one tentative explanation (see 'Male preponderance, pathogenesis', p. 240).

AGE AT ONSET

The age of onset in various series is evident from the data given in Table 1.7. In the series studied by Manzoni *et al.* (1983b), approximately 80% of patients had their first attack in the second to fourth decade (see Figure 1.2). The average mean age of onset in the various series is 31.5 years (Table 1.7). Dalsgaard-Nielsen (1970) found that migraine has a tendency to start around the time of sexual maturation. The mean age of onset of migraine in Ekbom's material (1970) was 15.6 years and the range was 3–35 years (mean for males, 11.9 years; mean for females, 17.1 years). The mean age of onset of cluster headache is thus considerably higher than that of migraine.

Ekbom (1970) found a slightly higher mean age of onset for male (27.8 years) than for female (25.6 years) cluster headache patients. It is, however, noteworthy that the age at onset in the female patients seems to show a bimodal distribution with a second peak in the post-menopausal period (from 50–59 years of age). Females with cluster headache starting in the post-fertility phase may constitute a particularly interesting group of patients, because of the atypical features, i.e. female sex *and* higher age of onset than usual.

Cluster headache may begin at any age. The youngest patient in Sutherland and Eadie's series (1972) was 6 years old. Kudrow (1980) has described a 3-year-

Table 1.7   Age at onset of episodic cluster headache

	Age (years)	
Authors	Mean	Range
Symonds (1956)	26.9	14–43
Friedman and Mikropoulos (1958)	28	11–44
Robinson (1958)	36.8	22–56
Bickerstaff (1959)	—	11–?
Duvoisin *et al.* (1961)	—	16–?
Nieman and Hurwitz (1961)	—	13–69
Balla and Walton (1964)	—	12–61
Hornabrook (1964)	—	20–60
Ekbom (1970)	27.5	10–61
Lance and Anthony (1971a)	—	<10–>60
Sutherland and Eadie (1972)	37.1	6–73
Kudrow (1980)	—	<10–>60
Pearce (1980)	—	10–>60
Heyck (1981)	35.6	10–60
Manzoni *et al.* (1983b)	28.9	2nd–7th decade
Mean of means	31.5	

old patient who since the age of 1 year had experienced left-sided supraorbital/ temporal attacks of headache, usually 1–2 per day and lasting 10–60 min. This may possibly be a case of early-onset cluster headache. It should, however, be noted that: (i) the patient was a female; and (ii) the headache seemed to be chronic and, if belonging to the cluster headache syndrome, it seems to be of the primary chronic variety. Apart from the unusual age of onset in this case, a primary chronic cluster headache in a female is rare. Furthermore, typical cluster headache attack-related features such as nasal secretion and conjunctival injection were absent, and lacrimation was only occasionally present. All these features represent strong reservations against the diagnosis of cluster headache. Terzano *et al.* (1981) described a 4-year-old patient, who since the age of 1 had experienced 1–2 daily episodes of right-sided, severe and short-lasting headache. The attacks were accompanied by lacrimation and ptosis on the symptomatic side. Supplementary examinations, including an electroencephalogram and a computer tomography (CT) scan, were all normal.

Cluster headache may also start at later ages; in Sutherland and Eadie's series (1972), 26% of patients had their first attack after the age of 50 years, and the age of onset was 73 years in the oldest patient.

PHYSICAL APPEARANCE

There is a clear preponderance of males in all large cluster headache series studied (see Sex Distribution; page 26). Moreover, males affected by cluster

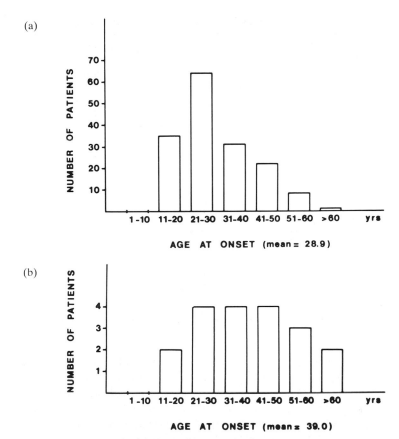

Figure 1.2 Age of onset of: (a) episodic cluster headache (*N* = 161; mean 28.9); (b) chronic cluster headache (*N* = 19; mean 39.0). (Reproduced from Manzoni *et al.* (1983b). Courtesy of *Cephalagia*.)

headache have a particularly masculine physiognomy and physique (Graham *et al.*, 1970; Graham, 1972, 1975). Characteristic traits are thick, coarse skin on the face, partly with a *peau d'orange* appearance, and marked wrinkling of the forehead and face, with deep furrows. The patients are often tall, well-built, athletic males, giving the appearance of hypermasculinism and physical robustness. Facial telangiectasia and a plethoric appearance may also be part of the picture. Even in the female patient there may be a 'masculine' appearance, with a square, well-creased face. These physical characteristics of cluster headache patients have been termed the 'leonine' appearance (Graham *et al.*, 1970).

Such special physical characteristics do not seem to be specific to cluster headache. For example, Graham mentions that patients with peptic ulcer may have deep, vertical furrows in the brow, and so may patients with broncho-genic carcinoid tumours. Telangiectasia has also been observed in another disorder in the cluster headache syndrome, chronic paroxysmal hemicrania (Sjaastad *et al.*, 1980), particularly on the eyelids and usually more emphasized on the symptomatic side.

Such hypermasculinism has also been noted by other clinicians. We have seen several such patients (see, for example, Figure 1.3). It has been said (Kudrow, Rapoport and Sheftell, personal communication) that paramedical personnel working in headache centres in the USA where a number of cluster headache patients are seen, are able to pick out prospective cluster headache patients, on the basis of their appearance, at a prediagnostic stage.

Patients with cluster headache are frequently heavy smokers and apparently drink more alcohol than healthy controls (Graham, 1975; Kudrow, 1980). However, even cluster headache patients who do not smoke or drink tend to have this characteristic appearance, according to Graham (1975). The *significance* of the leonine appearance is uncertain (see later).

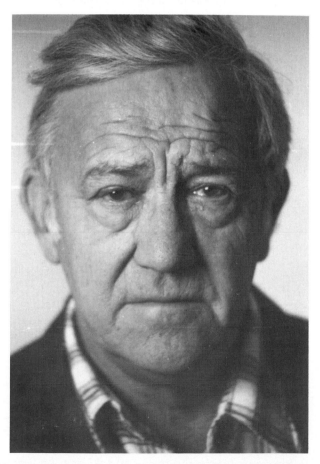

Figure 1.3 A 62-year-old cluster headache patient, with multiple and deep furrows in forehead and face ('leonine' appearance, as described by Graham (see text)).

MENTAL HABITUDE

The psychological characteristics of cluster headache patients have fascinated many investigators in this field. Graham (1975) has formulated the expression the 'leonine-mouse syndrome' to typify the psychophysical make-up of these patients. By this, Graham means to emphasize his clinical impressions that, although a hypermasculine external appearance (see Physical Appearance; page 28) is common in patients, their mental structure does not necessarily conform with this appearance. Whilst the exterior bears witness to masculine vigour and ruggedness, the mental picture of these patients does not live up to these expectations: they have the psychological and personality structure of a 'mouse'. Graham (1975) depicts the structure of the 'mouse cluster headache personality' in this manner: these patients are ambitious, hard-working individuals, 'go-getters', with great dependency needs, and an inability to disclose feelings of anger, guilt and inadequacy. Steinhilber *et al.* (1960) added some further typical personality characteristics: these patients are 'perfectionistic, rigid, conscientious, and meticulous'. Graham believes that this personality structure may play a role in the pathogenesis of the headache. Or, in Graham's own words: 'They push and push until they break with symptoms or reach the goal and drop exhausted into a cluster of headaches'.

These are clinical impressions. But are they borne out by psychological tests? The Minnesota Multiphasic Personality Inventory (MMPI) and Thematic Apperception Tests have been carried out by Graham's group (1975) (see also Harrison *et al.*, 1975) and indicate that these patients are similar to migraine patients but deviate from control individuals. They seem to exhibit obsessive, compulsive behaviour and perfectionism. They show an inability to admit or express feelings. Furthermore, they have high scores for hysteria, dissociative behaviour and 'conversion patterns'. As for depression, there was no deviation from controls. Steinhilber *et al.* (1960) also used the MMPI and compared cluster headache patients (*n* = 50) with an inhomogeneous group of headache patients (*n* = 50). A rather high prevalence of abnormal personality profiles — that is, hypochondriasis and hysteria — was found, in that 60% of both headache groups showed prime codes indicating scores on one or more of the clinical scales exceeding 2 standard deviations (SD) above the mean for the normal population. In addition, the *profiles* of the two groups were rather similar. Both groups demonstrated a 'conversion V' pattern with large scores on the 'hypochondriasis' and 'hysteria' scales and a relatively lower score for 'depression'.

Kudrow and Sutkus (1979) carried out MMPI tests on 41 cluster headache patients, a control group of 30 individuals, and also on patients belonging to other headache groups: 'scalp muscle contraction headache', migraine, 'mixed' headache, post-traumatic headache, and what they term 'conversion cephalalgia', a total of 217 patients. There appeared to be a great similarity between the scores for migraine and cluster headache patients. Neither female nor male cluster headache patients scored higher than controls on the scale for compulsive–obsessive behaviour. Although cluster headache patients did score higher than control individuals on some scales, scores of 65 (which is considered the upper limit of normal) were not obtained.

Cuypers *et al.* (1981) compared 40 cluster headache patients with 49 migraine patients (both common and classic migraine), by means of the Freiburg Personality Inventory, a personality test questionnaire comprising 212 items, which in terms of validity and information value is said to be comparable to the MMPI. Essentially similar findings were made in the two main groups. However, cluster headache patients had moderately elevated scores for 'anxiety' and slightly diminished scores for masculinity. Adler *et al.* (1987) feel that cluster headache patients are 'depressed', and claim that it is incorrect to ascribe the depression (as well as the suicidal thoughts) entirely to pain. They do not feel that there are conversion reactions in these patients as a group.

The accumulated evidence thus does not give credence to the view that cluster headache patients as a group differ essentially from other headache groups as far as psychologic habitude is concerned. Solitary cases—and there may be a good number of them—may show psychopathological traits, and bizarre behaviour may be part of the picture during an attack. In this context, it should be remembered that to have acquired cluster headache must be considered the tragedy of a lifetime. The enormous suffering caused by this headache soon modifies the life and life-style of the victim, at least in the worst cases. Although most patients manage—and some even manage well—to live with this disorder, not all do. Bizarre behaviour in cluster headache such as trance-like states, transvestism, fugues, cries and aggressive behaviour (Graham, 1975) is probably best interpreted as a *consequence* of the disorder. The suicidal ideas of these patients can also probably best be explained on this basis.

Another possibility is that the disorder may affect the cerebral areas that 'govern' behaviour and personality traits, so that changes in the personality can conceivably occur transitorily during the bout or even the paroxysms. The possibility that more permanent, discrete, organic cerebral changes may be acquired over the years as a consequence of the disease process *per se* cannot be refuted. If 'central' in nature, cluster headache may even from the beginning, as a prerequisite, be combined with minor, discrete, cerebral dysfunction.

There is good reason to believe that most patients with cluster headache would have managed the stresses and chores of life as well as anybody else had they not had their headache attacks. An indication that this is so is that, during remissions, cluster headache patients seem to manage well.

Marchesi *et al.* (1989) studied the prevalence of various types of headache in a population of 160 depressed patients. Cluster headache was diagnosed in two patients (1.2%) and migraine and tension headache in 22.5% and 24.4%, respectively, of cases. The figure for cluster headache is somewhat higher than would be expected in the population as a whole. Due to the small sample size, conclusions should be drawn from these data only with great caution.

An interesting aspect of the study by Cuypers *et al.* (1981) is that the patients showed *less* masculinity than normal. This trait in the autopathography may indicate that the patients are not so interested in living up to a masculine role as was suggested by Graham (1975). It should also be stressed that the refinement of the tests applied may not be adequate for detecting discrete and specific psychopathologic traits.

HORMONAL INFLUENCE IN FEMALE PATIENTS

There is a clear male preponderance of cluster headache patients (see Table 1.6). Furthermore, in many female cluster headache patients there may seem to be atypical traits. We have isolated a group showing a distinct symptomatology—chronic paroxysmal hemicrania—mainly from the group of female chronic cluster headache patients (Sjaastad and Dale, 1974, 1976). Heyck (1981) contends that in his eight female cluster headache patients, the headache 'never took such a severe course as often seen in men'. Other investigators, such as Lovshin (1961) and Peatfield *et al.* (1982) also believe that atypical cases are more common among women. There is, nevertheless, a consensus that, although atypical traits may be shown by many female cluster headache patients, females can have cluster headache *as such*, and not only a variation on the theme. Is there any special influence of sexual development on cluster headache?

Whilst migraine tends to start around the time of sexual maturation (see, for example, Dalsgaard-Nielsen, 1970), cluster headache seems to start, on average, somewhat (10–15 years) later in life. There is a consensus that *menstruation* as such has no influence on the tendency to cluster headache attacks (Horton, 1941; Heyck, 1976; Ryan and Ryan, 1978; Ekbom and Waldenlind, 1981), in clear contradistinction to the case in migraine.

Caskey (1966) noted the influence of *pregnancy* on cluster headache attacks in one patient. Ryan and Ryan (1978), without giving any figures, stated that the *majority* of female cluster headache patients will notice a remission of their headaches during pregnancy and a return of symptoms immediately on delivery.

Ekbom and Waldenlind (1981) found that eight female cluster headache patients (of 34 female patients) who had cluster headache before pregnancy had had a total of 13 pregnancies. Six of these eight patients experienced a remission of their headache during pregnancy. They also found that cluster periods started on delivery, as had been demonstrated previously in chronic paroxysmal hemicrania (Sjaastad *et al.*, 1980). The patients, therefore, generally seem to be most sensitive to the hormonal changes that occur during pregnancy.

A further finding by Ekbom and Waldenlind (1981) is that female cluster headache patients tend to have rather fewer children. This was most pronounced in those married women who contracted cluster headache as nulliparae ($n = 17$). In this group, the frequency of childbirth was significantly lower (mean number of childbirths 0.8; range 0–3) than in Swedish women as a whole and in matched migraine patients. In female patients contracting the disease after pregnancy ($n = 5$) the mean number of childbirths (2.6; range 1–5) did not differ significantly from that in the Swedish female population as a whole. Of course, when subgroups of female cluster headache patients are dealt with, the data base is relatively small and this must be kept in mind when searching for the reason for the seemingly reduced fertility in those who contracted cluster headache early in life. The possible infertility may be linked to hormonal dysfunction in this headache. Alternatively, the infertility may have psychological causes: it may be that, owing to the tragedy of having developed cluster headache, a patient's attitude towards her husband and/or the future bringing up of a child may change.

There are gaps in our knowledge regarding the role of oral contraceptive pills in female cluster headache patients. Ekbom and Waldenlind (1981) did not find that the use of such pills differed quantitatively from that in the Swedish female population as a whole. As for the influence of oral contraceptives on the tendency to develop bouts and paroxysms, only anecdotal reports exist.

The role of the *menopause* is also uncertain: it is clear that cluster headache may continue after menopause. It is even evident that a *de novo* cluster headache (cluster headache-like picture?) may arise in post-menopausal women (Peatfield *et al.*, 1982). Heyck (1981) found that in two of his eight female patients the onset of headache was after menopause. Ekbom and Waldenlind (1981) found that in 8 of 34 female cluster headache patients the headache started after menopause (mean age of onset 65.5 years). The influence of menopause on the frequency and severity of bouts and paroxysms is not known. Is there usually an alleviation, or is there a tendency for attacks to continue as before? This would certainly be interesting information to have.

TRIGGER POINTS

Horton (1956b) found no trigger zones such as those that are found in trigeminal neuralgia (probably during the cluster period). Horton *et al.* (1939) frequently found marked tenderness on pressure over branches of the external and common carotid arteries. In our attempt to distinguish chronic paroxysmal hemicrania and cervicogenic headache from cluster headache, we have made a thorough search for cluster headache trigger points in the neck, nape of the neck area, and back of the head. Although some soreness may be present over the C_2/greater occipital nerve area in cluster headache, the discrepancy *vis à vis* the other headache forms is striking. Bing (1952) found that attacks could be triggered by pressure on the infraorbital nerve. This finding probably attests more to the variant nature of the headache he described than to characteristic features of cluster headache.

2

Episodic Cluster Headache

TEMPORAL ASPECTS: VARIOUS DEFINITIONS

A paroxysm refers to an *individual attack*, which usually lasts no more than 1–2 h. A 'bout', 'cycle' or *cluster period* refers to a relatively circumscribed time-span within which an accumulation of single paroxysms occurs. A bout is usually of some weeks or months duration. The period between the single paroxysms in a bout is referred to as the *interparoxysmal* or *interictal period*. A *remission* indicates the relatively or absolutely symptom-free period between two cycles or bouts.

CLINICAL APPEARANCE

THE 'UPPER' AND 'LOWER' SYNDROMES

Ekbom and Kugelberg (1968) have, on the basis of pain distribution, divided cluster headaches into 'upper' and 'lower' syndromes. The intensity and nature of the pain in the two groups were similar, and the *maximal* pain in both groups occurred in the same areas—that is, in the ocular/supraorbital areas. However, in the upper group, the pain radiated into the forehead, temporal area, vertex and occipital area and, in a small number of cases, into the upper jaw but not down to the upper teeth. In the lower group, the pain radiated into the jaw, mandible and neck.

Some investigators have tried to use this categorization in their clinical studies (see Table 2.1). In the total data, the upper type is slightly dominant. As to the relative importance of the two subgroups, however, there is a marked variation between series. In one series (Pearce, 1980), the upper group outweighs the lower one by a factor of 2.7, whereas in another series (Manzoni *et al.*, 1983b) the lower type outweighs the upper type. This discrepancy is rather remarkable and it may mean that, even in the hands of experienced clinical

Table 2.1 Relative frequency of the 'upper' and 'lower' types of episodic cluster headache

	Upper type		Lower type		Total
Authors	No.	%	No.	%	No.
Ekbom (1970)	55	52	50	48	105
Pearce (1980)	69	73	26	27	95
Manzoni *et al.* (1983b)	71	44	90	56	161
Total	195	54	166	46	361

investigators, the definitions of what belongs to one group or the other are so vague that clearly diverging results will be obtained.

Many clinical variables were similar in the two groups. For some variables, however, the frequency differed: gastroduodenal ulcer, attack-related hyperhidrosis of the ipsilateral side of the forehead, and a partial Horner's syndrome (Ekbom, 1970) were found more often in the lower than in the upper syndrome. Ipsilateral swelling of the temporal artery was, however, encountered more often in the upper syndrome. The frequency of various, presumably 'autonomic' symptoms and signs in Pearce's (1980) and Ekbom's (1970) series is shown in Table 2.2. A marked difference exists with regard to Horner's syndrome. Whereas in Ekbom's series a striking preponderance of Horner's syndrome was found for the lower syndrome, only a moderate preponderance was found in Pearce's series. As for the other autonomic features, there were some moderate discrepancies between the upper and lower syndromes.

Table 2.2 The relative frequency (%) of various autonomic symptoms and signs of 'upper' and 'lower' episodic cluster headache

	Upper		Lower	
	Ekbom[a] (N = 55)	Pearce[b] (N = 69)	Ekbom[a] (N = 50)	Pearce[b] (N = 26)
Conjunctival injection	78⎱	85	90⎱	89
Lacrimation	80⎰		84⎰	
Nasal congestion	67	35	68	35
Horner's syndrome	0	17	85	27
Photophobia	73	59	64	54
Nausea/vomiting	6	1	4	0

[a] Data partly from Ekbom and Kugelberg (1968) and partly from Ekbom (1970).
[b] Pearce (1980).

Ekbom and Kugelberg (1968) concluded that these various clinical expressions of cluster headache are due to a topographical difference in the involvement of carotid artery segments during an attack: the external carotid artery being mostly involved in the upper syndrome, and the internal carotid artery in the lower syndrome.

I am somewhat sceptical about this classification, and even more so about the interpretation of the findings, which cannot be taken at face value. The interpretation is based on the popular theory of the time that pain in cluster headache is caused by dilatation of the carotid artery or its branches (e.g. Friedman and Mikropoulos, 1958), a theory that is not now generally accepted. The authors postulate, as did Kunkle and Anderson (1960, 1961) and Nieman and Hurwitz (1961), that the dilated internal carotid artery compresses the sympathetic plexus around the artery during the attack, giving rise to Horner's syndrome. According to these assumptions, the sweat glands to the face are spared, since the sympathetic fibres innervating them were believed to run along the external carotid artery. This should explain the preserved, ipsilateral facial sweating during the attack. The mechanism underlying the sweating may, however, be a different one (see Sweating; page 212).

The occurrence of Horner's syndrome in 17% of the cases in the upper-syndrome group in Pearce's (1980) series is remarkable. If this finding is correct, it disproves the very basis of the original reasoning about the origin of Horner's syndrome in cluster headache: the upper syndrome, according to Ekbom and Kugelberg, should be associated with *external* and not with *internal* carotid artery pathology. The existence of a 'partial' Horner's syndrome would certainly be hard to explain on the basis of the external carotid artery being affected. A further critique of this view is given elsewhere (see Pathogenesis; page 230).

Is there then any advantage to this subclassification? It is rather obvious that, at present, we cannot attribute the *different* pain manifestations in the two syndromes to involvement of *different parts of the carotid artery tree*. There are apparent difficulties attached to a proper classification into upper and lower cluster headache cases from a clinical point of view, and few clinicians have used this classification. Because of the interinvestigator differences in the rating of these patients, it may be difficult to exchange meaningful information based on such a subclassification. The rationale for this subclassification, if any, is probably of more interest academically than practically.

BOUT, CYCLE OR CLUSTER PERIOD

A bout is a period in which there is an accumulation of solitary paroxysms, the individual attacks appearing daily or almost daily. Such a period lasts for some weeks or months, and often begins and ends rather distinctly. By arbitrary definition, a bout does not last longer than 12 months; if symptoms continue for 12 months or more, the syndrome is termed *chronic* cluster headache; the border for chronicity should possibly be lowered (see Chronic Cluster Headache; page 269).

The cycling of cluster headache was described clearly enough by Harris (1936) who, after having studied a total of 23 patients, stated that 'there may be three or more recurrences every twenty-four hours for periods of six to eight weeks yearly'. It is remarkable that Horton himself did not clearly appreciate the cyclical nature of this headache. This unawareness of certain critical facts was probably one of the major reasons for his recommendation of histamine treatment for cluster headache: he attributed the improvements observed to the treatment rather than the natural course of the disease (see Treatment: Histamine desensitization; page 130). The cyclical nature of cluster headache has also been emphasized by Ekbom (1947), Kunkle *et al*. (1952), Symonds (1956) and Kunkle (1982). The non-cyclical variety of cluster headache is dealt with later (See Chronic Cluster Headache; page 269).

Duration of bouts

Bouts are of greatly varying duration. The intraindividual variation may be considerable but is usually by no means as marked as the interindividual one. However, because of considerable variation in the single patient we should differentiate between the shortest and longest bouts and those of usual (average) duration. Manzoni *et al*. (1983b) found that in 78% of cases the bouts lasted 1–2 months on average (Table 2.3). Thirteen (8%) of 161 patients with episodic cluster headache had experienced at least one cluster period exceeding 6 months in duration. All of them were males, and the mean age of onset in these cases was higher than the mean for the whole series, i.e. 43.7 vs. 28.9 years. In Ekbom's (1970) series, 91% of the episodic cases had bouts lasting 2–12 weeks.

Sutherland and Eadie (1972) searched for the longest cluster periods and found that of their episodic cases, 50% had experienced periods lasting between 5 and 13 weeks and 4% had experienced episodes lasting >26 weeks.

At the lower end of the scale, Ekbom (1970) classified 3.4% of his cases as having bouts of 1-week duration, and 3 of 48 episodic cluster cases in Lance and Anthony's (1971a) series were classified as having bouts of '2 or less' weeks duration. Sutherland and Eadie (1972) specifically stated that bouts lasted down to 10 days in their material. In Kudrow's (1980) series, however, the duration of cluster periods varied from 1 to 11 months.

In view of the above, the question arises of how short a single cluster period may be. It is of course impossible to formulate an exact definition of what constitutes a bout or cycle. Sometimes there may be episodes of daily paroxysms for a few days. It may be appropriate to term short-lasting episodes with paroxysms lasting 3–6 days 'minibouts', and those lasting for 1 week upwards 'regular bouts' (Sjaastad, 1986c; Sjaastad *et al*., 1988e). Patients with mini-bouts seem to have 'regular' cluster headache characteristics, with autonomic changes and unilaterality of the headache without side shift. All our cases were

Table 2.3   Cluster headache, episodic form: duration of bout and remission

Authors	No. of patients	Bout (weeks)	Remission (months)
Kunkle *et al.* (1952)	30	Days to weeks	2–24
Symonds (1956)	17	1–10 in 88%	2–120
Friedman and Mikropoulos (1958)	50	6–8 in 50%	Usually 7–18 (range 3–60)
Robinson (1958)	20	>3 in 80% (range 1–12)	<6 in 45%; <12 in 80%
Duvoisin *et al.* (1961)	32	4–10 (usually)	—
Hornabrook (1964)	21	<3 in 90% (days to several months)	Range <1–300
Ekbom (1970)	105	1–>12; 4–12 in 72%	—
Lance and Anthony (1971a)[a]	60	2–12 in 73%	—
Sutherland and Eadie (1972)[a]	58	<12 in 68% (range 1.5–>52); <26 in 87%	Range $\frac{1}{3}$–168
Heyck (1976)	48	11–43 in 85%	Range 8–72
Kudrow (1980)	500	Median approx. 8	≤24 in 81% median: 7(M); 12(F)
		Range 2–>32	Range 1–240
Manzoni *et al.* (1983b)	161	4–8 in 78%	—

[a]The series also contained some cases of chronic cluster headache.

males (*n* = 6). It may be that mini-bouts can last for only 1 or 2 days. There are also cases of mini-bouts occurring only over prolonged periods (Sjaastad *et al.*, 1988e). Often, but not invariably, there is a co-existence of mini-bouts and 'mildness' of cluster headache (Sjaastad *et al.*, 1988c).

Frequency of bouts

Ekbom (1970) found the following frequency of bouts: <1 per year, 13%; 1 per year, 40%; 2 per year, 31%; 3 per year, 8%; and >3 per year, 8%. In other words, 87% of the patients had at least 1 bout per year.

Lance and Anthony (1971a) found a bout frequency of 1–2 per year to be the most usual pattern in 59% of the episodic cases. It should be emphasized that the frequencies cited are based on retrospective information and probably on individual averages. The intraindividual variation in frequency is not evident from such data. In some of our cases, cluster periods occurred as often as once a month or even more frequently. However, there may be several years between cluster periods (see Remission).

Is there a seasonal variation of bouts?

Seasonal variation of bouts was suggested by Horton (1956a), and later by, for example, Balla and Walton (1964) and Hornabrook (1964). It was believed that cluster headache was more prevalent in the spring–autumn period, as for peptic ulcer disease. Since gastrointestinal ulcer may have the same type of seasonal variation, an explanation of the suspected increased frequency of gastroduodenal ulcer in cluster headache patients was also thought to have been found.

These statements seem to have been based on rather circumstantial and retrospective evidence. To be reliable, studies should be carried out prospectively. Similar reservations have been reported by Sutherland and Eadie (1972), who state: 'We have encountered patients in whom at first the clusters seemed to have a regular seasonal incidence, but in instances where it has been possible to follow these patients over several years the season of occurrence has often changed'. With this reservation in mind, they found that fewer cluster episodes seemed to begin in the Australian autumn and early winter than at other times; that is, 22 cluster periods started during the summer, 3 during the autumn, 14 during the winter, and 15 during the spring. Ekbom (1970) found no clear predominance of spring–autumn onset of cluster periods: in 56% of cases such periods *mainly* started during the autumn or spring. Neither Manzoni *et al.* (1983b) nor Lance (1982) found any definite evidence of a seasonal peak with regard to the onset of bouts. Cluster periods thus seem to start at any time of year, with an only moderate degree of fluctuation in frequency from one season to another. There does not seem to be any *major* spring or autumn predominance of onset. Another question is whether there still may be a tendency for cluster periods to start in certain seasons in certain patients. In a recent study, Kudrow (1987) found some evidence that there is an accumulation of bout onset during the lightest and the darkest periods of the year. A large international study is currently under way which is aimed at elucidating the influence of weather conditions on bout generation (Nappi *et al.*, 1989).

Number of cluster periods experienced

Data on the number of cluster periods experienced have apparently only been given by Sutherland and Eadie (1972): 29% of their patients were seen during their first bout, 39% had experienced 2–5 bouts, whereas 16% had experienced 6–10 bouts, and 5% more than 10 bouts. It should be emphasized that 10% of the patients who had experienced more than one bout would give no exact information on the number of bouts. Figures obtained in the middle of the disease process have only a limited bearing on what will happen in the course of a life-time. The average duration of pre-study untreated headache in the series studied by Sacquegna *et al.* (1987) was 12.6 years (range 3–44 years).

The lack of prospective studies in this field is deplorable. A good-sized group of patients in whom reliable retrospective information is available should be closely followed up to a high age in order to elucidate the life history of this disease.

Bout-provoking factors

As mentioned above, there is some evidence to indicate that there not infrequently is a *seasonal* variation in the onset of bouts. Some authors have mentioned a spring–autumn predominance, just as in peptic ulcer disease (Symonds, 1956; Friedman and Mikropoulos, 1958; Balla and Walton, 1964). It has, therefore, been queried whether factors related to seasonal changes (e.g. temperature changes, amount of daylight and climatic changes) could be influential in bringing on another cluster period (Symonds, 1956).

Several investigators (e.g. Graham, 1975; Kudrow, 1980; Adler *et al.*, 1987) postulate that *psychological events*, such as stress, anxiety, 'tension', a 'new' situation, a feeling of insecurity, or 'exhaustion', can trigger bouts of cluster headache. This view is doubted by others (e.g. Symonds, 1956). In our own series there were instances when attack series could seemingly have been elicited by psychological factors. However, in the very same patients, stress of an even higher level was tolerated at other times without any attacks occurring. At still other times, bouts started in the same patients without any apparent external provoking factors (Sjaastad, 1987a).

The presence of psychological factors at the onset of a bout may possibly be explained as mere coincidence. There is an alternative explanation which seems more plausible. In the attack-free interval between two well-defined bouts, there are sometimes minor, although clearly observable, clinical symptoms, even though they do not reach the level of paroxysms/bouts. Such symptoms may possibly indicate that the situation is labile at the time, and a new episode may or may not develop. The extra force or impetus needed to manifest the cluster headache may be small in this situation. The situation may be analogous to that when the patient is approaching another bout: he may be extremely vulnerable to many kinds of stimuli. During such periods, even psychological factors with their somatic accompaniments, such as autonomic nervous engagement, blood-pressure increase and catecholamine changes, may be sufficient to set off a bout. Under such circumstances the cluster period might have started in any case, being only delayed in comparison with what was actually the case under the given circumstances. The significance of psychological factors in such a situation may easily be overestimated.

Another factor believed to provoke bouts (Graham, 1975) is viral infection. Graham has repeatedly observed the onset of cluster periods to be temporally associated with a herpes simplex affection. Graham speculates whether activation of this virus or other viruses in cranial nerves (or the central nervous system) may make the patients unusually susceptible to noxious stimuli.

In conclusion, the significance of bout-precipitating factors remains somewhat speculative at present.

REMISSION

A remission, or remission period, is a period of absolute or relative freedom from attacks between two well-defined bouts. Pain reminiscent of mild attacks during the cluster phase sometimes appears during remission. Sometimes there is only slight discomfort. These episodes have the same localization as the usual pain attacks but may be short-lasting and are usually not accompanied by the autonomic phenomena associated with regular attacks. The episodes vary in duration, but are frequently relatively short-lasting and the pain mild.

There is a fleeting transition from the clear-cut pattern of a combination of sharply delineated cluster periods and long-lasting remissions to the chronic forms. The duration of remission is an inverse function of the frequency and partly also of the duration of the bouts.

The remission period has most frequently been reported to last from 2 months to 2 years (Kunkle *et al.*, 1952). In Kudrow's (1980) series of 428 patients, the remissions lasted between 1 month and 2 years in 81% of the cases and between 6 months and 2 years in 62% of the cases, while in 67% of the cases the duration was 12 months or less. There is a wide variation in the duration of remissions (see Table 2.3).

The *longest* individual interval between bouts was looked into by Sutherland and Eadie (1972). Adequate data were available in 34 of 58 cases. Of these patients, 44% had experienced intervals of 1–5 years duration; only 15% had experienced an interval of >5 years duration.

Long-lasting remissions have been observed. Thus, Sutherland and Eadie (1972) observed remissions lasting between 10 days and 14 years, whilst Symonds (1956) found remissions to last between 2 months and 10 years. Balla and Walton (1964) had one patient (among 28) with a remission period of 11 years. Kudrow (1980) has described two patients who had only two cluster periods each, 20 years apart. Heyck (1975) mentioned a patient who in the course of 40 years had only three bouts, each being characterized by severe symptoms of a few weeks duration, and with no pain whatsoever in the intervening periods. Hornabrook (1964) reported a patient with a remission of 25 years duration, and Graham (personal communication, 1984) has observed a remission of >30 years. In such cases, the disorder, however awesome it may have been, may almost or even totally have been forgotten by the patient, when it suddenly again strikes out of the blue.

Interindividual variation in remission duration is generally greater than the intraindividual variation. Intraindividual variation may, however, be considerable as, for example, described by Symonds (1956): a patient with almost annually occurring bouts for 16 years then had a remission period lasting for 8 years. We have seen a patient who experienced annual or bi-annual bouts for approximately 15 years, followed by an approximately 4-year remission and then one of the most severe and long-lasting bouts ever experienced (of approximately 5 months duration).

At the low end of the scale, there is no clear definition of the duration of remission. Sutherland and Eadie (1972) mention 10 days, and Kudrow (1980) mentions 1 month.

The wide range of duration of remission will infringe upon the definition of chronic cluster headache and that of a bout. Ekbom and de Fine Olivarius (1971) proposed that there should, at the lower end of the spectrum, be at least 2 attacks per week. In the extreme, this would mean that if, for example, a chronic patient had only one attack during one particular week, their symptoms would have to be defined as two cluster phases with an intervening headache-free period (remission) of 1 week. We have seen a most irregular course in one of our cases with painful and pain-free periods intermingling continuously, the painful periods dominating on the whole. However, the patient experienced some short (1–3 weeks) interposed, relatively symptom-free periods. During these periods, the patient usually had minor, slightly fluctuating pain sensations on and off, occurring in the areas usually affected. A similar course has been described by Heyck (1975) in five patients showing permanent symptoms for 3–9 years. Headache-free periods of 10–14 days duration were interposed along the time axis. Such cases provide problems of definition. Do the attacks still represent one and the same bout, i.e. is it a chronic cluster headache case, or are there many bouts along the time axis?

The best solution is to take a flexible attitude. If the attack pattern continues as previously, being interrupted for 1–1.5 (2) weeks at irregular, rare intervals, we could probably classify this headache as one cycle. If, however, both a prolonged headache-free interval occurs and the tendency to attacks on the whole seems to have changed, then the patient has probably been through a remission period, and a 'new' bout is now occurring. If a remission lasts for more than 2 (?) weeks, it would probably be most correct to classify the subsequent period of attacks as a *new* cluster period. These proposed limits are of course arbitrary, and they may have to be changed if and when the underlying pathological process of cluster headache is uncovered. Then, we may know when the pathological process is active and when it is at relative rest. Until then, terms that are as precise as possible should be used.

THE SINGLE ATTACK

The attack is characterized by the pain and the associated phenomena. The pain is characterized by its severity, its nature, its unilaterality, its localization and its duration.

Pain localization and distribution

Pain in most instances *starts* retro-orbitally, periorbitally, supraorbitally (in the forehead), or temporally. The pain may also start in the face. Only a few patients experience the initial pain in the ear region, occiput, neck, scapular

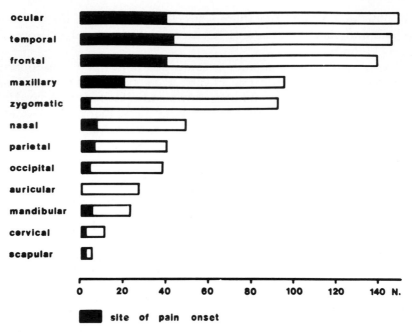

Figure 2.1 Distribution of pain at onset and at maximum (open bars) in episodic cluster headache. (From Manzoni *et al.* (1983b). Courtesy of *Cephalalgia*.)

area, or whole hemicranium (Sutherland and Eadie, 1972). Many patients localize the *pain maximum* behind the eye. According to Manzoni *et al.* (1983b) this is the case in >70% of patients. Sutherland and Eadie (1972) arrived at similar figures. On direct questioning as to the point of maximum pain, most patients put one finger in front of the eye on the symptomatic side and another directly above the middle part of the zygomatic arch, and state that the point is where the extended lines from the two fingers meet. Even when the pain starts in other areas, it will eventually spread to and mainly be felt in this area.

Although the maximum pain is usually in the ocular area at the height of an attack, the pain may be felt over a wide area—the temporofrontal area, cheek, mandibular angle, upper jaw, and roof of the mouth, including the teeth (Kudrow, 1980); even the lower teeth and, on rare occasions, the ear, occiput, neck, whole hemicranium, and ipsilateral shoulder and arm may be involved. The difference between the distribution of pain at onset and at maximum pain in a large series is shown in Figure 2.1.

Character of the pain

The descriptions of the pain given in various reports are summarized in Table 2.4. The pain is partly described as pulsating ('throbbing' or 'pounding'), and partly as having non-pulsatile qualities, more like a pressing, boring pain. There seems to be some consensus that the pain is *mostly* of a non-pulsating

Table 2.4 The type of pain associated with episodic cluster headache

Authors	No. of patients	Quality of pain[a] (%)
Hornabrook (1964)	21	Boring, tightening, squeezing
Heyck (1976)	48	Stabbing, partly burning or pulsating
Ekbom (1970)	105	Boring, pressing (47); burning (43); dull (12); pulsating (10)
Robinson (1958)	20	Burning, boring, throbbing
Manzoni *et al.* (1983b)	161	Throbbing (42); stabbing, burning (16); 'mixed' ('vascular' and 'neuralgiform') (29); unclassifiable (13)
Sutherland and Eadie (1972)	58	Throbbing, burning, aching
Graham[b]	>500	Deep, steady, boring, knife-like pain; occasionally throbbing
Symonds (1956)	17	Sharp, vicious, stabbing, throbbing, shooting
Horton (1961)	1402	Constant, excruciating, burning, boring
Lance and Anthony (1971a)	60	Throbbing, burning, boring, piercing, tearing, screwing
Kudrow (1980)	500	Boring, burning, sharp
Friedman and Mikropoulos (1958)	50	Stabbing, piercing, knifelike (56); throbbing (38); sharp (30)

[a]The total percentage exceeds 100 in some series because some patients described several pains of different quality.
[b]Personal communication.

type (e.g. Lance and Anthony, 1971a; Graham, 1975). Only 10% of Ekbom's (1970) patients had a pulsating pain. However, Manzoni *et al.* (1983b) found a throbbing and pulsating pain in 42% of cases and a 'mixed' pain (i.e. 'vascular' and 'neuralgic') in 29%. The pain is sometimes described as 'deep' and not as 'superficial'—for example, 'deep behind the eye'.

The frequency with which a 'stabbing' or 'piercing' quality has been described varies greatly (16–56%). Short-lasting 'jabs and jolts'-like exacerbations (Sjaastad, 1979; Sjaastad *et al.*, 1979, 1980) also occur in cluster headache, most frequently in the area where the most severe pain is usually located. In particular, they seem to occur at the beginning and end of a single paroxysm.

A residual soreness in the painful area may persist for some time after an attack. It usually diminishes somewhat but may persist until the next attack. Some patients complain of a hypersensitivity to combing their hair and to touching the skin in the head region on the symptomatic side. This feeling may be pronounced during exacerbations and may persist between paroxysms.

There are usually clear-cut paroxysms within a bout. With the passage of time, the delineation of solitary attacks in some patients may be reduced, being substituted by more long-standing and moderate pain. However, still there is clearly a fluctuation and, as a consequence, exacerbations reminiscent of previous *attacks* occur. In two patients with long-standing, typical episodic cluster headache we have observed a fairly continuous low-grade headache during bouts in recent years. One of these patients also experiences rather frequent solitary attacks during remission phases (see Abortive Attacks).

Pain severity

Although the attack consists of various components, the level of pain is a good indicator of the severity of the individual attack and is usually the only feature that the patient himself is concerned about.

The onset of attack is usually rather sudden; the diminishment of pain at the end of an attack may be as sudden as or less sudden than the start. It may be a few minutes before the pain reaches its maximum and there may be some fluctuation in severity even at the pain maximum. When the pain is at its maximum, it is usually excruciatingly severe, and often at the level of being almost unbearable (Symonds, 1956). The expression 'suicide headache' (Horton, 1961) has been used to characterize the degree of headache. Clinical investigators in this field have invariably been impressed by this formidable, intolerable pain, as shown by the following descriptions: 'often one of the most severe forms of human suffering' (Sutherland and Eadie, 1972); 'Histaminic cephalalgia is probably the most severe type of head pain that we know' (Ryan and Ryan, 1978).

Not all attacks are of the same severity, however. In a single patient, pain may be at any level from very slight to excruciatingly severe. In other words, during the bout there may be moderate attacks, sometimes only just noticeable. Such attacks may even be hard to discern from the background pain that may persist between the attacks in the bout.

Attacks generally tend to be more severe in the middle of the cluster period, the attacks at the beginning and end being more moderate. However, there certainly are exceptions to this rule. Russell (1981) observed the severity of attacks in a total of 77 attacks (in 24 patients, 22 males and 2 females; one patient having primary chronic cluster headache). The patients were without medication (and alcohol) for at least 48 h before the study, and only spontaneously occurring attacks were recorded. The patients graded the severity of the pain on a five-point scale (0 = no pain, 3 = moderate, and 5 = very (extremely) severe pain). The maximum pain was characterized as moderate to very severe in 78% of attacks, whilst approximately half of the attacks were graded 1–3 (Figure 2.2). There was a tendency for attacks that started during waking hours to be milder (graded 1–2) than those starting during sleep (12 out of 38 attacks and 5 out of 39 attacks, respectively). A statistically significant positive correlation was found between attack severity on the one hand and the duration of maximum pain and the total duration of pain on the other.

Russell (1981) categorized patient 'activity' during an attack (in comparison with that prior to attack) as either increased, unchanged, or decreased. Patient activity increased during maximum pain in 78% of attacks, whereas it was equal in 21%, and decreased in 1% of attacks. Naturally, the activity increased more often during night-time than during daytime attacks: activity increased

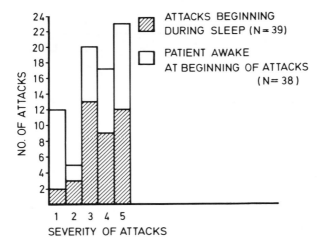

Figure 2.2 Severity (0 = no pain; 3 = moderate pain; 5 = extremely severe pain) of diurnal and nocturnal attacks in episodic cluster headache (see text for explanation). (From Russell (1981). Courtesy of *Cephalalgia*.)

during all night-time attacks, irrespective of attack severity. A significant positive correlation was found between the level of maximum pain and the increase in patient activity during attacks.

The intra-individual variation in attack severity, even within a relatively short time period, and the patient's response to it are clearly shown by Russell's (1981) study. The mildest attacks—that is, grade 1 attacks (16% of the 77 attacks)—occurred in 7 of the 24 patients. The majority of the attacks in these patients were characterized as moderate to extremely severe during the study period, and most of the attacks began when the patients were awake. The activity of the patients before the low-grade attacks did not differ from that before the more severe daytime attacks in the same patients. It is remarkable, however, that patient activity increased in connection with only one of the mild attacks, whereas it increased in 20 of 23 'very severe' attacks. The mild attacks were also clearly more short lasting than other attacks in the same patients.

We have recently (Sjaastad and Salvesen, 1986; Sjaastad *et al.*, 1988c, 1988e) obtained evidence that some patients only experience attacks of minor to moderate severity. These patients may or may not have bouts within the mini-bout category. These patients may seem to have 'regular' episodic cluster headache in other respects. These observations have somewhat changed our attitude towards the diagnostic criteria for cluster headache. They may also have some influence on the prevalence figures for this headache (see Prevalence of Cluster Headache).

Unilaterality of attacks

Cluster headache is, in principle, a unilateral headache without side alternation. Other headaches in this 'unilateral' group are chronic paroxysmal

Table 2.5   Laterality of pain in episodic cluster headache

Authors	No. of patients	Right (%)	Left (%)	Right and left (%)
Sutherland and Eadie (1972)	58	48	41	11
Ekbom (1970)	105	49	38	13
Lance and Anthony (1971a)	60	53	38	9
Manzoni *et al.* (1983b)	161	49	35	16
Kudrow (1980)	423	47	39	14
Friedman and Mikropoulos (1958)	50	Right > Left		?
Total	857	49	38	13

hemicrania, 'cervicogenic headache', 'hemicrania continua' (Sjaastad and Spierings, 1984), and probably also supraorbital neuralgia. This implies not only that the pain stays on the same side during a single paroxysm, but also that the pain usually recurs on the same side in other paroxysms in the same bout, and even in subsequent bouts. There are, however, exceptions to this rule.

McGovern and Haywood (1963) have described a case of side shift. Manzoni *et al.* (1983b) found a side shift in 16% of cases (see Table 2.5): 11% showed a shift between one bout and another, whereas 5% showed a shift of sides during a particular bout. There may even occasionally be a side shift during a single paroxysm (Sutherland and Eadie, 1972; Graham, 1975). Bilateral attacks have also been observed (Kunkle *et al.*, 1952; Graham, 1975; Sjaastad *et al.*, unpublished data). There may be a slight predominance of right-sided headache attacks (Table 2.5).

The attack does not consist solely of pain; there are also autonomic manifestations linked to the attack. It has generally been considered that these phenomena (such as lacrimation and rhinorrhoea) occur only ipsilaterally to the pain (Figure 2.3). However, quantitation of such phenomena during and between attacks has clearly shown that, although the abnormality during an attack is most marked on the symptomatic side, it is also present on the non-symptomatic side (Saunte, 1984a; Sjaastad *et al.*, 1985), but frequently at a subclinical level. We are, therefore, faced with a situation in which the pain is sensed on one side only, but in which the autonomic phenomena are bilateral (although asymmetric). We have termed this the 'bilaterality of cluster headache' (Sjaastad *et al.*, 1985). In my opinion, this is a major counter-argument against a solitary third neuron sympathetic dysfunction being the cause of, for example, the sweating abnormality observed in cluster headache (see Pathogenesis).

Bilaterality of cluster headache

In the vast majority of cluster headache cases, the headache manifests itself on one side only throughout life. The cause of this unilaterality remains unknown,

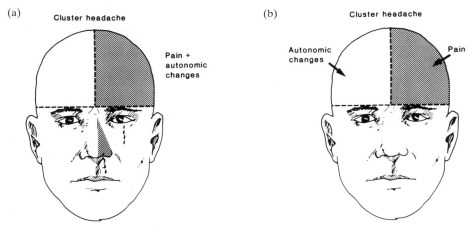

Figure 2.3 The inter-relationship of pain and autonomic symptoms and signs in episodic cluster headache. (a) The usual pattern: both manifestations on the same side. (b) The atypical pattern: autonomic phenomena on the side contralateral to the pain.

but it may have to do with *localized changes* near the midline of the brain (Sjaastad, 1988b) (see also Pathogenesis).

Cluster headache is thus, in principle, a unilateral headache without side shift; this is now recognized by the Headache Classification Committee of the International Headache Society (1988). However, the headache does change side in a fair proportion of cases, i.e. approximately 15% of the cases (see, for example, Manzoni *et al.*, 1983b). The prevalence of cluster headache may be around 7 per 10 000 (d'Allessandro *et al.*, 1986). The chances that a patient who has his first bout of unilateral cluster headache will get attacks on the other side in the future, therefore, seems to be around 200 times higher than the chances that a hitherto unaffected individual of corresponding age will get a unilateral headache of this type.

Bilateral pain in cluster headache (that is, pain occurring simultaneously on both sides during a solitary attack) is extremely rare. We have seen one such case: a 24-year-old man had bilateral headache during one entire cycle, whereas during other cycles the headache was confined to one side, either right or left. Other investigators have also observed occasional cases of bilateral pain. Graham (personal communication to the author) has observed three such cases (out of >600).

Evidence obtained in recent years substantiates the view that autonomic variables may be bilaterally affected in cluster headache. Corneal indentation pulse (CIP) amplitudes reflect the pulsatile part of the intraocular vascular bed. In the pain-free phase, the mean amplitudes were of similar size on both sides (23.6 and 23.0 u on the symptomatic and non-symptomatic sides, respectively) and clearly lower than the mean control value of 30 u (Hørven and Sjaastad, 1977). During an attack the amplitudes increased significantly on the sympto-matic side (mean 34.8 u), both when compared with the same side interparoxysmally and when compared with the opposite side during attacks (mean 28.3 u). In this context it is noteworthy that the amplitudes on the non-symptomatic side also increased significantly during attacks as compared with amplitudes on that side during the interparoxysmal period. The involvement thus seems to be bilateral, but most marked on the symptomatic side. The finding of a bilateral increase during attack, but with the most marked response on the symptomatic side, as with the CIP amplitudes, is also typical of other variables (see later), e.g. the results of pupillometric studies (Sandrini *et al.*, 1984) show the same trend (see Sural Nerve Stimulation and Pupillometry).

Therefore, with regard to the many associated autonomic factors, cluster headache seems to have a bilateral involvement. Concomitant with the pain activation, there seems to be a co-activation of the centres that regulate autonomic functions on the opposite as well as the same side. Theoretically, activation of the autonomically innervated organs on the side contralateral to the pain in cluster headache may take place in several ways. It is hardly likely that the activation of, for example, sweating is mediated through circulating substances (Sjaastad and Saunte, 1984). This activation *could* take place centrally, in an area where the regulating centres for the autonomic function of the two sides of the body are situated topographically close together; such an area is the hypothalamus. It is, however, also conceivable that a structure close to the midline or on both sides of the midline and on the 'periphery' could be the site of origin of bilateral symptoms; an example of such a structure is the cavernous sinus.

There seem to be two clear exceptions to this bilaterality: corneal tempera-ture (Hørven and Sjaastad, 1977) shows a much more marked increment on the symptomatic side during attacks (that is, means of 33.06°C before and 33.93°C during attacks) than on the non-symptomatic side, where the increment was almost non-existent (means of 33.09°C before and 33.11°C during attacks). Likewise, the intraocular pressure (Hørven and Sjaastad, 1977), which is moderately but clearly increased on the symptomatic side during attack (from 12.3 to 13.7 mmHg), does not increase on the non-symptomatic side (from 12.1 to 11.9 mmHg). These exceptions are so clear-cut that they are probably due to some special, underlying mechanism.

There seem to be other aspects to this bilaterality. A patient with a long-lasting, typical history of cluster headache had right-sided pain for approxi-mately the first 10 years of his disease (Sjaastad *et al.*, 1987b). Pupillometric and evaporimetric measurements indicated a sympathetic deficiency on this same side. However, for the next >6 years, his pain attacks were consistently on the left side, although the signs of sympathetic dysfunction were still more marked on the right side. This was also true for the autonomic findings obtained during the interictal period. During attacks, forehead sweating increased markedly on the *previously symptomatic side*, i.e. the right side. There thus seems to be a dichotomy between pain and autonomic phenomena in this patient (Figure 2.3).

Two separate lines of symptom production thus seem to lead to the pain and autonomic phenomena of cluster headache. This case seems to demonstrate that, if a cluster headache changes side, this does not necessarily indicate that the autonomic phenomena follow suit. Only the pain of the attack may change side. There may be an autonomic 'scar' left in the previous headache side, and this peripherally located scar may form a strong 'link' with the headache-generating focus (Sjaastad *et al.*, 1987b). The latter possibility is probably the most likely one.

There has recently been a further development along the same lines (Sjaastad *et al.*, 1988d): a 55-year-old male cluster headache patient had, during five bouts over the course of 11 years, always had the headache attacks on the left side. Autonomic abnormalities (a Horner-like syndrome and forehead sweating) were consistent with a pathological condition on the right (non-symptomatic) side. A dichotomy of pain and autonomic signs not due to change of side of pain localization—in other words, a *primary* dichotomy—thus seemed to be present in this case.

These cases may, at face value, seem to afford evidence in favour of a 'central' theory of cluster headache, but they do not prove it. The entire attack may still be 'peripheral' in nature. The *pain generation* in cluster headache is even likely to be peripheral in nature.

Duration of attacks

The duration of the single attack varies intraindividually, although usually not to the extent that it varies interindividually. The duration of attacks seems to some extent to be a function of the phase of a given cluster period. Generally, more short-lasting attacks are experienced at both ends of the cluster period, the middle part of the period being characterized by longer lasting attacks. But this is not always the case; short-lasting attacks may be interspersed between long-lasting ones in a given cycle (Russell, 1981). There is a significant, positive correlation between attack severity and duration (Russell, 1981).

Attacks may, in the extreme, last from 5–10 min up to 1–2 days (Robinson, 1958, Sutherland and Eadie, 1972; Graham, 1975). However, most attacks last for 0.5–2 h (Table 2.6). In the series of Manzoni *et al.* (1983b) this was the case in 73% of patients, the corresponding value in Ekbom's series being 63%. Only exceptionally do attacks last more than 3 h; thus in Lance and Anthony's series (1971a) they did so in only 3% of cases. In a survey of 500 patients (428 males and 72 females) Kudrow (1980) found that females tended to have longer attacks (average 90 min) than males (average 60 min).

Most data are based on patients' impressions, and partly even on retrospective information. Such figures are bound to be somewhat incorrect. Russell's (1981) observations were made prospectively (24 patients with a total of 77 attacks, the patients themselves triggering a marking system at the beginning and at the end of attacks). In Russell's series, 29% of attacks lasted ≤30 min,

Table 2.6 Some characteristics of attacks of episodic cluster headache

Authors	Attack duration (min)	No. attacks per day
Kunkle *et al.* (1952)	<120 (up to 420)	1–5
Symonds (1956)	10–180; usually <120	1–8
Friedman and Mikropoulos (1958)	30–120 in 86%; Range some minutes to 480	1–3
Robinson (1958)	5–480; usually 60–240	0.5–6; usually 2–4
Duvoisin *et al.* (1961)	15–180	1 per week to 4 per day
Ekbom (1970)	<30–180; 30–120 in 63%	<1–>3; 1–2 in 78%
Lance and Anthony (1971a)	Shortest 10–360, longest 15–480, usually 10–120	Usually 1–2 (up to 8)
Sutherland and Eadie (1972)	<30–>360; 30–120 in 50%; 30–360 in 80%	<1–6 ≤3 in 98%
Heyck (1976)	10–30 (120); occasionally several hours	Usually 2–6; occasionally ≤1
Kudrow (1980)	Usually 30–120[a]	
Manzoni *et al.* (1983b)	30–120 in 73%	Usually 1–2; range <1–5

[a]Females tend to have longer attacks than males (average 90 min, i.e. 30 min longer than males).

62% lasted ≤45 min, and 78% lasted ≤60 min. There was a tendency for the shorter attacks to appear during the daytime rather than during the night. Thus, 16 of 38 daytime attacks (42%) lasted ≤ 30 min, the corresponding figure for nocturnal attacks being 6 of 39 (15%) (Figure 2.4). These figures are statistically significantly different (χ^2 test with Yates' correction $p < 0.02$). An analogous situation was found for the severity of attacks. Consequently, there is a positive correlation between the duration and the severity of attacks.

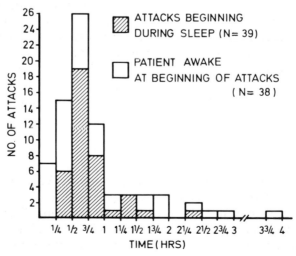

Figure 2.4 Total duration of episodic cluster headache attacks beginning during the night and during the day. (From Russell (1981). Courtesy of *Cephalalgia*.)

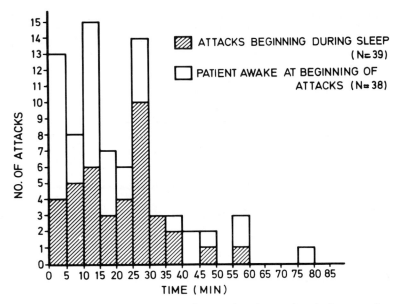

Figure 2.5 Duration of maximal pain of episodic cluster headache attacks. (From Russell (1981). Courtesy of *Cephalalgia*.)

The attacks usually consist of a middle plateau phase, with a crescendo phase before, and a decrescendo phase after. According to Russell (1981), the middle phase usually (80% of the cases) lasts up to 30 min (Figure 2.5), the foregoing and subsequent phases each usually (82% and 77%, respectively) last up to 15 min.

Nocturnal attacks seem to be more severe and long-lasting than daytime attacks. The severity and duration of nocturnal attacks are unlikely to be dependent only on a difference in sensitivity to pain during the night. It has long been claimed that there is a nocturnal preponderance of attacks in cluster headache (for a discussion of this, see later). Therefore, it may appear that cluster headache is a predominantly nocturnal disorder. This must of course not be taken to indicate that attacks of maximal severity do not occur during the daytime.

Attack frequency

In most cases, the frequency of attack ranges from <1 to 3 per 24 h (Table 2.6). It is not unusual for the attacks to skip 2–3 days in a row during a given bout, probably most frequently at the beginning or end of a bout. There may even be a considerable variation in attack frequency within a cycle. The interindividual variation in attack frequency appears to be larger than the intraindividual one.

In the series studied by Manzoni *et al.* (1983b) the most frequently observed attack frequency was 1–2 attacks per 24 h, the median 'usual frequency' being

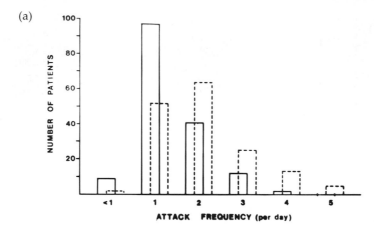

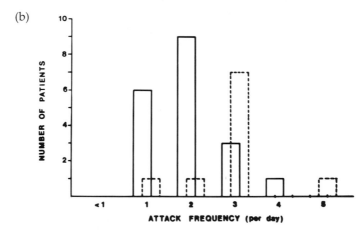

Figure 2.6 Attack frequency: (a) episodic cluster headache (*N* = 161); (b) chronic cluster headache (*N* = 19). (———) Usual frequency; (– – – –) highest frequency. (From Manzoni *et al*. (1983b). Courtesy of *Cephalalgia*.)

one attack, and the median 'highest frequency' being two attacks (Figure 2.6). The highest frequency observed in the series studied by Manzoni *et al*. (1983b) was 5 attacks per 24 h (Figure 2.6). The average attack frequency was somewhat higher in the chronic than in the episodic form. In Russell's (1981) prospective study, in which 77 attacks were monitored in 24 patients, a range of <1–4 attacks per 24 h was found, with a mean of 1.63. An attack frequency in the exceptional case of >6 per 24 h in episodic cluster headache has been reported by Lance and Anthony (1971a) and Ekbom (1970). It may or may not be of importance that these investigations were done in the period before the first description of chronic paroxysmal hemicrania (CPH) (1974). The attack frequency in cluster headache *may*, however, on rare occasions seem to be well within the range of that of chronic paroxysmal hemicrania. Thus Bogucki and

Niewodniczy (1984) have described a patient having a clinical picture consistent with cluster headache (probably the chronic variety), in whom there was an attack frequency exceeding 25 per 24 h. Another case with a relatively high attack frequency, described as cluster headache, rather definitely belongs to the chronic paroxysmal hemicrania cycle—that is, to the pre-continuous (remitting) stage (Geaney, 1983).

Timing of attacks

Attacks may occur at any time during the day or night. It has been said that attacks of cluster headache occur more frequently during the night than during the daytime. It is somewhat unclear, however, whether this is true if 'night' is defined as the hours of sleep only—that is, approximately one-third of the 24-h period (see later).

With regard to the circadian rhythmicity of the syndrome, it was claimed right at the beginning of the cluster headache story that attacks can occur with clockwork regularity in a single patient (Horton, 1941; Ekbom, 1947; Symonds, 1956) (Table 2.7). In a solitary case, this may be so at least for a limited time, usually within a given bout or part of it; the attacks may then occur for a prolonged time at the same time of night or day. Within the next bout, there may be no such tendency, or attacks may appear at set, but quite different, times. Even within a given cycle, the fixed times may suddenly change to other fixed times for unknown reasons, or the abrupt change may be temporally associated with small changes in the environment or the person's habits. We have observed several cases showing quite fixed times of attack, the attacks occurring both during the night and in the daytime. The fragility of this temporal pattern became evident when we were in the process of measuring corneal indentation pulse amplitudes, intraocular pressure and corneal temperature during *spontaneously* occurring attacks. Some patients had their attacks at regular times, for which reason we would stand by at such times in order to make the measurements. When the patients knew that we stayed in the hospital with that objective in mind, be it during the day or night, the attacks would *not* occur; as a matter of fact, the timing of attacks for that cycle had been broken. Attacks would then start coming at other, regular times. There is little doubt that within a given cycle the intraindividual variability in the timing of attacks during the 24-h span frequently may be clearly less marked than the interindividual variation. When several cycles are followed in the same individual, this difference tends to lessen. Prospective studies of spontaneous attacks are clearly needed in order to obtain the *complete* picture of the timing of attacks.

Abortive attacks, in the remission period and otherwise

During remissions, there may be an absolute (Symonds, 1956) or relative (Duvoisin *et al.*, 1961; Balla and Walton, 1964) freedom from pain and attacks.

Table 2.7 Nocturnal and diurnal occurrence (%) of attacks of episodic cluster headache

Authors	No. of patients	Definition of 'night' hours	Timing of attacks					
			Total diurnal	Nocturnal mainly	Nocturnal only	Total nocturnal	Clockwork regularity	During relaxation
Horton (1941)	72	6 p.m.–6 a.m.	5	94	85	95	+	
Robinson (1958)	20			10	12			
Friedman and Mikropoulos (1958)	50	'Night'	52	36		48		
Hornabrook (1964)	21	6 p.m.–6 a.m.	0			100		
Ekbom (1970)	105	11 p.m.–6 a.m.	38	53	9	62		
Lance and Anthony (1971a)	60	'Night'	47			53	47	29
Sutherland and Eadie (1972)	41	6 p.m.–6 a.m.	25			75		87
Russell[a] (1981)	22	6 p.m.–6 a.m.	35			65		+
		9 p.m.–10 a.m.	25			75		
		'Sleep'[b]	49			51		
Manzoni et al.[c] (1983b)	180	6 p.m.–6 a.m.	52			48		+

[a] Prospective study. The patients were not on drugs that could influence the attack frequency. The attack frequency was also 'monitored'.
[b] Defined as the time between 'lights off' and awakening.
[c] Prospective study.

The complaints during remission may be of various degrees: reminiscences of attacks, or just a fleeting, transient feeling of discomfort, interspersed in the otherwise symptom-free interregnum. Occasionally, there may be a more long-lasting soreness in the painful area. These manifestations may occur at any time, even at night, and they occur in the usual localization. The pain is usually moderate or weak, rather short-lasting and does not seem to be accompanied by the usual autonomic phenomena of the attack such as conjunctival injection, lacrimation, and rhinorrhoea (Ekbom, 1974a); at other times the pain is of considerable strength. There seem to be cases that continue to behave in this manner for a long time. At times, attacks may occur for a couple of days or more, giving the impression of a 'mini-bout' (see Duration of Bouts). There may be a fleeting transition to chronic cluster headache.

Duvoisin *et al.* (1961) reported that many patients experienced infrequent, and usually minor attacks between the cluster periods. They also emphasized that, although the clustering phenomenon was well developed in most patients, it was not so well delineated in others. Hornabrook (1964) also observed that paroxysms occasionally were isolated events. Ekbom (1970) described patients who initially had only sporadic attacks, the cluster pattern developing over time; he found abortive attacks in 56 of 70 patients. Mild attacks and even abortive attacks may also appear in the cluster period, most frequently at the beginning and end of the cluster period, when the nitroglycerine induced attacks may often be relatively moderate (Ekbom, 1970). Such attacks may, however, also occur in the middle part of the cluster period, in which attacks are generally severe (Rusell, 1981).

The evidence that attacks in remission periods may be unaccompanied by autonomic phenomena may be important. This could indicate that the attacks are so mild that 'autonomic mechanisms' are not activated. It could also be that the autonomic signs occur at a subclinical level. It is possible that the activation of autonomic mechanisms is required if a real bout is to be brought on and, if these remain unactivated there will be only solitary attacks and mini-bouts. Remission-phase attacks—and, for that matter, mild attacks occurring during the bout—should be studied closely. Admittedly, however, a study of the rather elusive attacks that occur during the remission phase may be a tough task.

Nocturnal attacks. Is there a noctural preponderance of attacks?

Horton originally stated that only cluster headache would make its victim awaken, jump out of bed and pace the floor. He later stated (Horton, 1952) that 'tension headache' could also awaken the patient at night—but a tension headache sufferer would not jump out of bed. Neither of these statements seems to be absolutely true any more: patients with chronic paroxysmal hemicrania also typically develop nocturnal attacks and are awakened. Some, but apparently not all, chronic paroxysmal hemicrania patients (Stein and Rogado, 1980) also pace the floor during attacks. Nightly awakenings due to headache are also found in tension headache, as stated by Horton (1952) and occasionally in 'hemicrania continua' (Sjaastad and Spierings, 1984). Some patients with 'cervicogenic headache' (Sjaastad *et al.*, 1983c) may also be awakened at night.

In a given cycle, attacks are frequently predominantly nocturnal at the onset, when they tend to be relatively short-lasting and of relatively moderate severity. The attacks become diurnal as the cycle progresses. However, there are variations on this pattern, since there are patients who are rarely, or even never, awakened at night.

The tendency to nocturnal attacks seems to be a typical phenomenon in cluster headache. But do the nocturnal attacks really outnumber the diurnal ones? There is a clear lack of a uniform definition of 'nights' in the pertinent literature; for example, one half of the 24 h, the hours of darkness, the hours of sleep, and so forth. This clearly hampers the comparison of the various series. For the elucidation of this problem, a definition of what is meant by 'night' is mandatory.

For several of the series, it has not been mentioned whether the patients were receiving any medication at the time of study and, if so, in particular, what percentage of the patients received prophylactic therapy. For example, Symonds (1956) recommended prophylactic night doses of ergotamine tartrate, which might have significantly influenced the outcome of the study. A further disadvantage is that several of the studies are partly or wholly *retrospective*. The headache, although it is agonizing and certainly engages the patient, is not the only and sometimes not even the main interest of these patients. The veil of forgetfulness will, therefore, partly dull the memory of cluster periods that are many months or several years in the past. Clearly, the best way to obtain adequate and reliable data would be to study only current cluster periods, in a prospective fashion and in the absence of any medication. The most exact type of recording is, therefore, to record every attack on a time chart for every day in one (as done in the study by Manzoni *et al.* (1983b)) or more cluster periods. A detailed recording done over a shorter section of a cluster period (one or several days), as done by Russell (1981), is also valuable in this respect. A major advantage of Russell's study was the use of a digital clock with a marking system that could be activated by the patient at the very beginning and end of the attacks. In this manner the length of the attacks could be timed exactly.

There are pertinent observations from the early literature: Symonds (1956) observed that in 12 of 17 patients (71% of the patients) the attacks were 'mainly nocturnal', with a tendency for the attacks to occur during the day only if their frequency became more than one in 24 h. Friedman and Mikropoulos (1958) stated that 'the occurrence of paroxysms at *night only* was found in 12 percent', while those who showed a nocturnal *predominance* of attack constituted 36% of the total group (Table 2.7). In other words, almost 50% of their sample presented a nocturnal predominance of attacks. None of these investigators defined exactly what they meant by 'night'.

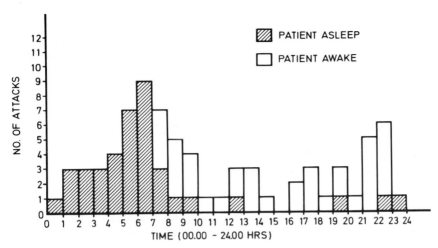

Figure 2.7   Time of onset of attacks of episodic cluster headache (*n* = 77). (From Russell (1981). Courtesy of *Cephalalgia*.)

In general, nocturnal attacks seem to outnumber diurnal attacks in the various series (Table 2.7) if 12 'night' hours are compared with 12 'day' hours. Thus, in Sutherland and Eadie's study (1972), in which 'night' was defined as the time span from 18.00 h to 06.00 h — in other words, *not* corresponding to the hours of sleep — there was a clear nocturnal preponderance. Nocturnal attacks even seem to outnumber diurnal attacks when a definition more in accordance with the actual sleeping period is used. This was the case in Ekbom's (1970) series, in which 'night' was defined as lasting from 23.00 h to 06.00 h (that is 7 h, or less than one-third of the day and night). It should be noted, however, that this study was based on personal interviews and that the category 'nocturnal mainly' makes up a large percentage (53%) of the entire group. This group may contain a number of diurnal attacks.

Russell found that, whichever definition of night he used, there was a nocturnal preponderance; however, this was minimal, when 'hours of sleep' was used (51%) (Table 2.7). If, however, a more strict definition of 'night' (from 23.00 h to 06.00 h) is used in conjunction with Russell's data then the following findings are made: 22 out of 77 attacks (29%) occurred during sleep. Or, if an 8-h period is used (23.00 h to 07.00 h), 31 attacks (40%) occurred, and all during sleep (Figure 2.7). There thus does not seem to be any *definite preponderance* of 'nocturnal' attacks in absolute figures, if the night is defined as one-third of the 24 hours.

If, however, the *relative frequency of attack per time unit during the hours of night sleep* is compared with the relative frequency of attacks during the hours of wakefulness during the day, the results will be different. The frequency of attacks per hour during the night — that is the period 23.00 h to 07.00 h — is 3.9 for Russell's *whole* series. The corresponding figures for the remainder of the 24 h is 2.9.

Table 2.8   Diurnal and nocturnal occurrence of attacks of episodic cluster headache

	Occurrence (%)	
	Russell (1981)	Manzoni *et al.* (1983b)
Mostly or exclusively nocturnal attacks	59 (m = 53, e = 6)	12
Mostly or exclusively diurnal attacks	35 (m = 11, e = 24)	47
Approximately even numbers of daytime and night-time attacks	6	41

m, Mostly; e, exclusively.

Manzoni *et al.* (1983b) found slightly more attacks during the day than during the night (a 'night' to 'day' ratio of 0.94), when night was defined as lasting 12 h (from 18.00 h to 06.00 h) (Table 2.7).

The results of the studies done by Russell and of Manzoni *et al.* cannot be compared directly because of the difference in design. The design in Russell's type of study gives the overall frequency for every hour during the 24 h period for the entire material which is, of course, less useful for interindividual comparison. Plotting the hours when attacks most commonly occur in all patients, as in the study done by Manzoni *et al.*, is also a useful method for making interindividual comparisons. Considering single patients Manzoni *et al.* found that only 12% of the patients had attacks mostly or exclusively at night, whereas 41% had nocturnal and daytime attacks on an equal basis (Table 2.8).

Until proven otherwise, the results of the studies of Russell and Manzoni *et al.* will have to be accepted: *Probably more attacks occur during the daytime than during the night. However, the frequency of single attacks per hour seems to be substantially higher during the night than during the daytime.*

Manzoni *et al.* (1983b) found that there was a nocturnal peak between midnight and 2 a.m. (see Figure 2.8) and another marked peak between 1 and 3 p.m. (when almost one-third of the patients had their attacks) and a smaller peak between 8 and 9 p.m. Russell (1981) found a markedly different pattern (Figure 2.7) with no 'midnight' peak and no early afternoon peak as in Manzoni's patients. Manzoni *et al.* have explained the discrepancy between their own findings and those of Russell in the following manner: 'Almost all the patients' in the Italian series had a break in their working hours from 1 to 3 p.m. Russell also found that daytime-onset attacks had a tendency to start during hours of relaxation. This may or may not be the entire explanation for the observed discrepancy in diurnal pattern. It seems that more research is needed before the timing of attacks is fully understood.

Behaviour during attacks

Cluster headache patients generally prefer to assume an erect rather than a reclining position during attacks. This is so typical that it could almost be

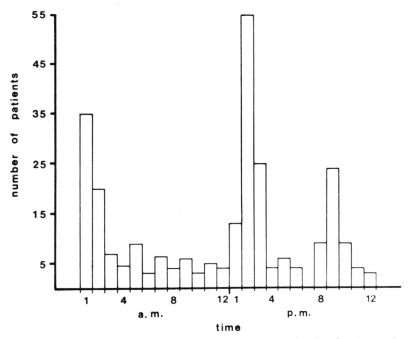

Figure 2.8 The timing of episodic cluster headache attacks. Predominant times are recorded for each patient (who may have more *than one* peak each). (From Manzoni *et al*. (1983b). Courtesy of *Cephalalgia*.)

included among the diagnostic criteria. Some patients claim that they feel some alleviation if they can walk about. Manzoni *et al*. (1983b) observed that 80% of the 145 patients seen under at least one cluster headache attack were restless and agitated, constantly moving around. Ekbom (1970) found that only 3% of patients preferred to lie quite still in the recumbent position during an attack; 10% preferred the recumbent position but were unable to lie still, whereas 29% favoured the sitting position, and 58% paced the floor. Russell (1981) found that 'patient activity' increased during an attack in comparison with pre-attack activity in 78% of cases, was unchanged in 21%, and decreased in 1%. Patient activity invariably increased during nocturnal attacks and increased in 55% of daytime attacks. There was a significant positive correlation between increased patient activity and the severity of maximum pain.

Patients tend to isolate themselves during an attack, in their office, in their den, or in the lavatory. Moreover, each patient develops his own routine, adapted in accordance with place and situation, and his own set of techniques in a vain attempt to ease the pain: some bang their head or their knuckles against the wall, some crawl on the floor, some are in constant motion and behave in a frantic manner, refusing to be touched, caressed, or consoled. Some try to place the head in certain positions, which some contend may help a little, but there does not seem to be any uniformity with regard to the preferred position. Some prefer the slightly extended position, some the slightly flexed position. Some have an entire ritual, in which, for example, the making and drinking of coffee is one of the activities. Some scream and cry, and some even become violent during attacks (Graham, 1975). Bizarre behaviour may also be seen. Thus, Graham (1975) has described trance-like states, amnesia, transvestitism and fugues in connection with particularly bad attacks.

The pain is so terrible, so terrific, so excruciatingly severe (Graham, 1975; Kudrow, 1980) that it at times seems unbearable. Most patients have, therefore, considered suicide, and this headache has indeed been termed 'suicide headache' (Horton, 1952). However, few patients have committed suicide, one reason for this probably being that there are usually good periods in between attacks which the patients learn to appreciate. One of Graham's (personal communication) patients committed homicide when another person, in an attempt to comfort him, came up to him during an attack. Opinions are divided concerning the reasons for this bizarre behaviour. It may be due to the severity of the pain, it may have a psychological basis, or it may be due to a combination of these two factors.

Associated phenomena

The frequency of associated phenomena given in various reports vary considerably, which is probably due to a large extent to the different ways in which data were collected. It is important to know whether the attacks have been observed by the patient himself only, by his family, or by his physician. The power of self-observation cannot be expected to be very good when pain is excruciating. For example, the frequency of conjunctival injection on the basis of self-observation will probably be far too low. The severity of attacks is also of importance, since there are probably differences between severe and less severe attacks in terms of the frequency of the associated phenomena. There may also be differences between spontaneously occurring and provoked attacks in these respects. The figures reported for various series for most variables are thus probably minimum figures. While associated phenomena usually *accompany* an attack, they may occasionally precede it (Graham, 1975; Sjaastad, unpublished data). However, falsely high figures may possibly arise in a given situation: the frequency of certain symptoms and signs, such as nausea and vomiting, may partly be a function of drug ingestion. Rubbing of the eye on the symptomatic side, in a vain attempt to lessen the discomfort, may eventually give a falsely positive 'conjunctival injection'. A major obstacle to comparing the different series is the definition, or rather the lack of definition, of the pathological phenomena. Needless to say, interstudy differences in the rating of criteria may produce large differences in results with regard to factors that are difficult to evaluate such as facial oedema, flush and conjunctival injection.

Table 2.9   Frequency (%) of various autonomic signs in episodic cluster headache

Authors	Lacrimation	Conjunctival injection	Rinorrhoea (R)/ Nasal stuffiness (S)
Duvoisin *et al.* (1961)	78	Frequent	R + S 38
Hornabrook (1964)	29	38	R + S 38
Heyck (1976)	Pathognomonic	Pathognomonic	R + S mostly present
Ekbom (1970)	82	84	R + S 68
Robinson (1958)	95	95	R + S 95
Manzoni *et al.* (1983b)	84	58	R 43; S 48
Sutherland and Eadie (1972)	62	45	R 7;[a] S 37
Symonds (1956)	50	50	S 35
Lance and Anthony (1971a)	82 (5[b])	45	R 15[a] (1.7[b]) S 47 (7[b])
Kudrow (1980)	84	78	R + S 72
Friedman and Mikropoulos (1958)	80	50	R + S 88
Mean of means	73[c]	60	R + S 67 R 22 S 42

[a]One case with ipsilateral epistaxis during occasional attacks.
[b]Bilateral phenomenon.
[c]Mean except Hornabrook (77).

Lacrimation. Lacrimation is probably the most frequently occurring single observable accompanying sign of an attack (Table 2.9). Thus, Lance and Anthony (1971a) found lacrimation in 82% of cases, and there was a striking discrepancy between the frequency of lacrimation and the frequency of all other accompanying signs, including conjunctival injection. A similar, although less pronounced, difference was observed by Manzoni *et al.* (1983b). This difference may be real, but the reason for the discrepancy may be that lacrimation is easier to observe than the other manifestations. The mean frequency of lacrimation (Table 2.9) in the major series is 73% (or 77% if one exceptionally low value is deleted).

It has been observed *clinically* that the lacrimation is usually only ipsilateral to the pain; in Lance and Anthony's (1971a) series, lacrimation was found to be bilateral in only 5% of the cases. Blurred vision on the symptomatic side has at times been attributed to the excessive lacrimation on that side. That is unlikely to be a complete explanation of this phenomenon because blurred vision occasionally occurs in the absence of excessive lacrimation (Lance and Anthony, 1971a; Sutherland and Eadie, 1972) (see Blurred Vision). Quantification of lacrimation has been carried out (Saunte, 1983, 1984a).

Conjunctival injection. Conjunctival injection on the symptomatic side is one of the most characteristic signs of cluster headache. It is usually of a moderate degree and may be only segmental. Heyck (1981) has stated that conjunctival injection together with lacrimation are 'pathognomonic'. However, it is note-worthy that, although conjunctival injection occurs frequently, most investi-gators have found that lacrimation is a more consistent finding during attacks (Table 2.9). Lance and Anthony (1971a) found lacrimation in 82% of their patients and conjunctival injection in 45%. The corresponding figures for the series should by Manzoni *et al.* (1983b) are 84% and 58%. Two investigators have reported a higher frequency of conjunctival injection than of lacrimation: Hornabrook (1964), who found 29% lacrimation and 38% conjunctival injec-tion; and Ekbom (1970), who found 82% and 84%, respectively. The mean frequency of attack-related conjunctival injection in the major series is 60% (Table 2.9).

Conjunctival injection is thus one of the cardinal features of a cluster headache attack. It is natural to see its origin and significance together with the intraocular circulatory changes, the temporal artery dilatation, and the skin temperature changes in adjacent areas.

Blurred vision. During a cluster headache attack, patients occasionally complain of blurred vision on the symptomatic side. Lance and Anthony (1971a) observed this phenomenon in 5 of 60 patients and even in patients not subject to excessive lacrimation. To the best of my knowledge, it has not been checked whether *visual acuity* is actually reduced during such episodes. Since the blurring is strictly monocular, the cause is probably to be found among other *local* pathological conditions. In this connection, the following observations should be noted:

1. reduced monocular vision is also a complaint of some patients with chronic paroxysmal hemicrania;
2. both chronic paroxysmal hemicrania and cluster headache give rise to intraocular circulatory changes during attacks, more markedly so on the symptomatic than on the non-symptomatic side (Hørven *et al.*, 1971b, 1972; Hørven and Sjaastad, 1977). The increased intraocular pressure and the circulatory changes that probably occur during an attack may poss-ibly play a role in the cause of visual disturbances. In other words, the pathology of the monocular, visual disturbance of the attack may be within the globe of the eye or within the orbit. The underlying *cause* of the *ocular/orbital* pathological changes may, however, reside retro-orbitally; and
3. patients with cervicogenic headache also seem to have reduced monocu-lar vision during an attack (Sjaastad *et al.*, 1983c). It is not known what the corneal indentation pulse amplitudes and intraocular pressure are like during attacks of cervicogenic headache.

Photophobia. Photophobia seems to be one of the most frequently occurring accompaniments of attacks. The frequency of photophobia, however, varies widely between the various series: Sutherland and Eadie (1972) found photophobia in only 5% of their cases, whereas Friedman and Mikropoulos (1958) found it to be present in 22%. On the other hand, Ekbom (1970) and Kudrow (1980) found photophobia in 69% and 72% of their cases, respectively. The *nature* of the photophobia is most unclear. Some of our patients localize their photophobia to the symptomatic side only. It may be secondary to the circulatory changes in the eye (see Conjunctival Injection); it may, however, be a consequence of supersensitivity phenomena.

Rhinorrhoea and nasal stuffiness. Nasal stuffiness is a rather frequent symptom (Table 2.9) during attacks, but is not always present. Nasal stuffiness appears to occur more frequently than does rhinorrhoea. Lance and Anthony (1971a) found relative frequencies of nasal stuffiness and rhinorrhoea of 47% and 15%, respectively, whilst Sutherland and Eadie (1972) reported 37% and 7%, respectively. The initial phenomenon during an attack seems to be a local swelling of the nasal mucosa, perhaps in particular of the turbinates. Depending on the severity and duration of the attack, nasal symptoms may be restricted to plugging of the nose or, if the attack is protracted and severe enough, nasal secretion may follow. The combination of rhinorrhoea and a blocked nostril was, on average, found in 67% of cases (Table 2.9).

Few investigators have mentioned that nasal symptoms may be bilateral. Lance and Anthony (1971a) found clinical signs of bilateral blockage in 7% of their patients and of bilateral nasal secretion in 2%. Saunte (1984a,b) has quantified the nasal secretion occurring between and during spontaneously occurring attacks. Nasal secretion increased bilaterally during attacks, with a mean symptomatic to non-symptomatic side ratio of 1.3. As compared with the basal secretion the attack-related secretion increased by a mean factor of 1.9 on the symptomatic side.

According to Barré (1982), nasal congestion is also a typical trait of nitroglycerin induced attacks. In particular, the inferior turbinate on the symptomatic side increases markedly in size (up to double its normal size). This contributes to the nasal obstruction. The middle turbinate on the symptomatic side also markedly increases in size.

Sutherland and Eadie (1972) and Lance and Anthony (1971a) have both reported ipsilateral *epistaxis* during the attack in one case.

Rhinorrhoea often accompanies lacrimation during a cluster headache attack. For this reason, the prevailing view seems to be that the nasal secretion is in fact a reflection of the lacrimation on the same side, the tears being partly forwarded to the nares (e.g. Kunkle and Anderson, 1961). This facet of the cluster headache attack has, therefore, been made the object of a special study in our laboratory (Saunte, 1983, 1984a). Coloured fluid (fluorescein) was instilled into the conjunctival sac of control individuals in the supine ($n = 13$) or sitting position with the head in an upright position ($n = 10$). In case cluster headache patients differ from control individuals in this respect, a few patients with cluster headache were also studied, outside attack. The route of the coloured fluid was recorded at various time intervals by means of Schirmer's test tapes on the nasal septum and at the bottom of the nasal canal. In addition, cotton swabs were applied in the nasopharynx. The coloured fluid was only found in the nasopharynx and not on the test tapes in the anterior part of the nose. The condition could be essentially different *during* an attack of cluster headache, tears being, for example, propelled in the anterior direction owing to local oedema formation. In this case there would have to be *two* abnormalities as far as lacrimation during an attack is concerned: increased lacrimation and drainage of tears along unusual pathways. This possibility seems somewhat unlikely, but has not been fully examined.

There are two other lines of observation that have a bearing on the origin of nasal secretion during attack. Lance and Anthony (1971a) and Sutherland and Eadie (1972) found that lacrimation occurs far more frequently (in 82% and 62% of cases, respectively) than nasal secretion (in 15% and 7% of cases, respectively) (Table 2.9). This indicates that, even during an attack of cluster headache tears usually flow in a direction other than towards the nares. Lance and Anthony (1971a) also observed cases of nasal secretion, but without tearing, a finding that corroborates our strong belief that we are dealing with two separate phenomena. The fact that our patients were also studied in the supine position during the attack and even then (see later) showed clearly increased nasal secretion (from the *anterior* part of the nose) indicates that there is attack-induced rhinorrhoea of endogenous, nasal origin. The inference may, therefore, be made that *although rhinorrhoea and lacrimation frequently co-exist, they probably are two separate, independent manifestations of the cluster headache attack.*

Prominent temporal area and forehead vessels. Horton *et al.* (1939) mentioned swelling of temporal vessels in their first report. Ekbom and Kugelberg (1968) noted swelling of the ipsilateral temporal artery in 6 out of 9 patients with the 'upper' syndrome (67%) but in none of 14 patients with the 'lower' syndrome. They concluded that 'the underlying vascular' process can presumably be ascribed mainly to the external carotid artery in the upper syndrome and mainly to the internal carotid in the lower syndrome. Lance (1982) found a 'prominent, tender temporal artery' in 10 and 'prominent veins in the forehead' in 2 of a total of 60 patients. We have observed dilated vessels on the symptomatic side during occasional attacks in several patients (Figure 2.9). Symonds (1956) mentions that the ear on the symptomatic side in one of 17 patients having a prominent temporal vessel was redder and hotter than the contralateral one.

Oedema. While some 'vascular' phenomena, such as conjunctival injection, frequently occur during an attack, other vascular phenomena, such as oedema, seem to be rare. Some clinical investigators, like Sutherland and Eadie (1972), have indicated that *ptosis* may be only just apparent in some cases, being due to the pure mechanical effect of oedema of the upper eyelid, and they also

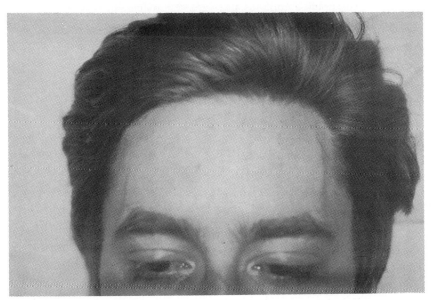

Figure 2.9 Bulging vessel in the left temporal region during a left-sided attack of episodic cluster headache. This patient had attacks on the other side during other bouts and during the early phase of the present bout. At times he had bilateral pain attacks.

mentioned that there is 'occasional swelling of the face . . . due to local vasodilatation'. Lance (1982) also mentioned that 10% of his patients get 'puffiness around eyes' during an attack (Table 2.10).

We too have seen oedema of the eyelid and in the periorbital area on the symptomatic side in cases that we believe belong to the cluster cycle. We cannot give any frequency figures, but *overt* oedema is certainly a rare phenomenon in cluster headache. Oedema, mostly of the ocular region, seems to occur more frequently in chronic paroxysmal hemicrania and in other vaguely defined, unilateral headaches. 'Cervicogenic' headache (Sjaastad *et al.*, 1983c) is also accompanied by facial/forehead oedema at times. Oedema in these conditions is probably subclinical in many cases.

The real frequency of oedema in these conditions will, therefore, not be known until more refined techniques for its clinical detection are available. Even if it is overt, the rating criteria are so poor that assessments will be purely subjective. For example, photographs are probably unsuitable for demonstrating such changes and are hardly likely to be scientifically convincing enough unless the oedema is marked. We, at least, have been unable to obtain photographs that would convince others that facial oedema really was present (which is *one* objective of such efforts). We have, in recent years, at the suggestion of Prof. F. Lembeck, tried to develop a method for the quantification of oedema based on the fluorescent properties of vibramycin. It has not been possible, so far, to make this test clinically applicable.

Table 2.10   Autonomic symptoms and signs (%) in episodic cluster headache

Authors	Nausea (N)	Vomiting (V)	Facial oedema	Facial flush
Duvoisin *et al.* (1961)	28	9	Sometimes	—
Hornabrook (1964)	19	10	—	—
Heyck (1976)	10	Rare	—	17
Ekbom (1970)	19	5	—	Lacking
Robinson (1958)	20	10	10	5
Manzoni *et al.* (1983b)	40	—	—	—
Sutherland and Eadie (1972)	N + V: 21		—	Occasional redness of ear (Horner)
Symonds (1956)	24	12	—	1 case red/hot ear
Lance and Anthony (1971a)	43	15	10	20
Kudrow (1980)	54	—	?	Lacking
Friedman and Mikropoulos (1958)	N + V: 28		1 case, periorbitally	—
Pearce (1980)	—	1	—	—
Mean of means	29	9	7	14

The possible occurrence of oedema and extravasation is of considerable scientific importance for the understanding of the pathogenesis of this condition.

Facial flush. Several investigators have observed facial flush during spontaneous attacks (see e.g. Hardman and Hopkins, 1966; Curless, 1982). Few investigators, however, have reported exact figures of the frequency of facial flush, they merely have mentioned that it does occur (Table 2.10). Heyck (1981) reported flushing in 8 of his 48 patients (17%) during spontaneously occurring attacks, whereas Lance and Anthony (1971a) observed flushing in 12 of their 60 patients (20%). Flush has also been observed during spontaneously occurring attacks by Jelenczik (personal communication, 1984). Because of the vagueness of this phenomenon, the average frequency given in Table 2.10 should be viewed with some reservation.

Lance seems to have been influenced by Ekbom and Kudrow's (1979) note, in which they claimed that facial flush is not present during attacks. Lance (1982) thus later stated: 'but the general impression given to the observer at the height of the attack is one of pallor', even though he only had observed 'pallor of face' in 2 of his 60 cases, and 'flush' in 12 of them. This dualistic attitude is also taken by Graham (1975), who states that the 'face may become markedly flushed sometimes, only on the side of the headache', or it may 'grow ashy pale'. It should be emphasized, however, that Ekbom (1970) to a not inconsiderable extent studied attacks provoked by nitroglycerine, and it has so far not been convincingly demonstrated that such attacks are identical to spontaneously occurring ones. Ekbom and Kudrow (1979) thought that flush may be due to rubbing of the skin during the attack.

Facial flushing is not an infrequently occurring feature of 'cervicogenic' headache (Sjaastad *et al.*, 1983c). However, we have also observed diffuse facial redness in ocular and infraocular areas in a few cases which we believe belong to the cluster cycle. We cannot express any views as to the frequency of this phenomenon since we have carried out no systematic observations, but we believe that it is a rare phenomenon. Nor can we refute the possibility that the flush is caused by rubbing the skin in some (all?) cases, although it has been our impression that it was not. Heyck (personal communication, 1980) was convinced that the flush in most of his cases was not caused by rubbing.

Again, the lack of clear rating criteria constitute a great barrier towards obtaining more accurate information. Further studies are clearly indicated before the dispute concerning flush in cluster headache can be settled.

Nausea, vomiting, diarrhoea and anorexia. In his early reports, Horton (1941) claimed that nausea/vomiting were almost non-existent during attacks. His views on this changed considerably over the years. da Silva (1974) found nausea/vomiting in only 5.5% of his patients. A slightly different picture has evolved from most later studies. Ekbom (1970) found that 19% of his patients had nausea and 5% had vomiting as well, whereas in the series studied by Manzoni *et al.* (1983b) 40% of patients complained of nausea (Table 2.10) and Kudrow (1980) found nausea in 54% of his cases. *Vomiting* is a rare accompaniment of the cluster headache attack; that is, in most series it was present in <10% of cases (Table 2.10). Vomiting seems to occur mainly (only?) when the attacks are particularly long-lasting or severe, or both.

The difference between migraine and cluster headache is, nevertheless, clear in this respect, in that in Ekbom's (1970) comparative study 70% of migraine patients had nausea and vomiting.

Lance and Anthony (1971a) have recorded the frequency of *anorexia* among their chronic headache patients as 3%. *Diarrhoea* is, in our experience, an infrequent symptom during attack periods. We have seen one such patient; Lance and Anthony (1971a) reported two cases out of 60 patients.

Salivation. Several investigators have mentioned salivation during attacks as a sign of cluster headache. Thus, in a case report, Horton (1952) stated that 'thick mucus formed in the mouth'. Graham (1975) has also noted this, and states that 'excessive amounts of thick saliva may be produced', and 'salivation—very marked manifestations'. Some of our patients also told us that they had abundant and thick saliva during attacks. Later, when we started *quantifying* salivation and requestioned the patients, we were told that salivation was characterized by being thick and viscous rather than by being abundant.

Solomon and Guglielmo (1985) have tried to assess retrospectively the salivation during attacks. They claim that an 'increased quantity of saliva' is present in 8% of the cases (12 out of 146 cases), whereas 'no change in salivary secretion' was present in 83%. They have even proposed, still from retrospective data, that it is possible to distinguish two more groups: one group having 'decreased quantity of saliva' (8%) and one group having normal quantity with increased viscosity' (1%).

As far as I am concerned, a retrospective quantification—and even characterization—of salivation is hardly a field in which much exact information is going to be obtained. However, a quantitative study on salivation has been done (Saunte, 1983, 1984a).

Convulsions and paraesthesiae during attacks. Horton (1961) observed 'convulsive seizures' at the height of the pain attack in five patients. 'Extensive investigations' disclosed no source of these manifestations. Sutherland and Eadie (1972) described a patient who during a 'particularly persistent cluster of attacks' observed that the foot contralateral to the side of headache would twitch involuntarily in some attacks. Furthermore, Lance and Anthony (1971a) observed a patient who had 'unilateral carpal spasm' of a few minutes duration on three occasions.

There is no particular reason to believe that the Australian cases are at variance with ordinary cluster headache, and these observations are hard to reconcile with the hypothesis that cluster headache is merely a disorder of 'extracranial vessels'.

In two of Sutherland and Eadie's (1972) patients, paraesthesiae occurred in the face and limbs on the side contralateral to the head pain during some attacks.

Bradycardia. Bradycardia during attacks was noted by Kunkle and Anderson (1961) in two of 98 cases. Jacobsen (1969) reported on a 64-year-old male patient who was observed during 10 cluster headache attacks. During the inter-paroxysmal period, the pulse was 52–68 beats/min, whereas during the attack, the pulse rate varied between 40 and 48 beats/min. It is noteworthy that intravenously injected atropine (0.4 mg) did not change the heart rate in this case. Bruyn *et al.* (1976) reported an even more marked bradycardia in a 47-year-old male, ranging from 20 to 44 beats/min as against a usual heart rate of 66–70 beats/min in this patient.

Electrocardiac investigations in cluster headache are dealt with elsewhere (see Electrocardiographic Rhythm Disturbances During Attacks).

Unusual symptoms during attacks. Lance and Anthony (1971a) have mentioned 'polyuria' in four of their cases, 'lumps in the mouth' (whatever that might be) in two, and 'vertigo and mild ataxia' in four cases.

PARTLY ATTACK-INDEPENDENT COMPLICATIONS AND CONSEQUENCES

HORNER'S SYNDROME

Horner's syndrome (Horner, 1869) (or, to be more cautious at this stage, a Horner-like picture) can frequently be observed on the symptomatic side.

Table 2.11 Presence of 'Horner's syndrome' (%) in episodic cluster headache: clinical observations[a]

Authors	Horner's syndrome during cluster period	Persistent Horner's syndrome
Robinson (1958)	—	5
Duvoisin *et al.* (1961)	16	—
Nieman and Hurwitz (1961)	22	20
Ekbom and Kugelberg (1968)[b]	0: 'Upper' syndrome	—
	84: 'Lower' syndrome	18[c]
Lance and Anthony (1971a)	32	—
Sutherland and Eadie (1972)	—	7
Heyck (1976)	44	4
Pearce (1980)	17: 'Upper' syndrome	—
	27: 'Lower' syndrome	—

[a] Hardman and Hopkin's (1966) data have not been used because in their case material there was a sex ratio of 1:1 (questionnaire material).
[b] Partly studied during *induced* attacks.
[c] Data from Ekbom (1970).

Miosis and ptosis were mentioned by Eulenburg as early as 1878 as a feature in 'hemicrania angioparalytica'. In his early reports, Horton did not mention Horner's syndrome (e.g. Horton, 1939), but in later communications he mentioned it as a sign of cluster headache. Thus, Horton in 1952 stated: 'Horner's syndrome is not uncommon in this type of case'. Later, he says, 'Horner's syndrome is common; it may disappear after a given series of attacks has ceased or may persist indefinitely' (Horton, 1961). In Nieman and Hurwitz's (1961) series the frequency of Horner's syndrome was 22%. There is apparently a great variation (see Table 2.11) in the frequency of occurrence of Horner's syndrome in clinical series of cluster headache patients.

Ekbom and Kugelberg (1968) have attempted to categorize cluster headache into 'upper' and 'lower' syndromes (see Tables 2.1 and 2.2 and The 'Upper' and 'Lower' Syndromes). They proposed that the underlying abnormality in these subgroups is to be found in certain segments of the arteries, i.e. in the external carotid artery for the upper and in the internal carotid artery for the lower syndrome. They found Horner's syndrome only in the lower syndrome (see Tables 2.2 and 2.11). Ekbom returned to this problem in 1970 when he stated that 19 of 104 patients presented with signs of a 'partial' Horner's syndrome (17 males and 2 females), and all of them belonged to the lower type. Heyck (1976), however, found Horner's syndrome in 11 of 48 patients with the upper syndrome and in 7 patients with the lower syndrome. Three patients with Horner's syndrome were classified as having a 'combined type' of the upper and lower syndromes. Likewise, Pearce (1980) found Horner's syndrome in cases of the upper syndrome (Tables 2.2 and 2.11). This may indicate that *a*

Horner-like picture is an integral part of cluster headache as such, and *not,* of a subgroup of it.

When trying to assess from a clinical point of view how frequently Horner's syndrome occurs in cluster headache, one encounters problems of definition. What is meant by 'anisocoria', by 'ptosis' and 'anhidrosis'? For each of these factors there have been great problems of definition. To deal with the anisocoria first, Del Bene and Poggioni (1987) and Del Bene *et al.* (1985) have defined anisocoria as a difference between pupil diameters of more than 10%. An accurate way of defining anisocoria, although of limited value in *clinical* practice, would be to measure the pupil size by pupillometry. The sensitivity of the pupillometer is, however, so high (0.03 mm resolution) that most control individuals will have anisocoria. Smith *et al.* (1979) found that 95% of 150 healthy individuals of both sexes and aged 18–67 years had a difference of 0–0.7 mm between the pupil diameters, irrespective of which pupil was the larger. In other words, 5% of controls had an anisocoria exceeding 0.7 mm. In our own series ($n = 124$) (Antonaci *et al.*, 1989), an anisocoria of >0.6 mm was present in 7% of cases and an anisocoria of >0.7 mm in 2.4% of the cases, irrespective of which pupil was the larger. The most marked anisocorias could be discerned by the observer in dim light with the naked eye. One possible approach to a definition of anisocoria would, therefore, be the lowest level of difference in pupil width that the naked, unaided eye might be able to discriminate. Boniuk and Schlesinger (1962) in their study of Raeder's syndrome (Raeder, 1924) defined anisocoria as at least a 1 mm difference between the pupils. Strict definitions have not been used in the clinical cluster headache series; the figures given should, therefore, not be accepted at face value. This fact also hampers interseries comparison. The figures for Horner's syndrome in attacks of cluster headache, based, as they frequently are, partly on patients' observation and partly on findings in provoked attacks, cannot be expected to reflect the true occurrence.

The Horner-like findings are apparently partly periodic (Table 2.11). If persistent, they may appear to be more pronounced during the bout. If obtained by competent observers, the figures given for the pain-free state should *a priori* be a closer representation of the occurrence of marked anisocoria. A comparison with a relatively large control series shows that a Horner-like picture in cluster headache is frequent (Salvesen *et al.*, 1988a; Antonaci *et al.*, 1989).

In some cases the cluster headache changes side from one cluster period to another. In such cases, the 'Horner signs' may remain on the 'old' side, like a 'scar' (Figure 2.3). Whether there may, in addition, be minor signs of sympathetic deficiency on the 'new' side may be next to impossible to assess clinically, since the only criterion that can be used in this evaluation is the asymmetry.

The term 'partial' Horner's syndrome has been used to characterize the Horner-like findings typical of cluster headache (see Ekbom and Kugelberg, 1968; Ekbom, 1970; Lance, 1982). This term is used to indicate that only *two* components of the typical Horner syndrome—that is, the miosis and the drooping eyelid—might be present, whilst a third characteristic, the anhidrosis, was found to be lacking or even to be replaced by hyperhidrosis (Ekbom, 1970; Heyck, 1976, 1981). Sometimes, even the ptosis seems to be moderate (Heyck, 1981) or even lacking. While sweating can be quantified, it is difficult to *quantify* ptosis. A certain amount of ptosis is, nevertheless, at times a definite component of cluster headache attack. Nieman and Hurwitz (1961) in a series of 50 cluster headache patients found 11 patients with Horner's syndrome. Nine of these had ptosis, and three had ptosis without miosis. Jaffe (1950) has claimed that miosis is a constant feature of Horner's syndrome, while ptosis is not.

With refined techniques, such as evaporimetry during body heating, it has recently become possible to demonstrate that hypohidrosis (but *not* anhidrosis) is generally present in the forehead on the symptomatic side outside of attacks (Sjaastad and Saunte, 1982; Saunte *et al.*, 1983b). The *hyperhidrosis during the attack* (which is subclinical in many cases) does not alter this fact (see later). The three major components of Horner's syndrome may, therefore, be present in many cases of cluster headache (Sjaastad, 1985a) and the term 'partial' Horner's syndrome may, therefore, not be appropriate.

Kunkle and Andersson (1961) and Nieman and Hurwitz (1961) hypothesized that the dilated internal carotid artery during the attack compresses the sympathetic plexus around the artery, giving rise to a Horner's syndrome. According to these assumptions, the sweat glands to the face should be spared, since they supposedly run along the external carotid artery. In their opinion, there would be a third-neuron sympathetic lesion in cluster headache. The situation with regard to the sympathetic fibres should then be rather similar to that in Raeder's (1924) paratrigeminal syndrome. These problems are discussed further in the sections dealing with the particular components of Horner's syndrome (forehead sweating (evaporimetry) and miosis (pupillometry)).

A remarkable finding has been reported by Barré (1982): within 2 min of nasal application of cocaine, the miosis could be aborted. The normalization of the pupil even seemed to precede the resolution of the pain slightly.

In conclusion, it should be emphasized that, although some aspects of cluster headache may clinically greatly resemble Horner's syndrome, it may still be different from it. Similarity does not necessarily indicate identity, and these symptoms of cluster headache may still indicate a 'pseudo-Horner' picture.

GASTRODUODENAL ULCER AND GASTRIC ACIDITY

The evidence that histamine plays a fundamental role in cluster headache pathogenesis includes an increase in gastric acid secretion in cluster headache patients outside attacks. According to Horton (1956b), the situation would be as follows:

> During spontaneous and induced attacks it seems evident that histamine is released from the shocked tissues in the region of the pain and accounts for most local phenomena. The increased acidity of the gastric contents indicates absorption of this agent in the blood stream and is *comparable to that which is induced by the subcutaneous injection of known amounts of histamine*. A relationship between acute duodenal ulcer and histaminic cephalalgia has been observed. Other biological agents may be liberated in the region of the pain (the italicization is mine).

Ulcers are said to occur more frequently in cluster headache patients than in the population at large. Graham (1972) found 22 cases of peptic ulcer in 100 patients. Ekbom (1970) found ulcer in 15 of 105 patients. Ekbom's patients underwent radiographic examinations. Heyck (1981), however, found ulcers 'clinically confirmed' in only 3 of 48 patients. Moreover, in two of these cases the ulcer antedated the headache by far. Kudrow (1977) has also claimed that there is an increased occurrence of peptic ulcer in patients with cluster headache.

I do not feel convinced that the evidence demonstrates conclusively an abnormally high frequency of ulcer in cluster headache. Nor have I been impressed by the occurrence of ulcers in my own patients. It is not always clear whether the figures given concern the *actual* frequency of ulcer or the frequency during a life-time. In the latter case the figures for ulcers in the control population seem to be rather high. To be convincing, a blind study of the occurrence of ulcers in cluster headache patients should be carried out (including the X-ray examination) and must include a control group. Even if an increased prevalence of gastrointestinal ulcer in the cluster headache group were found, it will be an open question what fraction may be ascribed to the heavy intake of drugs.

Relevant studies of gastric acidity in cluster headache are few and far between. Graham *et al.* (1970) observed increased gastric acid secretion in 50% of his patients ($n = 16$) after histalog stimulation, occasionally with levels in the Zollinger–Ellison range. A large-scale, systematic study of gastric acidity during and between bouts and paroxysms ought to be conducted. Since most attacks occur during the night-time, the night acidity levels will be of greatest interest. The level of gastric acid secretion will need to be compared with that in a control population. Even if increased acidity should prove to be a regular accompaniment of the cluster headache cycle or paroxysm, this fact may be interpreted in the diametrically opposite manner, as done by, for example, Kunkle *et al.* (1952): 'Any gastric hyperacidity during an attack can plausibly be attributed to the known non-specific effect of a stress situation'. The tendency to ulcer formation may accordingly be viewed from the same angle. It should again be emphasized that the great variety of drugs (some of which are ulcerogenic) ingested by cluster headache patients may be of importance in this connection.

ATTACK PROVOCATION

In many cases it is difficult to observe an actual attack of cluster headache because attacks are frequently nocturnal and those that do occur during the daytime may be so sporadic and short-lasting that they evade the observation of the clinician. To compensate for this obvious drawback from a diagnostic point of view, various provocative tests have been introduced, such as the histamine test (Horton *et al.*, 1939) and the nitroglycerin test (Peters, 1953). The provocation agents used have in common that they are vasoactive, and even vasodilatory, agents. Graham (1975) has observed that even tyramine can provoke attacks.

NITROGLYCERIN TEST

Nitroglycerin (1–3 mg sublingually) has been extensively used as a provocative agent in tests done by Peters (1953) on 100 headache cases, including 19 of cluster headache. The test was carried out with the patient in the supine position. Peters stressed that with this test, patients would get an immediate, generalized, throbbing headache, just like healthy individuals (Figures 2.10 and 2.11). This headache is generally mild and is not of diagnostic importance, whereas the later-appearing headache is. The late headache appears after 30–50 min in >50% of cluster headache cases (Ekbom, 1970) (see Figures 2.10 and 2.11). Drummond and Anthony (1985) found an average latency of 44 min. Peters found that nitroglycerin and histamine were approximately equipotent

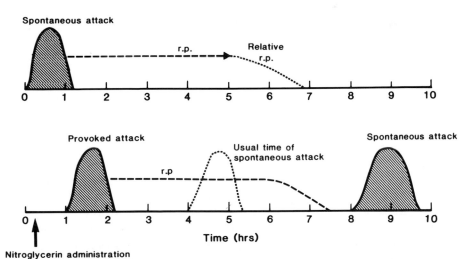

Figure 2.10 Cluster headache and nitroglycerin test: the temporal relationship between the refractory period and spontaneous and nitroglycerin-provoked attacks. During the 'relative' refractory period (r.p.), a 'latent' attack may be provoked. (From Bogucki.)

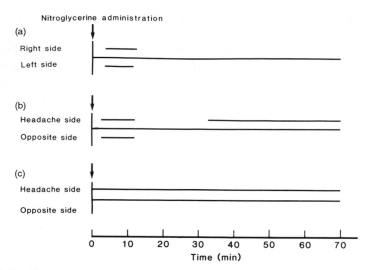

Figure 2.11 Response to nitroglycerin. (a) Healthy individuals: short-lasting bilateral headache. (b) Cluster headache: in addition to the short-lasting, initial pain similar to that observed in healthy individuals, there is a late long-lasting pain on the symptomatic side. (c) Cervicogenic headache: immediate onset of long-lasting headache on the symptomatic side. We do not know how frequent this pattern is in cervicogenic headache.

in precipitating cluster headache attacks (79% and 75%, respectively), whereas nitroglycerin was much more effective than histamine in provoking migraine headache (71% vs. 28%). Remarkably, both the nitroglycerin and histamine tests were negative in tension headache. Horton (1956b, 1957) also used nitroglycerin (1.3 mg) as an attack-provoking agent but did not find it as satisfactory as the histamine test, although it did frequently precipitate an attack.

Ekbom (1970) carried out the nitroglycerin test in the following manner. Ideally, no vasoconstrictor agent had been taken by the patient before the test, and at least 8 h ought to have passed since their last attack. Nitroglycerin (1 mg) in tablet form was given sublingually. If a unilateral pain 'identical' to the ordinary one occurred within 90 min, the test was said to be positive. The mean latency period before appearance of attack was 41 ± 3 min (standard error), with a range of 12–72 min. Ekbom was able to provoke attacks in all of his 28 patients, in the acute phase. During remission, nitroglycerin is ineffective. It is also ineffective during successful prophylactic treatment and is usually negative some hours after an attack (the 'refractory period', see Figure 2.10), and a provoked attack may postpone the onset of an expected attack (Figure 2.10). Barré (1982) found a 100% response rate in 12 experiments (1.0 mg nitroglycerin sublingually), the mean latency time being 46 min. He noted, however, that, although the character of the induced attack was generally the same as that of the spontaneous one, there was a tendency for the induced pain to be more widespread than the spontaneous one. This may be an important observation. Nasal congestion was a typical trait in nitroglycerin induced attacks. The inferior turbinate swelled and could double in size, and the middle turbinate also swelled, but to a lesser extent. This contributed to the nasal obstruction.

Drummond and Anthony (1985) provoked a pain attack in 68% of their 22 patients studied during a bout.

The available information suggests that this test is not specific for cluster headache, because it may also precipitate attacks of migraine (Peters, 1953; Dalsgaard-Nielsen, 1955). Furthermore, Hildebrandt and Jansen (1984) have applied the test in cases of vascular malformations of the upper cervical roots (C2/C3) (see Figure 2.11). The test reproduced the pain attacks even in these cases, but *not* after surgical removal of the malformation. Although these results are preliminary, they indicate that this may be a valuable test for pain reproduction, but the test does not have *absolute* power so that it cannot be used to make a differential diagnosis of unilateral headaches (see Figure 2.10). More work is clearly needed in this area.

The mechanism underlying the nitroglycerin provocation of attacks is unknown. Nitroglycerin (and histamine) may stimulate the release of arachidonic acid conversion products. Bogucki and Kozubski (1985) carried out nitroglycerin tests on cluster headache patients in the cluster cycle before and after indomethacin treatment (75–100 mg day^{-1} for 3 days). Attacks were provoked in all nine cases before and after indomethacin, and the average latency time between drug administration and the occurrence of pain was of the same order of magnitude in the two groups. This study does not, therefore, provide any evidence for prostaglandin involvement in the nitroglycerin precipitation of attacks.

Later, Rozniecki *et al.* (1989) found that nitroglycerin causes a more significant degranulation of basophil cells *in vitro* in patients in the cluster phase ($n = 32$) than in controls ($p < 0.001$). They suggest that vasoactive substances, like histamine and serotonin are released from the basophil cells and cause the attacks.

Recent studies by Kudrow (1989) in nine patients in the cluster phase have indicated that nitroglycerin might give rise to a small decrease in SaO_2 which may mediate the provoked attack.

HISTAMINE TEST

Horton himself used the histamine test early in his cluster headache investigations (Horton *et al.*, 1939; Horton, 1941). Horton first experimented with doses of 0.1–1.2 mg histamine subcutaneously (probably histamine acid phosphate; histamine base = histamine disphosphate × 0.362), but further refinement of the test resulted in a standard dosage of 0.35 mg histamine base subcutaneously (Horton, 1956b). The test should preferably be carried out with the patient in the supine position (Horton, 1956b). According to Horton, the ideal test situation is as follows: the patient should be in a cycle, but should be neither in a well-defined attack nor in a period of slight pain or a refractory period after an attack.

After histamine administration, there is an *early* physiologic histamine-induced headache in both cluster headache patients and non-headache control individuals. This headache is transitory, moderate to rather severe and of bifrontal, throbbing character, appearing within 1–5 min of histamine adminis-tration and lasting 5–10 min. This headache is not associated with the usual autonomic accompaniments of cluster headache attacks. Horton termed this response 'histamine headache', and he felt that this was intracranial in origin. However, in the cluster headache patient there will, in addition, be a *late* pain, usually after 20–40 min but no later than 1 h after histamine administration. The late headache is unilateral, the spontaneously occurring headache seem-ingly being reproduced. The late headache was believed to be chiefly extra-cranial in origin. Horton stressed the importance of using this *late* response and not the early one as an index of cluster headache. Some authors (e.g. Stern, 1969) have, despite Horton's recommendations, apparently used the *immediate* headache as a diagnostic test.

The histamine test was positive in 75% of the cases in the series studied by Peters (1953). In Horton's study it was positive in more than 60% of cases with a dosage of 0.35 mg histamine base. Gardner *et al.* (1947) were, however, only occasionally able to provoke cluster headache attacks in this manner. The histamine test was also carried out by Robinson (1958): in only 1 of 11 cases did he fail to reproduce the pain.

Robinson also considered a positive response to be pathognomonic of the disorder. Likewise, Horton (1956b) claimed that the late response 'occurs only in cases of histamine cephalalgia'. Peters' (1953) demonstration of precipitation of migraine attacks with histamine shows that this does not seem to be the case. Peters found the test to be negative in 'tension headache'.

The various intricacies and the apparently relatively low accuracy of this test as well as the high reliability of the nitroglycerin test seem to make the latter test preferable from a diagnostic point of view.

Infusion of histamine gives rise to a headache (Krabbe and Olesen, 1980), which can be remedied with histamine H_2 blocking agents. The fact that H_2 blockers are ineffective in cluster headache (but active in the aforementioned experiment) does not exclude the possibility of histamine involvement in cluster headache. Infused histamine may be more easily accessible for this type of drug than histamine formed or liberated during the course of a disease process.

IDENTITY OF SPONTANEOUS AND PROVOKED ATTACKS

Ever since the early days of Horton's work it has been said that provoked attacks (mostly by histamine) are identical to spontaneous ones. Whether attacks initiated in this manner really are *identical* to the spontaneously occurring ones is a crucial question. Such an identity has never been demonstrated beyond doubt. Even if this is the case, the provocative agents (histamine as well as nitroglycerin) may hypothetically initiate various metabolic processes. These other metabolic processes may be responsible for phenomena associated with this type of attack, but not for generating the pain itself. Accordingly, results obtained during provoked attacks may or may not be representative of what happens during a spontaneously occurring attack. If provoked attacks are used to study attack-related biologic factors, one may possibly be faced with a situation in which the actual factor studied is a direct metabolic consequence of the provoking agent used and not of the attack *per se*. If, therefore, the pathologic finding is attributed to the attack itself, one may easily be on the wrong track. Until it has been proved that nitroglycerin and histamine induced attacks are identical to the spontaneously occurring ones, it is mandatory that every factor studied in induced attacks be verified in spontaneously occurring attacks. For these reasons, our group has only studied spontaneously occurring attacks of cluster headache.

When trying to assess whether there is an identity or not, the situation of the patient, on whose statements one depends to a large extent, is also crucial: it should be appreciated that it is very difficult to be a patient in such a test situation. It may be difficult for the patient to point out the exact differences between what he feels during spontaneously occurring and precipitated attacks. The patient does not know what the salient and crucial features are in the view of the investigator, and if the question asked is slightly leading, like: 'Does this headache remind you of the one you usually have?', the easiest answer is 'Yes'.

One example of a precipitated headache that probably does *not* correspond to the usual one is that reported by Horton (1941): the patient (case 2), a 32-year-old woman, had left-sided attacks 'associated with swelling about the left eye, drainage from the nose'. *Four minutes* after the subcutaneous injection of 0.3 mg histamine acid phosphate, she got a pain in the left supraorbital region which she stated was of the same type as the usual pain, except that it was milder. *Both eyes began to water, and the lids became swollen.* Even though the histamine test response appeared after only 4 min, the attack was typified as a characteristic one. Furthermore, the provoked attack does seem to have traits that separate it from the spontaneous ones: 'the *lids* became swollen' (only the lid on the symptomatic side was swollen in spontaneous attacks); and *bilateral* lacrimation occurred during the provoked attack but was not mentioned in connection with the spontaneous attack.

There are also other observations at hand which, to a certain extent, indicate that spontaneous and provoked attacks are not identical. One such indication is a study done by Nelson *et al.* (1980) on cerebral blood flow. They found that the mean cerebral blood flow was increased in cluster headache attacks induced by histamine. In spontaneous attacks the blood flow was mostly normal (in three of four patients). It should, however, be noted that, more recently, Krabbe *et al.* (1984) found more or less normal cerebral blood flow, even in precipitated attacks of cluster headache (the attacks were provoked by alcohol, occasionally in combination with nitroglycerin). In Barré's (1982) study, spontaneous and provoked attacks seem to have differed in terms of the extent of the pain experienced.

To interpret the results of the histamine test correctly, it probably is mandatory to have considerable experience and a critical, 'objective' attitude both on the part of the investigator and on the part of an observant, alert patient. Even with this combination, the interpretation is not always easy.

The *latency* of the late-appearing headache is of particular interest: the intermediary steps in the process that eventually lead to an attack following administration of the vasoactive substance seem to be time-consuming. Substances may have to be produced/released to initiate the pain process. The effect does not seem to be the *direct, vascular* one of histamine, such as the one studied by Pickering (1933) and Wolff (1972). It has been speculated that gastric acid constituents could be intermediates in the provocation process, since both alcohol and histamine have a marked gastric acid producing effect (Graham, 1975). The situation may be far more complicated, however, since nitroglycerin, which apparently does not have such a pronounced effect on gastric acid secretion, also provokes headache in a predictable fashion.

It may still be that spontaneous and precipitated attacks are identical in all relevant aspects. Only time will show. Until more adequate information on this subject has been collected, one must exercise extreme caution in interpreting results obtained on attacks precipitated in this manner.

INFLUENCE OF ALCOHOL

It has long been recognized that alcohol is not well tolerated during the cycle, whereas during remission patients tolerate alcohol to the same extent as healthy individuals. Horton (1956b) mentions that approximately 40% of the patients observed that alcohol precipitated attacks and refrained from its use. da Silva (1974) specifically mentioned that attacks could have been precipitated by alcohol in 8 of his 18 cases (44%) during the symptomatic period. There is probably also a dosage factor with regard to alcohol, in that minor dosages may be noxious, whereas larger dosages remove the inclination to attacks. This might be an observation of some significance but may be difficult to use in the clinical approach to diagnosis. Alcohol seems to be a triggering factor more frequently in the chronic than in the episodic variety. However, chronic use of alcohol may reduce the number of attacks in the chronic form. This fact has apparently represented a problem in some of the chronic cases, as has been noted in one of the first descriptions of the chronic variety (de Fine Olivarius, 1970, 1971).

DIAGNOSIS AND DIFFERENTIAL DIAGNOSIS

THE DIAGNOSIS

The cluster phenomenon itself is an important diagnostic hallmark. It is so important that a diagnosis is difficult or impossible to make unless a temporal pattern—that is, that more than one bout has appeared—has been established.

First and foremost, cluster headache is a *unilateral* headache. We have made a rough grouping of headaches based on laterality (Sjaastad and Saunte, 1983) (Table 2.12). The side localization is such an important feature of a headache that it is frequently advisable first to ask a headache patient about the *localization* of the pain: Is it global? Is it unilateral and, if so, does it change side? Various unilateral headaches that may pose differential diagnostic difficulties versus cluster headache are dealt with later. However, there are also vague, less well known, and partly unclassified unilateral headache pictures that may be mixed up with cluster headache and confuse the situation.

In the diagnostic process it is essential that typical features other than the unilaterality are heeded. We have hitherto believed that the pain had to be of a formidable, *excruciating severity*, at least at times, to be in conformity with a diagnosis of cluster headache; an invariably moderate headache would usually not be compatible with this diagnosis. However, the severity of pain of cluster headache may, like many other clinical factors, follow a Gaussian distribution pattern. We have in recent years observed a series of 'mild' cluster headache cases (Sjaastad *et al.*, 1988c). We have, therefore, had to modify our views on the severity of cluster headache. There will be *nocturnal* attacks in most cases. In a large series, Ekbom (1970) found that daytime only attacks occurred in ≤8% of cases. The index of suspicion with regard to other diagnostic possibilities must certainly be raised markedly if only daytime attacks occur. The same applies if the patient is a *female*.

The accompanying ipsilateral *autonomic phenomena* are also most important diagnostic guidelines. As outlined elsewhere (see Tables 2.9 and 2.10), not all the autonomic stigmata are present in every case, i.e. one or more of these traits may be lacking in any particular case (Sjaastad and Haggag, 1987). However, I cannot recall a single case in which all autonomic features were constantly

Table 2.12 A rough categorization of headaches[a]

Type	Example
Global (or holocranial) headaches	Tension headache
Hemicranias *with* side alternation	Migraine
Hemicranias *without* side alternation	Cluster headache

[a] From Sjaastad and Saunte (1983). Courtesy of *Cephalalgia*.

Table 2.13   The main clinical features of episodic cluster headache: the *combination* of these five criteria affords strong evidence for the presence of cluster headache

Unilaterality of headache
Male sex
Clustering of attacks
Autonomic phenomena
Excruciating severity of pain

lacking. Perhaps this may occur in the early phase (see Abortive Attacks).

For diagnostic refinement, we at times include in our diagnostic arsenal the testing of intraocular pressure, corneal indentation pulse amplitudes, and occasionally also quantitation of nasal secretion and lacrimation during and between attacks. We have also, on a rather regular scale, included pharmaco-pupillometry and evaporimetry in the diagnostic procedure (see elsewhere). In the routine case, it is not necessary to use these tools in the diagnostic process and, admittedly, only few centres have access to these techniques. However, in the doubtful case, and in the process of drawing the line between cluster headache and headaches infringing on its borders, such tools are of importance. The presence of a Horner-like pupillometric pattern is in conformity with a cluster headache diagnosis. Diagnosis of cluster headache is not always easy, despite what was claimed at an early stage (Eszenyi-Halasy, 1949). Finally, it should be emphasized that, clinically, there probably are no *pathognomonic* signs of cluster headache. The main features of the syndrome are listed in Table 2.13.

DIFFERENTIAL DIAGNOSIS

Differential diagnostic considerations are greatly aided if the history is sufficiently long to enable the recognition of the long-term pattern. The clear fluctuation over time of the typical cluster pattern is, as far as we know, manifest in the overwhelming majority of cases. The differential diagnostic possibilities vary a great deal between a patient experiencing his first bout and a patient who has experienced several bouts.

There are *non-cluster headache* patients having a symptomatology *similar* to that of cluster headache. We have seen several such cases of both sexes in our material. In such cases, the paroxysms tend to be less clearly delineated, the interparoxysmal stages are less exempt from pain than is usual in cluster headache, and the bouts are less clearly discernible. The location of the pain may also differ slightly from that typical of cluster headache, and the extent of pain may vary. Such headaches have not yet been classified satisfactorily.

Table 2.14 Common misdiagnoses of episodic cluster
headache

Trigeminal neuralgia
Sinusitis
Migraine
'Psychogenic headache'
Chronic paroxysmal hemicrania
Cervicogenic headache

Some headaches that may be confused with cluster headache are post-traumatic and post-surgical (surgery of teeth, face, forehead, etc.) conditions. In some instances, one may be dealing with so-called atypical facial neuralgia (see p. 102). We suspect that cases of 'cervicogenic headache' (Sjaastad *et al.*, 1983c, 1984), which have only been diagnosed to a very moderate extent in the West, may often have been included in the diagnostic category of cluster headache.

The cluster phenomenon *per se* seems to be non-specific: it is also found in the early stages of chronic paroxysmal hemicrania and other headaches (Sjaastad *et al.*, 1988a). Chronic paroxysmal hemicrania in its 'pre-chronic' ('non-continuous', remitting) stage shows a cluster pattern, but the attacks are more short-lasting and frequent, and the temporal pattern differs from that of cluster headache. It may, however, be that hemicrania continua in the pre-chronic stage has a similar pattern, which *may* be confused with episodic cluster headache (Sjaastad, 1987d; Sjaastad and Tjørstad, 1987). However, too little information is available on this subject at present. Trigeminal neuralgia may also fluctuate to a large extent (e.g. Lance, 1982), but the attacks are short-lasting, and trigeminal neuralgia is more of a face pain than a head pain.

Some of what appear to be the commonest misdiagnoses are outlined in Table 2.14. The 'headache profiles' presented by Graham (1963) are helpful as rough outlines in the differential diagnosis.

Unilateral headaches

I discuss first the other unilateral headaches (and partly face pains) with a recurring pattern, such as chronic paroxysmal hemicrania, cervicogenic headache (Table 2.15) and trigeminal neuralgia.

Chronic paroxysmal hemicrania. Chronic paroxysmal hemicrania (CPH) was originally separated from cluster headache proper, and cases of CPH have probably to some (a large?) extent previously been diagnosed as ordinary cluster headache. At least, this was the case with our first two CPH patients. It is, therefore, reasonable to assume that this differential diagnosis still poses

Table 2.15 Differential diagnostic elements in recurrent unilateral headache

	Intensity of pain	Male (M)/female (F) preponderance	Treatment of choice	Frequency of attacks	Duration of attacks	Nocturnal waking due to attacks	Presence of cluster phenomenon
'Cervicogenic headache'	+(+)	F	Operative? NSAIDs?	+	+++	0(+)	–
Hemicrania continua[a]	+(+)	M < F?	Indomethacin	Chronic stage: none	Chronic stage: continuous	0(+)	–
Episodic cluster headache	+++	M	Prednisone, lithium, ergotamine, methysergide	++	++	+++	++
Chronic paroxysmal hemicrania	+++	F (M = F?)	Indomethacin	+++	+	++	'Modified'

[a] Another indomethacin responsive headache (see Chapter 4).

some problems. The diagnosis of CPH is dealt with in detail in Chapter 4, p. 309. Here I only state the principal features of CPH.

A multiplicity of incapacitating, relatively short-lasting attacks of unilateral pain prevail, and there is a special temporal pattern (Table 2.15). The daily number of attacks is usually considerably higher than in cluster headache. The lowest individual maximum of daily attacks compatible with a diagnosis of CPH was originally arbitrarily set at 15 in patients showing the fully developed condition (Sjaastad *et al.*, 1980). As more information became available, this border had to be lowered. In recent years we have carried out indomethacin trials on patients having an attack frequency of ≦4 per 24 h. At the upper border, Bogucki and Niewodniczy (1984) have shown that even a frequency of paroxysms of >30 (each lasting for up to 20 min) seems to be compatible with a diagnosis of cluster headache. It should be emphasized, however, that diagnoses other than cluster headache may be considered in such cases. The clinical suspicion of CPH increases if the patient is female, and if the headache has *never* changed side. The attacks at the height of the fluctuating curve are usually excruciatingly severe and frequently awaken the patient at night. But, in the 'pre-CPH' (non-continuous, remitting) stage—*the stage at which one should try to make the diagnosis*—the attacks may be milder. The ultimate clinical, diagnostic test is the *absolute* response to an adequate dose of indomethacin. Other supplementary diagnostic tests are described in the section on CPH. The prophylactic drugs used in cluster headache (e.g. ergotamine, methysergide and lithium) are generally of no use in CPH.

Trigeminal neuralgia. Trigeminal neuralgia is a rare disorder, possibly even rarer than cluster headache (Penman, 1968; D'Allessandro *et al.*, 1986). Trigeminal neuralgia occurs more frequently in females than males, but not to an extent to make this feature particularly helpful in the differential diagnosis. The age of onset is of significance in the differential diagnosis since 60–80% of cluster headache patients start getting attacks before the age of 40 years. Trigeminal neuralgia, however, rarely starts before 40 years of age, the *mean* age of onset in some series being in the 50s (e.g. Lance, 1982).

Whereas the pain in cluster headache is localized in the oculofrontotemporal area, the pain in trigeminal neuralgia is usually localized along the area of sensory distribution of the second and third branches of the trigeminal nerve. In trigeminal neuralgia, one will accordingly in the great majority of cases encounter a pain below and not above the eye; in other words, the patient has a face pain and not a head pain. I have only seen one definite case of solitary first branch neuralgia (in a woman). The pain localization is, therefore, an important differential diagnostic aspect. Furthermore, there are typical trigger zones in trigeminal neuralgia, and these are usually located within the distribution areas of the affected branches, i.e. in the lower part of the face.

Unilateral autonomic phenomena like those observed in cluster headache, such as miosis and lacrimation, are not usually found in trigeminal neuralgia. Nocturnal awakening from pain seems to be much more frequent in cluster headache than in trigeminal neuralgia. Ergotamine has no effect on the pain of trigeminal neuralgia, in contradistinction to the case in cluster headache. Carbamazepine is highly effective in trigeminal neuralgia, whereas it is inactive in cluster headache. Furthermore, the histamine provocation test is said to be negative in trigeminal neuralgia (e.g. Hanes, 1969).

Another characteristic trait of trigeminal neuralgia is the brevity of attacks, each attack usually lasting only a couple of seconds, but sometimes up to a minute or so. In the bad periods, there is a multiplicity of attacks per day in trigeminal neuralgia, as opposed to the case in cluster headache. There may be a clustering of attacks in trigeminal neuralgia, but the tendency to clustering is usually not as marked as in cluster headache.

The latter trait is, in addition to the severity and unilaterality of the pain, almost the only similarity between the two headaches. The differential diagnosis should, therefore, not be difficult. Nevertheless, Sutherland and Eadie (1972) have reported that 21% of their cluster cases had been given a diagnosis of trigeminal neuralgia by the referring physician. The diagnostic standard on a worldwide basis may have been considerably upgraded in the intervening period.

'Cervicogenic' headache. A clinical picture at times resembling cluster headache may arise from the neck. We have termed headaches of this type cervicogenic headache (Sjaastad *et al.*, 1983c). Headache stemming from the neck has hitherto been probably the most difficult and by far the most neglected differential diagnosis in Western countries. Our own interest in this field has brought forth a clinical headache picture that is rather similar to the one described by Hunter and Mayfield (1949).

The headache is strictly unilateral and occurs on the same side, although in such a manner that when it is at its maximum it may occasionally also be felt as a slight pain on the opposite side. The pain is usually initially felt in the nuchal and retroaural areas. The maximal pain is frequently in the temporal/ocular region and forehead. Not infrequently, the pain descends into the ipsilateral shoulder or even arm. The pain localization may, therefore, be of some, but not of definitively discriminatory value in differentiating this disorder from cluster headache. The longitudinal pattern is usually rather different from that of cluster headache (Fredriksen *et al.*, 1987): first, the single attacks may be rather long-lasting (many hours to several days) and, second, there is no clustering of attacks: attacks appear at random in a spread-out fashion, usually spaced at intervals of days or longer (Table 2.15). The pain in cervicogenic headache is generally not so severe as that occurring in most cases of cluster headache.

There is a clear preponderance of female cases in cervicogenic headache (4–5:1), to the extent that it may be a point of differential diagnostic importance (Table 2.15). Facial sweating patterns, intraocular pressure and corneal indentation pulse measurements during and between attacks and pharmacopupillometry have disclosed characteristic differences between the two conditions (Fredriksen *et al.*, 1988; Fredriksen, 1988, 1989).

For various reasons (see below), it is strongly believed that this headache originates in the neck. Many patients with this condition have sustained a neck/head injury. There is frequently an ipsilateral shoulder and neck pain. There is reduced range of motion in the neck, and attacks—or a similar pain— may be precipitated by pressure against certain tender spots in the neck (especially over the C2 root and greater occipital nerve) or by the patient assuming certain neck positions. Furthermore, anaesthetic blocks of the C2/C3 roots on the symptomatic side cause partial or complete transitory alleviation of the pain (Hunter and Mayfield, 1949; Sjaastad *et al.*, 1983c). Hunter and Mayfield also sectioned the second cervical root on the symptomatic side and obtained relief of the pain. The latter findings have been interpreted as having been made in cluster headache patients, the operations having been carried out at the time when a spontaneous remission was approaching; the improvement following the operation was thus considered to be only apparent. I feel that this point of view is clearly wrong.

The anaesthetic blocks of the C2/C3 roots or the major occipital nerve may seem to be crucial, supplementary diagnostic tests, but these factors may, nevertheless, prove to be inadequate in distinguishing between the two disorders. First, we have not, for unknown reasons, obtained a 100% response rate with diagnostic anaesthetic blocks in suspected cases of cervicogenic headache. Second, Anthony (1985) has apparently observed 'arrest of attacks' in cluster headache with local steroid injection around the greater occipital nerve. The interpretation of Anthony's finding is certainly difficult; we have not been able to reproduce Anthony's results, nor have Bigo *et al.* (1989) or Solomon *et al.* (1989).

As is evident from the foregoing, the differential diagnosis versus cervicogenic headache *may*, in selected cases, present a problem. We have seen several cases in recent years in which we were not quite able, even after thorough diagnostic work-up to pinpoint the correct diagnostic category. The claim that indomethacin is sometimes a good treatment for cluster headache should also be viewed in this light. We suspect that cases of cervicogenic headache have, to a not inconsiderable extent, in the past been placed in the diagnostic category of cluster headache or various migraine groups and migraine subgroups like 'facial migraine'.

In spite of these obstacles, it is our firm belief that we are dealing with two distinct disorders. The deviating clinical traits and the findings on supplementary tests attest to this view. In the typical case, the differential diagnostic task should not be too difficult.

'Hemicrania continua'. In the chronic form, hemicrania continua does not seem to represent any differential diagnostic problems; in the early phase, however, it may do so (see Table 2.15, and Chronic Paroxysmal Hemicrania).

Spontaneous dissecting aneurysm of the carotid artery. West *et al.* (1976) have described a syndrome consisting of the following elements:

1. pain in the head, face, or neck on the ipsilateral side;
2. ipsilateral Horner's syndrome;
3. occasionally, contralateral neurological symptoms and signs; and
4. angiographic evidence of narrowing of the internal carotid artery, with findings consistent with dissection within the arterial wall.

Furthermore, in one of their patients, in whom the diagnosis was corroborated by surgical exploration, an arterial wall biopsy demonstrated changes typical of cystic mediae necrosis. They felt that this clinical constellation of symptoms and signs represented a distinct, recognizable syndrome.

In Fisher's (1982) series ($n = 21$: 11 men, 10 women), the ages fell within the range 30–60 years. The site of the disorder was almost invariably in the cervical part of the internal carotid artery. The characteristic pain of the dissecting aneurysm of the carotid artery is a single event, and the headache is apparently rather severe, but slowly progressing, steady, or throbbing, with a plateau of some length, and is most marked in the forehead and orbital area; 12 patients had additional neck pain and one had neck pain only. The headache was generally the presenting symptom. Ipsilateral sensory changes in the scalp were occasionally discovered. These features would usually be enough evidence to rule out a cluster headache diagnosis, even in the presence of Horner's syndrome. Mokri *et al.* (1979) have also indicated that the periorbital area is the site of pain.

Sometimes, however, there may be several attacks of incapacitating headache of rather short duration (for example, 30 min, as in case 6 reported by West *et al.* (1976)). In cases where there is a co-existing, ipsilateral Horner's syndrome, the diagnostic difficulties are obvious. The Horner's syndrome that occurs in such cases has been considered to be caused by direct pressure of the bulging artery on the stellate ganglion (West *et al.*, 1976).

The possibility exists that there is pressure on the sympathetic plexus around the carotid artery. In a substantial number of such cases, symptoms arise from the contralateral extremities. These are probably due to circulatory disturbances in the domain of the stenosed or occluded carotid artery. Such symptoms will make the diagnosis easier and may possibly also explain the Horner's syndrome (first neuron lesion). For the proper localization of the abnormality of Horner's syndrome in these cases it is important to know whether it appears separately or always in connection with *central*, contralateral phenomena. According to Mokri *et al.* (1979), the contralateral extremity phenomena may be lacking in the presence of Horner's syndrome. Pupillometry and evaporimetry in such cases ought to localize the sympathetic dysfunction precisely.

Recurrent erosion of the cornea. This condition may pose a real differential diagnostic problem versus cluster headache. Both the erosion and the pain are unilateral, may occur at night or, more typically, on awakening, and usually last for less than 1 h, all features strongly reminiscent of cluster headache. The pain attacks may also recur, although usually not in a typical 'cluster' pattern.

The symptoms are remarkably localized to the orbit, the patient frequently having the feeling that a foreign body is present in the eye. The pain of cluster headache is usually not so localized, and the patient does not have the feeling of a foreign body in the eye; he rather feels a pressure *behind* the eye. Corneal ulcers may be demonstrated by fluorescein staining of the cornea and slit-lamp examination during a pain attack. It may be impossible to demonstrate the ulceration even after a respite of only a few hours. It should be emphasized that corneal ulceration is a rare condition and the following important points in the differential diagnosis should be noted:

1. blepharospasm is a prominent symptom in corneal ulceration;
2. the pain is localized, and the attacks appear at night or, more usually, during the early morning hours; and
3. the presence of corneal ulceration can be demonstrated.

Glaucoma. Acute glaucoma should normally not lead to any serious differential diagnostic problems *vis à vis* cluster headache, even though the disorder is usually unilateral, and nausea, vomiting, and conjunctival injection often accompany the acute attack. The protracted pain, the blurred and fading vision, and the coloured halos around lights are symptoms of differential diagnostic importance. The pupil is usually mid-dilated on the symptomatic side, whereas it is rather constricted in cluster headache. The intraocular pressure is clearly increased; i.e. it is usually >40 mmHg. The intraocular pressure also increases on the symptomatic side during the paroxysm of cluster headache, when compared with both that in the pain-free interval and that on the non-symptomatic side during an attack, but on a 'far lower scale' (mean 13.7 mmHg, versus a mean of 12.3 mmHg between attacks) (Hørven and Sjaastad, 1977).

Chronic glaucoma may provide greater difficulties diagnostically, since the pain may be considerable and recurrent, particularly in the chronic closed angle type. The optic nerve head may show cupping after several attacks. Intraocular pressure is markedly increased during the attack but, unfortunately from a diagnostic point of view, the pressure may be normal between attacks.

The typical temporal pattern and the unilateral nasal phenomena of cluster headache attacks are important differential diagnostic aspects. A good case history is of invaluable diagnostic help. If doubt exists, measurements of intraocular pressure during symptomatic periods should solve the problem.

Temporal arteritis. Temporal arteritis was first described by Horton and Magath in 1932. It is a rare disease, possibly even more rare than cluster headache. Contrary to cluster headache, temporal arteritis affects the older generations, i.e. mostly individuals over 50 years of age. There is a female-sex preponderance. Systemic low-grade symptoms like night sweating, anorexia, weight loss, malaise, fever and muscular ache and stiffness, mostly in shoulders and hips, are almost always present in addition to the headache. The erythrocyte sedimentation rate is usually markedly increased and is almost invariably elevated during the active phase of the disease. Various arteries are affected apart from the temporal artery.

The headache is usually unilateral but may be bilateral. It is usually continuous, although somewhat fluctuating, and is usually moderate (to severe), but does not usually awaken the patient at night. The temporal artery is frequently tender and tortuous. Horton (personal communication, 1973) stressed that there is frequently a claudication pain on chewing. Although the headache is usually unilateral, the pain characteristics and the associated symptoms differ clearly from those of cluster headache. A temporal artery biopsy will often provide diagnostic information.

Ræder's syndrome. This syndrome was first described in 1922 by the Norwegian ophthalmologist J.G. Ræder (1924). Several cases were later described under this designation (e.g. Ford and Walsh, 1958; Toussaint, 1968; Mokri, 1982). Ræder's syndrome consists of ordinary 'Horner's symptoms', but without the anhidrosis of regular Horner's syndrome. In addition, there was a discrete lesion of one or more cranial nerves in all the original cases. It is remarkable that in the later reported cases there did not seem to be any cranial nerve involvement in addition to that of (obligatory?) discrete trigeminal nerve involvement (Boniuk and Schlesinger, 1962; Minton and Bounds, 1964). Boniuk and Schlesinger, therefore, proposed that cases of Ræder's syndrome be divided into two subgroups: cases with neuralgia, a 'partial' Horner's syndrome, and parasellar cranial nerve involvement (categorized as group I); and cases with neuralgia and a partial Horner's syndrome, but without any parasellar cranial nerve involvement (group II). The term 'Ræder's syndrome' should be restricted to those cases in which, in addition to the unilateral headache and a partial Horner's syndrome, there is also evidence of a minor affection of the trigeminal nerve as a minimum. If this is not done, patients with cluster headache may be classified as having Ræder's syndrome. Furthermore, unless this provision is made, the chances of including cases of spontaneous dissecting aneurysm of the internal carotid artery (and other disorders in that area) will increase (see Spontaneous Dissecting Aneurysm of the Carotid Artery).

Even with discrete fifth cranial nerval involvement only, the abnormality does not necessarily have to be in the paratrigeminal area. There may occasionally be moderate, ipsilateral, facial sensory loss in connection with the spontaneous dissecting aneurysm of the carotid artery. In other words, such aneurysms may give rise to a clinical picture similar to that of Ræder's syndrome, although the localization is quite different, i.e. it is in the cervical part of the internal carotid artery. The cranial nerve affection, especially if including more than one nerve, has a decisive localizing significance in this constellation of symptoms and signs, as has been pointed out by Ledermann and Salanga (1976) and Fisher (1982). Preferably, therefore, there should be involvement of more than one neighbouring cranial nerve to prove the 'paratrigeminal' location of the affection.

The status of Boniuk and Schlesinger's (1962) group II is, therefore, uncertain; the softening of the inclusion criteria as originally set forth by Ræder seems unjustified. What Ræder described was the 'paratrigeminal' localization of a process leading to a certain constellation of neurologic symptoms and signs. It should be emphasized that the localization was *proved* pathologically in one of his cases. Although he could not *prove* that the localization was the same in all his cases, by symptom analogy he believed that it was.

The sympathetic fibres may be affected anywhere along the sympathetic chain. It has been pointed out (Ledermann and Salanga, 1976) that a *Ræder-like picture* may originate in the internal carotid artery in the neck. Vijayan and Watson (1978) have suggested that Ræder's syndrome belongs to what they term the 'pericarotid syndrome'. Vijayan and Watson's suggestion is, however, clearly invalid for Ræder group I cases with involvement of cranial nerves.

In group I the cranial nerve involvement should solve the differential diagnostic problems. When comparing the symptoms of cluster headache with those of Ræder's syndrome, therefore, it will be with the group II patients (if such a group exists) that difficulties mainly arise. Whether there are differences between the pain characteristics of group II patients and cluster headache patients remains uncertain. In most reports on Ræder's syndrome the pain is rather poorly described. The pain of Ræder's syndrome (both group I and group II) seems to be in the same area as the pain of cluster headache. It seems, however, to be more *chronic* in character (lasting one to several days) than the pain of cluster headache, without a temporal pattern of relatively short-lasting clear-cut attacks and relatively longer remissions as in the episodic form of cluster headache. Shafar (1966) has described the pain as both long-lasting and moderate. It may be fluctuating over the course of the disorder (see e.g. Minton and Bounds, 1964). The pain does not seem to be as severe as in cluster headache. Several authors apparently believe that Ræder's group II is identical to cluster headache (see e.g. Heyck, 1981). Sutherland and Eadie (1972) are of the opinion that cluster headache is one possible cause of Ræder's paratrigeminal syndrome. One fundamental question then arises: Ræder described the *paratrigeminal* syndrome. In any disorder giving rise to the same symptoms as in the Ræder group II, the pathological condition for this group should also reside in the paratrigeminal area. Is, then, the primary abnormality of cluster headache localized in the paratrigeminal area? Although no proof for such an assumption is at hand, there is ample evidence in favour of such a view, and this has recently been summarized (Sjaastad, 1988b). Until further evidence for a co-localization of the cluster headache and Ræder's syndromes exists, one should be somewhat cautious before putting a sign of equality between these syndromes.

Tolosa–Hunt syndrome ('painful ophthalmoplegia'). Even though the site of the pathological lesion in the Tolosa–Hunt syndrome (Tolosa, 1954; Hunt et al., 1961) is in the vicinity of that of Ræder's syndrome, the symptoms differ somewhat in the two disorders. The pathological process in the Tolosa–Hunt syndrome is apparently localized somewhat more to the anterior in the cavernous sinus and its immediate surroundings than that of Ræder's syndrome. The pain characteristics have recently been outlined by Hannerz (1985). The headache is unilateral and periocular, as in cluster headache; it is intermittent or more continuous over a limited time; it does not appear in regular bouts; and it apparently does not have the autonomic accompaniments of cluster headache. The pain episodes have neither the explosive, excruciating quality of cluster headache nor their brevity. Characteristically, in contrast to cluster headache, cranial nerves 3, 4 and 6 and the first branch of the trigeminal nerve are affected in various combinations (see e.g. Hoes *et al.*, 1981). Occasionally, the oculosympathetic fibres are also affected, a trait reminiscent of Ræder's syndrome. A diagnostic test of some value is the X-ray demonstration of an affected superior ophthalmic vein and cavernous sinus (Milsten and Morretin, 1971; Muhletaler and Gerlock, 1979; Hoes *et al.*, 1981; Hannerz *et al.*, 1984, 1986). Moreover, the clinical response to steroids is a good diagnostic index for the Tolosa–Hunt syndrome. A picture similar to the regular Tolosa–Hunt syndrome, with visual impairment but *without* the cranial nerve affection, has recently been described. X-ray changes like those in the regular Tolosa–Hunt syndrome and a positive response to prednisone have also been demonstrated for this syndrome (Hannerz *et al.*, 1986). However, cluster headache is also characterized by pathological orbital phlebography findings (Hannerz *et al.*, 1987a) and a positive response to steroids. Painful ophthalmoplegia does not respond to the typical cluster headache drugs, like ergotamine, and it is not known to respond to lithium.

Carotidynia. Carotidynia is a term apparently first used by Fay. In 1932, Fay stated that: 'If the thumbs are placed on the common carotid arteries just below the bifurcation and the structures pressed back against the transverse cervical process with a rolling movement, a severe reaction of pain is produced on the side of the atypical neuralgia: This response I have termed 'carotidynia' . . .. Fay then claimed that he had found a positive response in 'almost every case' with pain around the eye and in the face, as in 'atypical facial neuralgia'. Fay thus seems to believe that carotidynia is a special phenomenon in 'atypical facial neuralgia'—more or less a mechanism for the production of pain, the carotid artery being rather sensitive to external stimuli. Glaser (1940) also referred to Fay (1932) in his review of 'atypical facial neuralgia'.

The development in this field has, however, led to a differentiation of related pictures: Roseman (e.g. 1967, 1968) has described a constellation of symptoms and signs that differs from the original description of atypical facial neuralgia (see Chapter 1). This variety of facial, neck, and head pain usually seemed to be a self-limiting disorder, with only one pain episode, and even this was short-lasting (a mean of 12 days (Roseman, 1967)). The pain was described as *unilateral*, dull, throbbing, or piercing, frequently moderate, and the neck pain seemed to outweigh the headache; but in several cases the pain spread to the face. There was no sex preponderance (Roseman, 1967). This seems to separate the picture from the usual 'atypical facial neuralgia' —in which there is a clear female preponderance. Clear tenderness is apparently found along a limited segment of the carotid artery (Lovshin, 1977), and 'Fay's test' is apparently always positive (Roseman, 1967). The ESR (erythrocyte sedimentation rate) may or may not remain normal throughout the course.

On the basis of these clinical descriptions it may seem that this type of carotidynia is a separate, distinct disorder. The focusing on the carotid artery itself, however, may be unwarranted. We also believed for a long time that in chronic paroxysmal hemicrania, the carotid artery itself was excessively tender to external touch (Sjaastad *et al.*, 1979). Over time, however, it became clear that the maximum tenderness in this area was over the adjacent transverse processes of C5 and C4. The observation that chewing/swallowing is also pain provoking (Roseman, 1968) may provide a hint that the retropharyngeal space is *one* possible source of pain (Fahlgren, 1986). It is of interest that head movements, coughing and so on aggravated the headache. This is reminiscent of *cervicogenic headache*. Conjunctival injection and lid oedema have also been mentioned as symptoms in carotidynia. The latter findings may also be reminiscent of cervicogenic headache and may seem difficult to explain on the basis of a solitary affection of the carotid artery. No Horner's syndrome has been mentioned. It is somewhat surprising that in some centres rather large series have been collected with this disorder (Roseman (1968), 33 cases; and Lovshin (1960), 100 cases), whereas in many neurologic centres such cases are not seen or, more correctly, not diagnosed. I have seen only one case in which this diagnosis was suspected, in spite of a continuous search for such cases (the type described by e.g. Roseman) over the years.

This type of carotidynia is not characterized by brief, excruciatingly severe and multiple attacks as is cluster headache. The differential diagnosis versus this variety should thus not present any great difficulty.

Raskin and Prusiner (1977) have described a somewhat different picture under the same heading, with recurrent attacks of pulsating headache over weeks, lasting for minutes to a few hours. In this clinical variety, there seem to be similarities to cluster headache. The localization of the pain, however, is usually different in the two disorders. The typical accompanying symptoms of the cluster headache attack seem to be absent (except occasionally conjunctival injection). The nosologic status of the latter variety seems to be highly doubtful, as far as I am concerned. Not only does the picture seem to differ from 'atypical facial neuralgia', but it also seems to differ from the carotidynia cycle, in that tender carotid arteries do not seem to be a prerequisite for the diagnosis. Therefore the justification for linking this picture to 'carotidynia' seems to be somewhat dubious. More research is clearly needed before this variety can be accepted.

Post-traumatic dysautonomic cephalalgia. This headache was first described by Vijayan and Dreyfus in 1975. It is clinically characterized by episodes of throbbing, unilateral headache, accompanied by ipsilateral facial sweating and mydriasis. All their patients seemed to have had a history of trauma to the anterior aspects of the neck (carotid sheath area). There also seemed to be evidence of an ocular sympathetic dysfunction on the symptomatic side in the headache-free interval, as evidenced by cocaine and epinephrine tests. During an attack, however, there were signs of ocular sympathetic *stimulation*, and a β-adrenergic receptor blocking agent seemed to counteract the tendency to attacks. This picture differs from episodic cluster headache, in which no mydriasis is present during the attack. This point may possibly serve as a clue in the differential diagnosis.

I am in doubt with regard to the proper status of this headache. The autonomic changes with a combination of dysfunction and over-function are hard to grasp. Previous minor traumas, although their thrust may have been in the specific area, may not necessarily have been disease productive. The alleged role of the trauma is in all cases conjectural. Furthermore, our experience with chronic paroxysmal hemicrania has led us to believe that the significance allotted to autonomic disturbances in general in the symptom production in headache has probably been considerably exaggerated. The effect of a β-receptor blocking agent in this headache does not necessarily imply that headache relief is a consequence of counteracting the alleged overactivity of the sympathetic system. β-Receptor blocking agents may simply relieve this headache because it is a migraine or a migraine-like headache. One might repeat endlessly what the late Raymond Greene once said: 'the effect of a drug in therapy does not prove the theory that underlies its use'.

The claim that β-blocking agents really took effect was not substantiated by double-blind studies, which would be mandatory in such a headache. The follow-up of Vijayan and Dreyfus's patients was not such that the *long-term* effect of the drug could be established. Moreover, there is no mention of attack-related mydriasis in one of the cases studied by Vijayan and Dreyfus, and in the other cases the anisocoria may be on the border of being physiological (only a macroscopic evaluation was carried out).

Another strange fact is that no similar or identical cases have been described by others in more than 15 years that have passed since Vijayan and Dreyfus's original description, even though a total of five cases were originally described. A description of such cases by other clinicians is mandatory for the acceptance of this syndrome. This lack of subsequent reports may be due to the relative looseness of the original description, the rarity of such cases, and also to some extent the lack of a follow-up study.

Costen's syndrome (temporomandibular joint dysfunction). This syndrome was first described by Costen in 1934. The symptoms of the syndrome were outlined as follows: impaired hearing, continuously or intermittently; 'stuffy' sensation of the ear; tinnitus; snapping noise while chewing; dull pain around the ear; dizziness (even attacks of prostrating severity); alleged 'sinus' symptoms; and burning sensation in throat, tongue and side of nose. The mandibular joint was tender on palpation. Other diagnostic criteria were mild deafness and dizziness that could be aborted by Eustachian tube inflation. The headache was described as severe and constant; however, although being an integral part of the picture, it was not the dominant symptom; it might even be lacking. It was localized to the vertex and occiput and behind the ear. The headache characteristically increased towards the end of the day (Costen, 1951), and it was usually unilateral. A diagnostic clue was said to be the presence of the *typical* headache in the absence of sinus or eye involvement, or after such symptoms had been corrected.

The temporal pattern and accompanying symptoms in cluster headache differ markedly from those of Costen's syndrome which is included in this section because some investigators have been fascinated by similarities between Costen's syndrome and 'atypical facial neuralgia'. Atypical facial neuralgia has many similarities with cervicogenic headache which *is* a differential diagnostic possibility in cluster headache. Furthermore, the pain of Costen's syndrome may also be unilateral, although hardly at the level of the pain experienced in cluster headache.

The primary malfunction in temporomandibular neuralgia has been supposed to originate within the joint itself. Costen (1951) later even claimed that the temporomandibular joint had in the meantime been gaining more recognition as a factor in producing facial neuralgias. There may well in some solitary, rare case be a relationship between temporomandibular joint dysfunction and headache (Ryan and Ryan, 1978). However, a scientific proof of a causal relationship between temporomandibular dysfunction and headache remains to be delivered. To show that a cause-and-effect relationship is probable, not to mention established, would demand thorough studies.

Costen's syndrome is an ill-defined disorder, so ill-defined that clinical series hardly can be expected to consist of an homogeneous population. The fact that vast clinical series of Costen's syndrome have been collected in some centres is in contrast to the fact that in other centres this condition is rarely or hardly ever diagnosed. I have not seen a single case in which I have been convinced of the diagnosis of 'Costen's syndrome'. I have seen cases of major malfunctioning of the temporomandibular joint on one side, even to the extent that the noise produced by chewing could be heard even at some distance, but there was no pain, even on chewing. Conversely, in a continued search over a long time I have not found any crepitation or local tenderness over the joints that could explain the headache on routine examination of headache cases.

More recent research seems to stress the significance of the periarticular musculature and not of the joint itself in the symptom generation in so-called Costen's syndrome. Any relationship of so-called Costen's syndrome to Sluder's headache and the 'atypical facial neuralgias' is dubious. Possibly, in the original descriptions of Costen's syndrome, atypical neuralgia cases may have been included.

Cluster-tic syndrome. The term cluster-tic was first used by Green and Apfel-baum in 1978. Solomon *et al.* (1985) gave the first detailed report of this syndrome based on four case histories in which two components seemed to be clinically present: cluster headache and tic douloureux. Additional cases of this syndrome have been reported (e.g. Klimek, 1987). The mean age of onset in Solomon *et al.*'s patients was 31.5 years, which is considerably lower than the mean age of onset of tic douloureux. There were *either* short-lasting paroxysms (lasting a couple of seconds to 1–2 min) with a hemifacial distribution, *or* relatively long-lasting, unilateral attacks, both types of pain appearing on the same side. In the latter case, the pain was of a burning or boring character, as in cluster headache, and was accompanied by autonomic symptoms. The short-lasting paroxysmal pain attacks were always located in the distribution area of the two lower branches of the trigeminal nerve. In *two* cases, typical paroxysms could be triggered by cutaneous and mucous membrane stimuli. The two components might appear dissychronously, but most of the time they occurred simultaneously. At times the components blended to the extent that it was difficult to separate them. The pain attacks in the early period appeared in clusters, later becoming chronic.

The nosologic status of this syndrome is at present not established. The question automatically arises whether this constellation of symptoms may represent the fortuitous co-existence of two relatively rare headache forms. The operative results (that is, liberation of vessels from the trigeminal nerve root; $n = 4$) with a dichotomy—the tic pain being relieved and the cluster headache pain only modified—may indicate different aetiopathogeneses of the two headache components. It would have been most valuable to have data on pupillographic findings, forehead sweating, intraocular circulatory/pressure variables, and nitroglycerin tests to ascertain whether, in these respects, the cluster part of the syndrome is consistent with ordinary cluster headache.

The presence of rather typical tics in the case history (*sine qua non* in this syndrome) should be of great value in the differential diagnosis with regard to cluster headache. The point of maximum pain of these tics corresponds to the two lower branches of the trigeminal nerve. Short-lasting pain episodes, so-called jabs and jolts (Sjaastad, 1979; Sjaastad *et al.*, 1979, 1980) are also part of the cluster headache picture, but in the latter these are located in the head and not the face; they tend to change localization, and the level of pain seems to be lower. If trigger zones are present, this of course is helpful in the differential diagnosis.

Similar or identical cases have also been described previously. Thus, Eadie and Sutherland (1972) described a woman who had typical cluster headache for 6 years before she had shock-like, momentary pains as in tic douloureux, with trigger zones. The latter pains also appeared in bouts and on the cluster headache-pain side. Trigeminal rhizotomy relieved the tic-like pain. Horna-brook (1964) has also described a similar patient. We have also seen such a case (a 60-year-old man) with ipsilateral (left-sided) attacks of episodic cluster headache and tics in bouts, at times with a temporal overlap.

Cluster vertigo. Sutherland and Eadie (1972) and Lance and Anthony (1971a) have observed cases of co-existing episodic cluster headache and vertigo. A disorder having these components has been described by Gilbert (1965, 1970). Gilbert suggested that there is vasodilatation in the inner ear (as an integral part of cluster headache as such) and, as a consequence thereof, an excessive endolymph production (resulting in the vertigo). The clinical description was kept broad, and the duration of the episodes and the interrelationship between the headache and vertigo episodes were only vaguely outlined. Apparently, the disorder was characterized by a clustering of vertigo and of headache (of a cluster headache type?). No information was given about the relationship between the rotatory component and the side of the headache. The disorder was observed in seven cases.

Cluster headache is, in general, not associated with episodes of vertigo. There should, therefore, be no difficulties in differentiating between cluster vertigo and cluster headache.

As far as I know, no descriptions other than the ones hitherto mentioned have been reported. None of the members of the International Cluster Headache Research Group ('Cluster Club') present at a meeting held approximately 10 years ago had seen cases reminiscent of this disorder. This may be due to the infrequency of the condition or to the vagueness of the delineation of the condition. Cluster vertigo is not recognized as an entity or a subgroup of cluster headache at present. A prerequisite for acknowledging this headache as a group is that other cases are discovered by other groups. For the time being it should be considered as being *sub judice*.

The main question to be answered is as follows: Is there an intimate, causal connection between the vertigo and the headache in these cases, or is it just an occasional occurrence of vertigo in patients with headache (or cluster headache)? The answer to this question is not known, and it would take a thorough investigation to find one.

Charlin's nasociliary neuralgia. Charlin's (1931) syndrome or nasociliary nerve neuralgia is, in all probability, rare. In addition to orbital or periorbital pain (pain between the bridge of the nose and the medial canthus), the syndrome consists of unilateral rhinitis and nasal secretion (*hydrorrée énorme*) accompanying the headache attacks and 'affection of the anterior part of the eye'. The pain was said to be severe (*d'une extrême violence*). The temporal pattern of attacks is not described in any detail so that no comparison can be made with cluster headache. This constellation could possibly also fit with the unilateral symptoms and signs of cluster headache. However, the ocular signs seem to exceed what is expected in cluster headache with corneal ulceration and, at least at times, a marked redness of the eye.

Cocainization of the nasal mucosa was stated to abort the pain, whereas 'ocular treatment' was of no avail. The pain also seemed to change side from one attack to another. These features do not correspond with the usual features of cluster headache. The nosologic status of this syndrome is highly uncertain, as is the pathogenetic mechanism. Heyck (1981) believes that the cases reported in the original contribution by Charlin (1931) were cases of iridocyclitis that have been misinterpreted. I have no personal experience with this syndrome and, for this reason, abstain from further comment.

Headaches that to a somewhat greater extent tend to be bilateral

Sinusitis. The pain in sinusitis may be bilateral but is not infrequently unilateral, depending on which sinuses are involved. The unilateral involvement may give rise to differential diagnostic problems versus cluster headache. The localization of cluster headache, with headache in the ocular and frontal area, and also the ipsilateral, nasal discharge contribute to this. Our experience in the past in Norway has been that most patients with cluster headache had been through one or more diagnostic sinus punctures before the correct diagnosis had been established. In recent years, this picture may have changed somewhat: the new generation of physicians seems to be able to make the cluster headache diagnosis correctly and quickly.

It is believed that the following points are of specific importance in distinguishing clinically between the two disorders.

1. In general, the pain in cluster headache is much more severe than the pain of sinusitis, where the pain is *usually* dull. The pain of sinusitis may, however, occasionally be severe. Nocturnal pain is rather rare in sinusitis (Ryan and Ryan, 1978). The sinusitis pain increases on bending forward.
2. Along the time axis, cluster headache is punctuated by separate, severe paroxysms, and in between no or only low-grade headache occurs. Sinus headache is usually more even and protracted, although fluctuations may occur.
3. The nasal discharge in cluster headache is clear and non-purulent, whereas in sinusitis it is usually purulent, and application of nasal decongestants may alleviate the pain.
4. There is local tenderness over the inflamed sinuses in sinusitis.
5. Ipsilateral lacrimation is typical of cluster headache and is said to be a rarer finding in sinusitis.
6. Horner's syndrome is not found in sinusitis.

It is usually a simple task to differentiate between these two disorders on the basis of pure clinical variables. In exceptional cases of retention sinusitis and no nasal discharge, the diagnosis may be more difficult. If doubt exists, an incontrovertible diagnosis can usually be made by means of supplementary tests like radiography of the sinuses (and the nitroglycerin test and CIP measurements, sweat patterns, etc.).

Migraine. Since cluster headache was originally singled out from the gross group of 'migraine', there should be some similarities between the two groups. In the headache classification of the World Federation of Neurology's Research

Group on Headache (1970), cluster headache was still classified as a subgroup of migraine. My view is that these two clinical headaches are *two distinct, separate entities*. Various reasons for this have been given elsewhere (see: Migraine and cluster headache: a continuum or separate nosological entities?).

The important *clinical*, differential diagnostic points are as follows: Cluster headache is, in principle, a *unilateral* headache, without side alteration, whereas migraine (at least migraine with aura) is, in principle, a headache *with* a side shift in cases where it is unilateral: The pain usually shifts side, either during the solitary attack or from one attack to another (Sjaastad and Saunte, 1983; Sjaastad *et al.*, 1989a). There are, however, exceptions to these rules in both groups. Contrary to cluster headache attacks, the *classical* migraine ('migraine with aura') attack has typical visual accompaniments (fortification scotomata, etc.) or other first-phase symptoms. Furthermore, migraine attacks are long-lasting (from 4–6 h to one or more days) as opposed to the relatively short-lasting cluster headache attacks. Migraine attacks usually occur much more rarely (1–4 per month) than cluster headache attacks, and in migraine the attacks generally do not cluster (the exception possibly being cluster migraine (see below)). Nausea and vomiting are frequent complaints in migraine (in 85% of the patients) but occur infrequently in cluster headache, particularly the vomiting (in approximately 15% of cases (Lance, 1982)).

However, lacrimation, conjunctival injection, and so forth are frequent accompaniments of cluster headache attacks but are rare to non-existent in migraine. Migraine patients prefer to lie down in a dark room at least during the most pronounced attacks, whereas cluster headache patients prefer to pace the floor. The fact that migraine is a 'female' disease and cluster headache a 'male' disease is also to some extent helpful in the differential diagnosis.

'Cluster migraine'. It has recently been proposed by various authors that there is a cluster migraine variety (see e.g. Kudrow, 1980; Nappi and Savoldi, 1983). In Kudrow's classification of cluster headache, cluster migraine is categorized as a cluster headache variety (see Table 1.1). Migraine and cluster headache may of course co-exist in one patient. Migraine patients cannot be expected to be immune from cluster headache and, conversely, cluster headache patients cannot be expected to be immune to migraine (Sjaastad, 1976). So, it goes without saying that the chance co-existence of the two disorders must be expected and does not justify a special designation. If such a term were to convey any essential meaning, the interconnection between the two disorders ought to be such that attacks of one sort influenced the attacks or attack pattern of the other, or vice versa.

Clinically speaking, this headache is most probably a *migraine* that clusters to some extent, and it should be termed accordingly. The term 'cyclical migraine' is probably the preferred term at this time, because it focuses on one main feature of this migraine variant: i.e. that it occurs in cycles. As specific variables were not tested in these individuals, it cannot be known whether they have any traits characteristic of cluster headache. The word 'cluster' in this connection may, therefore, be unfortunate, since it gives the connotation of cluster headache. The use of this special term is inadvisable, since, as far as we know, there is no more of a special connection between this migraine variant and cluster headache than between migraine in general and cluster headache. Much more information is, however, clearly needed in this field, before definite statements can be made. The therapeutic aspects of cyclical migraine may differ little from those of migraine.

Sluder's sphenopalatine ganglion headache. Sluder (1908) was the first to focus attention on pain manifesting itself mainly in the facial area—that is, a 'lower-half headache'. He believed that this headache was linked to a sphenopalatine ganglion abnormality and used cocainization of this ganglion both diagnostically and therapeutically. Eventually, be believed that many bodily ailments could be attributed to sphenopalatine ganglion pathology (Sluder, 1910, 1915). In the end the clinical picture became so confusing to clinicians that in most centres clinicians stopped using the term.

According to Sluder (1918) the characteristics of this headache are as follows:

> The neuralgic picture is pain in the root of the nose and in and about the eye, in the upper jaw and teeth (sometimes lower jaw and teeth) extending backward under the zygoma to the ear, frequently making earache and pain in the mastoid; but severest often at a point 6 cm back of the mastoid, extending thence to the occiput, neck, shoulder-blade, shoulder, breast, and when severe, to the arm, forearm, hand and fingers; with sometimes a sense of sore throat on that side. Rarer additions to this picture are itching of the skin of the upper extremity, taste disturbance (parageusia), a sense of stiffness and muscle weakness in the upper extremity and fortification scotomata. Mild cases are described as a sense of tension in the face and stiffness or rheumatism in the shoulders. It may appear as a constant pain with exacerbations, or it may stop and reappear cyclically as a migraine; or it may stop and reappear with stabbing sharpness as a tic.

Sluder (1910) also stated that: 'after the neuralgic manifestations have continued for some time (approximately four weeks) they begin to run irregularly, assuming the form of *migraine*, which may persist, even for years, *after all local inflammatory conditions have disappeared*' (the italicization is mine).

The pain was said to be rather severe at times (see e.g. Sluder, 1913). The pain and other constituents of the attack were rather vaguely described, so vaguely that it is next to impossible at present to find out what was actually observed. For example, it was not mentioned specifically how frequently the headache was unilateral and bilateral, but apparently both types of distribution existed. The headache could be located both orbitally, supraorbitally, in the face, or in the ear region, but most frequently it was occipital (see also Aubry and Pialoux, 1968). It thus seems to be located in the areas where cervicogenic headache also manifests itself.

The picture described by Sluder is hardly an homogeneous one (Bickerstaff, 1968; Heyck, 1975). Solitary cases belonging to diagnostic categories not described at the time (see Atypical Facial Neuralgia), such as cluster headache, might have been included. He also described 'fortification scotomata'. In all probability, however, there is a core of solid, clinical observations in what Sluder described, information that, unfortunately, later became swamped.

Whereas Sluder himself had diagnosed 60 cases 2 years after his first publication, a multitude of neurologists and even headache specialists have never seen a case of Sluder's headache (e.g. Grinker and Sahs, 1966; Biemond, 1970; Heyck, 1975, 1981). This discrepancy is so striking that it must have a rational explanation; it is not only due to chance. The symptoms may possibly have been somewhat distorted owing to Sluder's background as an otolaryngologist, so that it may be difficult to recognize the headache pattern. An example that may be mentioned is his emphasis on the 'motor disturbances affecting the configuration of the soft palate': 'The palatine arch on the affected side is often, but not always, higher than on the well side'. He also stressed the 'earache' in this syndrome.

According to Sluder, 'in every instance there have been definite indications pointing unmistakably to the ganglion'. In his own words: 'the pterygomaxillary fossa may be regarded as tantamount to an accessory sinus of the nose, in so far as it may be affected by contiguity'. Furthermore: 'In view of its close proximity to the mucous membrane of the nose and the several accessory sinuses, it is not surprising that the ganglion should be affected by inflammation in these cavities'. The point is made that these characteristic pains can be reproduced by a certain procedure (Sluder, 1910), i.e. mechanical or electrical stimulation of the sphenopalatine ganglion. Sluder felt that he could anaesthetize the ganglion by administering cocaine through the nasal wall, because the wall is so thin. In this way, he felt that he could alleviate the pain in sphenopalatine ganglion neuralgia. Later, he injected alcohol into the ganglion for more permanent relief. This therapy was largely discredited over the ensuing years and by the late 1920s was no longer considered an adequate therapy (Glaser, 1928).

It may just be unfortunate that Sluder tried to tie this headache pathogenetically to the sphenopalatine ganglion. No satisfactory evidence has been provided to demonstrate that a causal relationship between the two generally exists. In one patient operated on with the intention of removing the ganglion (Sluder, 1910), the pain was abolished even though the specimen removed contained no ganglion tissue (on histological examination?). This is not meant to imply that I reject the possibility that headache or facial pain may originate from the sphenopalatine ganglion. The pain and discomfort in the face of *some* patients may be due to a dysfunction of this ganglion. The clinical manifestations of headache stemming from this ganglion—if it exists—are not known. Some of my ideas concerning Sluder's headache are expressed in the section entitled Atypical Facial Neuralgia.

Even though headache was mentioned as a cardinal feature, 4 of 11 patients apparently did not complain of headache. Be that as it may, at least there are many features that distinguish this headache from cluster headache (as a group). The headache was at least partly located in areas atypical for cluster headache, and was usually clearly less severe than the headache of cluster headache, and it apparently did not show the typical temporal pattern of cluster headache.

Vail's 'vidian neuralgia'. 'Vidian neuralgia' is only briefly mentioned here because, clinically speaking, it is considered to be only a variant of Sluder's neuralgia. Vail (1932) himself stated this very clearly: 'Comparing the symptoms of the cases which I report here with the cases reported by Sluder, it will be seen that they are identical'. For symptoms and differential diagnosis, the reader is, therefore, referred to the above section on Sluder's headache. Vail contended that the clinical constellation of symptoms and signs described by Sluder was more likely to result from a vidian nerve than from a sphenopalatine ganglion affection. The vidian nerve is formed when the greater superficial petrosal nerve joints the greater deep petrosal nerve; it runs along the vidian canal and ends in the sphenopalatine ganglion. The fact that Vail found a female:male ratio of 28:3 in his material is remarkable.

'Atypical facial neuralgia'. Few headache syndromes seem to have caused more confusion than 'atypical facial neuralgia' (Frazier and Russell, 1924). A good *outline* of this headache was given by Fay (1932): 'The term atypical facial neuralgia has become *all inclusive* for those types of pain about the face and head which do not fall into the classification of true trigeminal neuralgia. It has been more commonly accepted as the type of lower half headache described by Sluder' (the italicization is mine). And he continues: 'The present concepts of this syndrome are so varied and the reports of successes and failures in treatment so numerous that confusion reigns on all sides as to its true nature'.

Fay (1932) thus claimed that Sluder's headache, 'atypical facial neuralgia', and 'lower-half headache' are identical terms, despite the apparent differences in the descriptions of the syndromes. Fay stated this in 1932, just after Harris' first description of migrainous (ciliary) neuralgia, and simultaneously with Horton and Magath's (1932) description of temporal arteritis, but clearly before Horton's description of histaminic cephalgia, and before the description of other headaches. It must, therefore, be assumed that there is some inaccuracy in the early descriptions of this headache (e.g. Heyck, 1981).

The clinicians who originally studied such cases claim to have established that these pains:

1. are not superficial (as in trigeminal neuralgia) but deep-seated;
2. do not follow the distribution of any specific nerves or nerve branches and do not extend to the periphery (Frazier and Russell, 1924); and
3. may be felt in extratrigeminal areas, such as the occipital area, neck, and shoulder.

A good description of the symptoms has been given by Glaser (1928, 1940), Glaser and Beerman (1938), Eagle (1942) and Martin (1942): the pain was described as *mostly unilateral* (as in McElin and Horton's (1947) series where 61 of 66 patients had unilateral headache), manifesting itself in 'the chin, along the nose, around the eye, over the brow, to the vertex or to the temporal region, in front of, in or through the ear and thence down into the suboccipital region. Occasionally, it entered the shoulder, rarely the body' (Glaser, 1940). The pain was described as being most pronounced in the orbital, supraorbital and the occiput/neck areas. The pain quality was described as aching, burning and throbbing. Valsalva manoeuvres, as when sneezing and blowing the nose, could provoke the pain.

Glaser (1928) claimed that there may be autonomic (sympathetic?) phenomena; that is, transitory oedema, erythema and flushing, lacrimation, and conjunctival injection. As to the severity of attacks, patients might occasionally be awakened at night. The duration of pain attacks was described as being long (>1 day in 41 of 66 cases, or 62% (McElin and Horton, 1947)). Sometimes the discontinuous pain became chronic (Friedman, 1969). Atypical facial neuralgia is thus a rather vague pain category; the pain distribution, attack frequency, and the duration vary considerably interindividually. The attack is usually considered to be rather oligosymptomatic, the pain by itself making up the major part of the attack.

The female preponderance was evident in the various early series being mostly 3–4:1. The age of onset was in youth to mdidle age (mean age of onset, 33 years (McElin and Horton, 1947)). It is also remarkable that a variety of surgical procedures that have been tried in cluster headache, have also been tried in this headache, including alcohol injection of branches of the trigeminal nerve, subtotal section of the sensory root of the trigeminal nerve, avulsion of the supra- and infra-orbital nerves, cocainization and injection of the spheno-palatine ganglion and cervical sympathectomies and stripping of the peri-arterial carotid plexus. All these procedures have been of little or no avail (Glaser, 1940).

Campbell and Lloyd (1954), who described 'atypical facial pain', which is presumably the same as 'atypical facial neuralgia', added a special feature to the clinical characteristics: precipitation of the head/face pain by neck movements, such as during sewing, reading, floor polishing or ironing. Awkward neck positions might, in other words, precipitate attacks. Relief could also be obtained by appropriate neck movements. The picture described by Campbell and Lloyd thus considerably resembles what we have termed cervicogenic headache (Sjaastad *et al.*, 1983c), one of the early descriptions of which (at least of *similar* cases) was probably given by Hunter and Mayfield (1949). If these assumptions are correct and if Campbell and Lloyd's cases are representative of atypical facial pain or neuralgia as a group, then there is considerable similarity between the atypical facial neuralgia and cervicogenic headache groups as such (Sjaastad, 1986d). This concerns the *mainstream* of the two disorders.

The differential diagnostic considerations versus cluster headache will accordingly, as far as the present author is concerned, be much the same as those concerning cervicogenic headache. The duration and number of attacks, the severity of the pain, the accompanying symptoms and signs, the sex

preponderance and the precipitation mechanisms distinguish these two headache forms from one another.

It is clear from this description that atypical facial neuralgia is not only a facial
pain; it enters the supraorbital area and may give rise to a *head pain*. It may also
be discussed whether the term neuralgia is appropriate (neuralgia then taken
in the usual sense of the term). The qualifying word 'atypical' makes the total
term more palatable. The reason why Glaser (1928) and others preferred this
term may have been that it is non-committal, in that it does not point to any
special aetiology or pathogenesis.

So-called atypical cluster headache—'cluster headache variant'. The term 'atypical
cluster headache' was used by Hørven and Sjaastad (1977) to describe symptoms clearly reminiscent of cluster headache, although atypical traits were
present. The supplementary test results, such as the corneal indentation pulse
amplitude test, the intraocular pressure, and the corneal temperature measurements (see pages 193–199) were also consistent with the cluster headache
syndrome. This group comprised various types of patients: for example, two
males showed marked interparoxysmal electroencephalographic changes
(slow-wave activity) during the bout; at the time we did not attempt to classify
these patients more specifically. Furthermore another patient had recurring
bouts of ipsilateral, retrobulbar neuritis, a partial factor XII (Hageman trait)
deficiency, and a bleeding tendency (Sjaastad *et al.*, 1976, 1988b)).

The terms 'atypical cluster headache' and 'cluster headache variant' have
recently been used in an unfortunate manner (see e.g. Diamond *et al.*, 1982).
According to Diamond *et al.*, the intention was to 'specifically redefine' an
atypical subgroup of cluster headache, 'cluster headache variant', the group in
their estimation being 'a group of indomethacin-responsive patients with some
combination of *"three specific vascular headaches"'*. Furthermore, 'There are *three*
symptoms that occur in various combinations in the patients we see: atypical
cluster headache, multiple jabs, and background vascular headaches' (the
italicization is mine). In other words, without any further documentation,
'multiple jabs' (probably another version of the original term 'jabs and jolts
syndrome' (Sjaastad, 1979; Sjaastad *et al.*, 1979)) is classified as a 'specific
vascular headache' without any kind of reservation.

The two expressions used both contain the term 'cluster headache'. Therefore, if they are to convey any meaning, there must be a *link* to cluster headache
in *some* way; otherwise the reference to cluster headache should be omitted.
The authors are most eager to demonstrate the *differences* between their
'syndrome' and cluster headache and to some extent they have succeeded in
this task as there appear to be several differences. The question, therefore, is
again asked: What is the link to cluster headache? The inclusion criteria are not
stated. Atypical cluster headache has not been defined (despite the authors'
claim that this was their intent), and the description is vague and indistinct.
But, according to the vague description given, the headache could be uni- or

bi-lateral. A strictly unilateral headache was found in only 28 of 45 of atypical cluster headache cases (that is, 62% of cases). The headache was of moderate severity, *most* patients not being awakened by nightly pain attacks, whereas nausea and vomiting occurred more frequently than did lacrimation. The headache varied in duration from a few seconds to an almost continuous headache. Perhaps the most astonishing information offered is that it is *not a requirement that the patients respond to indomethacin*: there was thus no indomethacin response in nine and only 'fair' response in four of a total of 54 patients.

There are *various types of headache that respond to indomethacin* (see the section on the so-called indomethacin-responsive headache, in Chapter 4). In my estimation it is important to differentiate between a *moderate response* and an *absolute response* to indomethacin because many cases of 'cervicogenic headache' respond to indomethacin or other NSAIDs, such as piroxicam (see e.g. Sjaastad, 1986d), but usually only to a moderate extent. This fact ought to be taken into consideration because cluster headache may be clinically confused with cervicogenic headache (see Cervicogenic Headache). A moderate response is a rather commonplace event in headache. The absolute effect of indomethacin, however, is so dramatic that it is surprising for those who witness it for the first time.

Such a response probably has some fundamental pharmacologic or metabolic implications. There may be headache conditions other than chronic paroxysmal hemicrania and hemicrania continua (Sjaastad and Spierings, 1984; Sjaastad *et al.*, 1984c) that respond to indomethacin in an absolute manner. However, in order to ascertain this, one must work in a structured manner. The partial indomethacin response may to some extent distinguish this headache from ordinary cluster headache, since indomethacin is generally not known to influence ordinary episodic cluster headache positively (Sjaastad and Dale, 1974).

The lack of refinement of the diagnostic criteria apparently has led to a confusion concerning various diagnostic categories. One can still discern features of CPH and the jabs and jolts syndrome in this melting pot. Within the mixtum compositum, there are probably cases of cervicogenic headache (Sjaastad *et al.*, 1983c; Pfaffenrath *et al.*, 1984a, 1988), a headache that is, as far as is known, probably entirely or largely without any ties to cluster headache. There also may be cases in this series that cannot be classified properly—small 'gems' that might have been discovered.

There seems to be little advantage, rationale or justification for linking this 'syndrome' with cluster headache. No attempt seems to have been made to establish bonds between 'the new headache syndrome' and ordinary episodic cluster headache. The authors could have made various investigations to try to establish such a relationship. For example:

1. *Intraocular pressure* and *corneal indentation pulse amplitude* measurements (Hørven and Sjaastad, 1977). These variables show a clear increase on the

symptomatic side during attacks if the headache in question is within the realm of cluster headache.

2. *Nitroglycerin test*: nitroglycerin and other similar substances are known to give positive results in a high proportion of the tests in cluster headache.

3. *Pupillography* has been used in recent years (Riley and Moyer, 1971; Fanciullacci *et al.*, 1982; Salvesen *et al.*, 1987b) to show that there are signs of a sympathetic deficiency on the pain side in ordinary cluster headache.

There are also several other tests, clinical examinations, and supplementary tests of older or more recent date (such as sweat examinations (Sjaastad, 1981; Sjaastad *et al.*, 1981; Saunte *et al.*, 1983b)) that might have been applied before 'defining' this 'syndrome'. Unfortunately, it does not appear that such efforts were made.

Even this summary critique of this 'syndrome' should convey a clear conclusion: before too much confusion is created, the use of these terms should be abandoned.

Hysteria—'psychogenic headache'. Hysteria has been mentioned as a differential diagnosis for cluster headache by various authors (e.g. Robinson, 1958). In his thorough analyses of hysteria, Merskey (1979, 1981) stated that pain, including headache, can result 'from a conversion mechanism or from an idea and as a result of thought processes'. Pain of this nature could then be viewed as a retreat into illness, as a temporary conflict solution, or maybe even as an expression of guilt.

Partly as a result of long-lasting and penetrating discussions with Professor Merskey, I have reason to believe that such mechanisms really can underlie head pain in man. However, it is difficult to understand how ideas and conflicts can produce a strictly *unilateral* headache in the absence of organic disease. The temporal pattern with, for example, a relatively abrupt onset, as well as the excruciating severity would also be difficult to explain if the origin were psychogenic. Merskey is of the opinion that unilateral headache rarely has a pure psychogenic background.

The diagnostic clues of psychogenic headache are supposed to be: the constancy, the non-fluctuating and generalized quality of the headache, as well as the apparent mildness of the headache despite the vivid and colourful description of the headache by the victims and their contention that it is severe (e.g. Peters, 1953). Psychological problems may make it difficult for the patient to tolerate pain. The pain attacks do not respond to cluster headache (or migraine) drugs such as ergotamine. A non-responsiveness to medication is said to be typical of psychogenic headache. Another clue to the diagnosis of such cases has been hinted at by Dexter and Weitzman (1970) (evidence from one patient only). 'Nightly attacks' in 'psychogenic headache' ($n = 2$) appeared more than 20 min after awakening. Psychogenic headaches may thus be associated with wakefulness and not with sleep, the latter seemingly being characteristic of cluster headache.

In conclusion, it seems highly unlikely that cluster headache could resemble anything like a 'psychogenic headache' (if such a headache exists).

SYMPTOMATIC CLUSTER HEADACHE-LIKE PICTURE

It is my firm belief that cluster headache is a disease in its own right, with its own, specific aetiology and pathogenesis. In accordance with this view, cases of *identical*, clinical manifestations, but a different aetiology/pathogenesis, are non-existent. Clinical cases showing a symptomatology *reminiscent* of cluster headache, even strongly so, but at variance with cluster headache from an aetiological/pathogenetic point of view have been described. The theoretical reason for the clinical similarity may be: that the *structures* involved in cluster headache proper and those involved in a condition similar to cluster headache are identical or adjacent (the pathological process being different); or, that the *mechanisms* involved may be similar, but the location of the process different. If *both* the location and the underlying mechanism were identical, one would of course have congruent disorders. The question of *referred pain* should also be paid some heed to in this context.

Disorders of the hypophyseal area, occipital/suboccipital region, as well as the cervical spine area have been reported to give rise to clinical pictures reminiscent of cluster headache (Table 2.16).

Disorders in the nuchal area

Elliott (1971) has described two cases where a cluster headache-like condition ('migrainous neuralgia') appeared to have been caused by penetrating wounds in the suboccipital region. In one case, removal of a metal fragment embedded deeply in the nuchal muscles, at the level of C1, apparently cured the unilateral 'frontal neuralgia' which had been present since the time of injury. The extent of the period from injury to removal of the foreign body was not specified. The temporal pattern of the headache, the possible associated autonomic symptoms, and the post-operative time of obervations were not mentioned. The headache was unilateral; the side of the wound must be considered to have corresponded to the side of the headache, although this was not specifically mentioned. A considerable similarity to cluster headache may be assumed to have been present in these case. However, under the description of the clinical picture of 'migrainous neuralgia' as such, Elliott (1971) mentions that the pain may 'last for hours or days at a time'. One may, therefore, wonder if also there may have been differences on clinical grounds between the two cases described and the ordinary picture of cluster headache.

Table 2.16 Symptomatic cluster headache-like picture

Authors	Case No.	Area of pain[a]	Area of lesion	Nature of lesion[b]	Convincingly described similarity with cluster headache	Atypical traits
Herzberg et al. (1975)	1	R temporal	R posterior parasagittal region	AV anomaly	No	Attack frequency: NM. Visual phenomena, etc.
Thomas (1975)	1	R eye, *above/behind*	R above ear soft tissue of the scalp	AV anomaly	Not quite	Duration: 'late evening and all night'
Mani and Deeter (1982)	1	L temporal–parietal	L occipital lobe	AV anomaly	No	Duration: 3 days
Kuritzky (1984)	1	R temporal; mandible/neck	C1–C2, foramen magnum R	Meningioma?	No	Localization of pain
Tfelt-Hansen et al. (1982)	1	L eye/temporal area	Hypophysis	Prolactinoma	Rather similar (cluster phenomenon?)	
Sjaastad et al. (1988b)	1	L eye/behind eye. Previous: R	Anterior communicating artery (+A1)	Giant aneurysm	Quite similar	Hageman factor and early onset (at 14 years), etc.
Greve and Mai (1988)	1	Frontotemporal: first bout L; second bout R	Anterior communicating artery	Aneurysm	Some similarity	No nocturnal attacks
Greve and Mai (1988)	2	R behind orbit, spreading frontotemporally	Left carotid artery	Aneurysm	Rather similar	No alcohol provocation. 10–15 min attacks and frequent attacks
Greve and Mai (1988)	3	L frontotemporal; max. eye	Suprasellar pituitary tumour	Prolactinoma	No	No nocturnal attacks
Levyman et al. (in press)	1	L orbital, supraorbital	Prepontine inferior clivus area, more to the left	Epidermoid tumour	For one type (out of three) types of pain	Female

(continued)

Table 2.16 *Continued*

Authors	Sex	Unilaterality[a]	Excruciating severity	Cluster phenomenon	Autonomic symptoms and signs
Herzberg *et al.* (1975)	F	R	NM	+	Previously[c] on R side. Presently: NM
Thomas (1975)	M	R	+(?)	+	Lacrimation (R)
Mani and Deeter (1982)	F	L	+	+	Nasal congestion/lacrimation (L)
Kuritzky (1984)	M	R	+	+	Conjunctival injection/lacrimation (R)
Tfelt-Hansen *et al.* (1982)	M	L	+	Not really	Conjunctival injection/periorbital oedema/nasal symptoms (L)
Sjaastad *et al.* (1988b)	F	L. Previously R	+	+	Lacrimation/nasal symptoms (L)
Greve and Mai I (1988)	M	L: first bout R: second bout	+	+	Congestion eye/conjunctival injection (R)
Greve and Mai II (1988)	M	R	+	+	Congestion eye/rhinorrhoea (R)
Greve and Mai III (1988)	M	L	+	–	Rhinorrhoea/lacrimation (L)
Levyman *et al.* (in press)	F	L	+	+	Lacrimation/rhinorrhoea/ptosis (L)

NM, not mentioned.
[a]L, left; R, right.
[b]AV, arteriovenous.
[c]During the early classical migraine-like phase.

Meningioma in the cervical spine

Kuritzky (1984) described a male patient, aged 68 years, with a meningioma of the cervical canal, at the level of the foramen magnum, stretching down to approximately C2 (Table 2.16). The meningioma was located on the right side and dislocated the cord to the left side. The headache was localized in the right temporal region, and the mandible and neck on that side and had been present for approximately 6 months. It was severe and nocturnal, leading to floor pacing, and usually of 1–3 h duration. There are also lacrimation and reddening of the eye on the symptomatic side. Conventional therapy, such as steroids, ergotamine, lithium and analgesics, was of no avail. The meningioma was surgically removed, and the patient was headache-free for the 20-months post-operative period of observation.

Does this case conform with the characteristics of ordinary cluster headache? The patient was rather old for the onset of regular cluster headache. Onset at that age takes place in only approximately 2% of the cases (Ekbom and Waldenlind, 1982). Next, there was no cluster phenomenon. The severity and distribution of the pain may imply cluster headache, although the pain of cluster headache is most typically located in the ocular/frontal and not the temporal region (and over the mandible). So, there are some atypical traits in this case, but the similarity with ordinary cluster headache is tangible.

Arteriovenous malformations

Three of the reports listed in Table 2.16 concern arteriovenous malformations. In the first case (Herzberg *et al.*, 1975), the similarity to cluster headache was only marginal (Table 2.16). The patient, a 55-year-old female, had attacks characterized by unilateral, pulsating headache of long duration (upwards of 24 h) and preceded by visual disturbances since the age of 16 years. Ipsilateral autonomic phenomena were present. The location of the headache was not described other than being 'unilateral'. The arteriovenous malformation was in the posterior parasagittal area on the side of the headache. Even if the attacks eventually tended to cluster, the pattern exhibited by this patient might seem to fit more into a pattern of cyclical migraine.

The second case (Mani and Deeter, 1982) is a 36-year-old female who had experienced unilateral (left-sided) pain attacks since the age of 22 years. The pain attacks were strictly unilateral, localized in the temporoparietal area, were of incapacitating severity, and were accompanied by lacrimation and nasal secretion. The attacks showed a nocturnal predominance and lasted from 2–3 h up to 3 days. The attacks occurred in clusters of 2–3 months duration. A large arteriovenous malformation, located in the left occipital lobe, was detected on a computed tomography scan and angiography. The malformation was surgically removed, and the post-operative period (not specified exactly, but probably of approximately 2 years duration) was apparently free of further 'cluster headaches'. The authors mentioned the following atypical features which prompted them to undertake supplementary studies in this case: the patient was female; the pain was located temporoparietally (instead of periorbitally); and the pain did not change side. The last-mentioned fact would strengthen, not weaken, the case for ordinary cluster headache. Another aspect mitigating against an ordinary diagnosis of cluster headache is the duration of attacks, i.e. up to 3 days. This case does not present the typical picture of ordinary cluster headache.

The third case is that of a 39-year-old male who had experienced two bouts of unilateral headache over the course of approximately 4 years (Thomas, 1975). The pain attack was located behind and above the eye and was accompanied by ipsilateral autonomic phenomena. The patient would pace the floor during the crises which appeared, at least partly, at night and were relieved by ergotamine. During the first bout, attacks lasted up to 2 h, whereas during the last one they lasted all night. The demonstrated arteriovenous malformation, in the soft tissue above the ear on the pain side, was not operated upon. Apart from the protracted duration of the solitary attack, the pain characteristics present in this case could conform with those of cluster headache.

Recently, another case of symptomatic cluster headache due to an ipsilateral arteriovenous malformation in the middle cerebral artery zone has been described (Testa *et al.*, 1988). This case concerns a female in whom no autonomic disturbances were observed. Thus, *two* essential factors of cluster headache were missing. Furthermore, the pain location—the occipital region and left side of the face—was atypical. What is left of the cluster headache picture seems to be severe, unilateral headache appearing in clusters, but initially occipital in location. The cluster phenomenon itself is probably non-specific (Sjaastad *et al.*, 1988a). The similarity of this case to cluster headache is, therefore, marginal. The authors, therefore, also wisely use the term 'cluster headache-like syndrome'.

In all the cases described above, the demonstrated arteriovenous malformation was on the side of the headache (see also Bruyn, 1984), which suggests, but does not prove, a cause-and-effect relationship. The localization of the arteriovenous malformation was, respectively: posterior parasagittal region, occipital lobe, and soft tissue in the scalp above the ear. Discontinuation of the pain attacks after removal of the arteriovenous malformation like in Mani and Deeter's case adds weight to the view that there was a causal relationship between the arteriovenous malformation and the headache. Such information does, however, not change the balance of evidence on the question of whether cluster headache proper could be caused by arteriovenous malformations.

Aneurysms

Three cases of cerebral aneurysm and a cluster headache-like picture are outlined in Table 2.16.

A patient with Hageman factor deficiency and a cluster headache-like headache (Sjaastad *et al.*, 1976, 1988b) also had a giant aneurysm of the anterior communicating/A₁ arteries. The following main characteristics of cluster headache were present in this case: unilaterality, excruciating pain, autonomic phenomena, and a typical cluster phenomenon. Furthermore, even the pain localization was in the 'correct' (ocular, retro-ocular) area, and the corneal indentation pulse amplitudes increased during attacks. The clinical constellation of symptoms and signs in this patient is so similar to that of the regular cluster headache picture that this case could readily have been put into the cluster headache category.

However, manifold atypical traits were also present, e.g. the age of onset (around 14 years), the duration of the solitary attack (up to 5–6 h), vomiting during severe attacks, female sex, and episodes of retrobulbar neuritis. The pain even shifted side over the years (Table 2.16). Together these features minimize the chances that one is faced with ordinary cluster headache in this case (Sjaastad *et al.*, 1988a). It seems unlikely that the retrobulbar neuritis episodes in such a case are caused by cluster headache (Toshuwal, 1986).

The role of the giant aneurysm in this picture seems dubious. Principally, its significance may be either: (1) a chance and, until its rupture, harmless co-existence with the cluster headache-like headache; or (2) the aneurysm played a role, possibly even a fundamental one, in the generation of pain in this case for many years, in which case the headache is *not* a cluster headache, but a headache similar to it. If this is the case, the location of the aneurysm is important. The location of the aneurysm was such that it did not impinge on some of the structures (e.g. the trigeminal nerve, the third cranial nerve, or the third-neuron sympathetic fibres) which could possibly mediate the pain or autonomic phenomena. Furthermore, pupillometry and evaporimetry definitely showed that there was no third-neuron sympathetic lesion pattern present in this case.

There may, however, be other mechanisms of pain production in this case. *Structures involved by the aneurysm per se*, i.e. the proximal part of the anterior cerebral artery (and/or anterior communicating artery), may have been of importance for the pain production. If the aneurysm created the pain in this case, the pain might have originated because of the intraluminal pressure exerted on the aneurysmal wall and/or the adjacent vessel wall. If this were the case, then these structures (the anterior communicating artery or the inferior part of the anterior cerebral artery) may be able to produce 'a pain identical to that of cluster headache' *per se*. There may even have been a traction on structures on the other side of the midline. Consequently, even the side shift of pain that occurred in this patient could be explained on this basis.

A sufficiently large number of cluster headache cases have been angiographed to support the conclusion that giant aneurysms (or even saccular aneurysms of a minor scale) in this area do not underlie the pain of cluster headache in general. The possibility exists that in this case we are faced with an abnormality clearly at variance with that underlying cluster headache patho-genesis, *but located in or close to the area where the pain of cluster headache per se originates.*

Another case involving an anterior communicating artery aneurysm has recently been described by Greve and Mai (1988) (see Table 2.16). The clinical picture was in many ways similar to that of cluster headache, being of excruciating severity and showing a cluster phenomenon. It is remarkable that even in this case the pain shifted sides between the two bouts.

Pituitary tumour

A 52-year-old male (Tfelt-Hansen *et al.*, 1982) had, since the age of 21 years, suffered form left-sided headache attacks, located in the oculotemporal area (Table 2.16). The attacks were of excruciating severity and of 0.5 to 2 h duration. Ipsilateral lacrimation, conjunctival injection and periorbital oedema accom-panied the attack, and there was tenderness of the superficial temporal artery. Attacks occurred in both the night and the day, and the attack frequency had increased so that in the preceding 4–5 years the patient had experienced one moderately severe attack per day and 1–2 severe attacks per week. Ergotamine seemed to have a beneficial effect on the pain. A large pituitary, suprasellar tumour was detected, infiltrating the left temporal region. Angiography demonstrated that the carotid siphon was stretched and displaced anteriorly. The tumour, a chromophobe adenoma, could only partly be removed, because of infiltration around the chiasm. The residual tumour tissue regressed on post-operative X-ray therapy. Nine months after the operation, the patient was treated with carbamazepine because of complex partial seizures. During the 2-year post-operative period, the patient did not suffer any attacks similar to the previous ones, but experienced mild attacks of generalized headache.

This patient did not seem to exhibit a *primary* chronic cluster headache pattern, the attack frequency for a long time apparently being too low for that. ('For many years, he would have approximately one or two attacks per month'). The patient did not actually exhibit a *secondary* chronic pattern either, because there was no typical cluster pattern prior to the chronic stage. This patient, therefore, seems to have approached the chronic stage in an atypical way, in that the number of attacks increased steadily. This factor *could* signal an organic disorder at variance with cluster headache. It should be noted that the patient also became impotent at the time his headache became chronic in character. Otherwise, there are many traits in this case that suggest cluster headache of the chronic variety.

It is possible that in this case there are two independent disorders, i.e. a cluster headache with a slowly developing headache, and a pituitary tumour. The apparent beneficial influence of the operation could be due to a non-specific result of the operation, which has also sometimes been seen after other operations in cluster headache. Admittedly, this possibility is somewhat far-fetched. A pain referred from the affected area may spread just to the ocular area. It is, therefore, a possibility that this cluster headache-like picture in its entirety was created by the tumour, in which case any relationship to genuine cluster headache is only apparent. An unanswered question in this case is the influence of carbamazepine. The authors correctly state that carbamazepine has no influence on cluster headache. However, their patient probably did not suffer from *cluster headache* proper, and it is not known what influence carbamazepine would have on the kind of headache this patient exhibited.

Two other cases with tumours in this area and a cluster-like picture have been described: one of Greve and Mai's cases (No. 3, see Table 2.16) had a suprasellar tumour of the pituitary gland; and Hannerz (1989) has recently reported a case of parasellar meningioma. A case of epidermoid tumour in the prepontine (just behind the dorsum sella turcica) has also recently been described. The patient apparently suffered from various types of pain, among which was one with similarity to cluster headache (Levyman *et al.*, 1991).

THE SIGNIFICANCE OF 'SYMPTOMATIC CLUSTER HEADACHE'

A constellation like those reported may theoretically have been brought about in various ways:

1. There may be a chance co-existence of ordinary cluster headache and another non-pain-generating disorder in close spatial connection with the central nervous system, or even within it. The clinical picture will then be one of 'pure' cluster headache. (A similar constellation of factors was present in our first case of chronic paroxysmal hemicrania where an aneurysm of the middle cerebral artery was detected on the symptomatic side. It was considered non-symptomatic and was not operated on. When indomethacin was given, the pain attacks disappeared completely.
2. Cluster headache as such may exist together with a symptom-giving lesion inside or closely related to the central nervous system. Although cluster headache as such is present, its manifestations could to some extent be modified putatively by the other disorder.
3. There is only *one* disorder in or in close relation to the central nervous system. If this disorder is localized in an area from which pain impulses are referred to the ocular area (e.g. the sella turcica area), it may give rise to differential diagnostic problems. The evolving picture will, however, be a *cluster headache-like picture*, and not a cluster headache. On removal of the primary pathology, the headache could eventually disappear.

The pathology demonstrated in the various cases does not underlie ordinary cluster headache. The *localization* of the pathology may nevertheless be of interest (Table 2.16). The localization of the demonstrated organic pathology in these cases varies; it was partly in the posterior parts, i.e. in the occipital lobe and in the upper cervical area. This is interesting in view of the increasingly recognized significance of the cervical spine in both cluster headache (Bogduk *et al.*, 1981; Bogduk, 1984; Anthony, 1985) and chronic paroxysmal hemicrania.

From a diagnostic angle, it would have been advantageous to have carried out diagnostic tests for cluster headache (e.g. corneal indentation pulse amplitude determinations, nitroglycerin provocation test, tests for latent Horner's syndrome, and evaporimetry) in such cases. Only in this way would it have been possible to determine as far as possible the similarity of the conditions described to cluster headache. The reported cases provide no proof that cluster headache as such originates in the central nervous system; rather they direct the attention towards extracerebral (but intracranial) structures.

POST-TRAUMATIC CLUSTER HEADACHE

Reik (1987) has reported four cases of what he considers to be post-traumatic cluster headache. All four cases developed the headache in rather close, temporal association with a moderate head injury. Admittedly, there are many traits pointing to genuine cluster headache in these cases: the patients were males; attacks appeared at night and were apparently severe; and attacks were accompanied by autonomic phenomena. The localization of the pain mostly seemed to fit with cluster headache. However, the cluster phenomenon may not have been as clear-cut in these cases as desirable. It should be stressed that even a rather close temporal association is no *proof* of a cause-and-effect relationship.

TREATMENT

Due to the special temporal characteristics of cluster headache, prophylactic treatment is more preferable in this instance than in, for example, migraine. If attacks occur at regular intervals it may be possible to use *planned* prophylaxis, i.e. to give the drug slightly in advance of the expected attack.

PROPHYLACTIC TREATMENT

Ergotamine

It was demonstrated early in the history of ergotamine that it is effective in migraine. Both migraine and cluster headache were considered to be 'vascular' headaches. This is probably the reason why ergotamine was tried also in cluster headache. Harris (1936) was probably the first to mention ergot alkaloids in relation to this headache. Horton (1941) briefly mentioned the use of ergotamine in cluster headache. In 1945, Horton *et al.* used ergot alkaloids (dihydroergotamine) in the treatment of cluster headache. From 1948, Horton used ergotamine tartrate. In 1952, Horton reported that suppositories of 2 mg ergotamine tartrate combined with 100 mg of a caffeine at bedtime

Table 2.17   Ergotamine prophylaxis: some rules to be followed

1. Dosage   Oral: 1–3 mg day^{-1}
                 Rectal: 1–4 mg day^{-1}
                 Parenteral: 0.25–0.5 mg up to 2 times daily

2. Use the *smallest* effective dosage

3. Medication should preferably be given at appropriate times
   before expected attacks and not twice or three times daily

4. Frequent discontinuations of medication in order to detect a
   spontaneous remission

frequently prevented nocturnal attacks. Ergotamine was also used by Ryan (1950).

In the meantime, Ekbom (1947) had used ergotamine tartrate tablets prophylactically in cluster headache. Tablets of 2 mg were administered 2–3 times daily. Using this regimen he obtained good results in 13 of 16 patients. Symonds (1952, 1956) treated patients with parenterally adminstered ergotamine tartrate, usually 0.25–0.5 mg, once or twice daily (at bedtime, and sometimes also in the morning) to prevent attacks. Since the attacks frequently occur during the night, bedtime medication was preferably used.

Around 80% of cluster headache patients seem to benefit from ergotamine when administered prophylactically by various routes of administration (Kudrow, 1980). If ergotamine is given as tablets on a regular prophylactic basis, there may be many break-through attacks which will have to be treated. A combination of a regular prophylactic medication and an attack treatment is one therapeutic alternative. If there is a known pattern of attacks, ergotamine may be given 1 h or so in advance of the expected attack in a sort of combined prophylactic/attack therapy, or in planned prophylaxis: the therapy is not given during the special attack but, on the other hand, the therapeutic measure is directed towards a particular, expected, forthcoming attack (Table 2.17). However, as far as I am aware, no investigations have been done to compare different treatment regimens of ergotamine.

In migraine, it may be advantageous to administer ergotamine rectally, because of nausea and vomiting. These features are usually not prominent in cluster headache and so there does not seem to be any particular advantage in administering ergotamine rectally for these reasons. However, the absorption from the various sections of the gut is another question. The bioavailability may be different in different forms of administration. Suppositories have been used by many investigators (e.g. Ryan, 1951).

The determination of ergotamine in plasma, whether by higher performance liquid chromatography (HPLC) and a fluorescence detection method, or a Rosenthaler immunoassay, is generally fraught with difficulty (Ala-Harula *et al.*, 1979; Ekbom *et al.*, 1981; Hovdal *et al.*, 1982). Ekbom *et al.* (1981), using HPLC with fluorescence detection, found a low biological availability after oral dosing of ergotamine in cluster headache patients. In a cross-over study on healthy volunteers, Bülow *et al.* (1986), compared the absorption from tablets and suppositories of 1 mg ergotamine. Only 29 of 160 blood samples contained detectable (i.e. >0.1 ng ml^{-1}) concentrations of ergotamine. However, only suppositories caused a significant reduction in a toe–arm systolic blood pressure gradient, measured by means of a strain-gauge technique (see also Tfelt-Hansen, 1986). On the basis of such indirect estimations, rectal adminis-tration may, therefore, seem superior to oral administration. In general, rectal or oral administration of ergotamine should be used initially; if ineffective, one may resort to parenteral administration of ergotamine for a short time, to get an idea whether the lack of effect is due to poor absorption. Ergotamine may be administered via other routes which at times may be advantageous, i.e. sublingually and by inhalation.

A single oral dosage of ergotamine should preferably not exceed 1 mg. It may be necessary to repeat the dosage up to 3 times daily. The suppository dosage should preferably not exceed 2 mg; and the dosage by this route should not exceed 4 mg in 24 h (see Tables 2.17 and 2.18). The total daily dosage should preferably not exceed 3–4 mg with these modes of administration. Huge dosages have sometimes been recommended (Stern, 1969), i.e. up to 8 mg orally per 24 h. The advantage of various additives (e.g. pentobarbital sodium, 60 mg) has also been tried out but with inconclusive results (Ryan, 1951). Sedation and sleepiness were frequently observed with these additives. Ergo-tamine is often combined with caffeine, which may enhance intestinal absorp-tion (Berde *et al.*, 1970).

The well-known adverse effects of ergotamine appear particularly when the dosage is high and the treatment period extensive. Nausea and vomiting, cold extremities, diffuse 'muscular' ache, and a general feeling of not being well are common complaints. Dizziness and numbness of the fingers may also occur. The adverse effects are not usually serious enough to interrupt the therapy (Stern, 1969).

If ergotamine treatment has been associated with freedom from attacks for 1 week, the drug should be discontinued to assess whether or not the bout is over (Table 2.17). If attacks reappear, ergotamine should be readministered until another attack-free week when it should again be discontinued. Considering the limited time-span of the cluster phase and if the rules listed in Table 2.17 are adopted, adverse effects should be rare, and major adverse effects ought to be more or less non-existent.

Methysergide

Methysergide was the first of the so-called serotonin antagonists to become clinically available, being introduced around 1960 (Sicuteri, 1959). Methyser-gide, however, has other properties, e.g. it is antihistaminic as well as anticholi-nergic. It is uncertain to what extent the antiserotoninergic property of this drug plays a role in its clinical effectiveness in headache. In migraine, for

Table 2.18 Remedies in current use for cluster headache

Remedy	Prophylactic ('P') or acute ('A') treatment	Also for chronic cluster headache	Preferred route of administration	Preferred dosage
Ergotamine	P/A	Yes[a]	Oral Rectal Parenteral	1–3 mg day^{-1} 1–4 mg day^{-1} 0.25–0.5 mg up to 2 times daily
Lithium	P	Yes	Oral	900 mg day^{-1} (600–1200 mg). Plasma levels should be determined
Prednisone	P	–	Oral	Initially 60–80 mg day^{-1}, tapering off to 25–10 mg day^{-1} rapidly. Total course <1 month
Methysergide	P	–	Oral	1–4 mg day^{-1}; never >6 mg day^{-1}. For only 4–6 months, then a break for 1–2 months
Pizotifen	P	Yes?	Oral	1.5–4 mg day^{-1}
Calcium entry blockers	P	Yes?	Oral	Dependent upon the brand
Oxygen	A	Yes	Inhalation	7 l min^{-1} for 10–25 min

[a]May be used during circumscribed periods. The same to some extent goes for prednisone and methysergide, but for these drugs the periods must be short and the surveillance close (see text).

instance, which has been termed a 'low serotonin syndrome' it may not be the antiserotoninergic properties that count. It has even been mentioned that it compensates for the reduction in whole blood serotonin.

Sicuteri (1959) has reported on prophylactically treated patients, as have Graham (1960), Harris (1961) and Rooke *et al.* (1962). Heyck (1960) described therapeutic success in eight cases, but he later (Heyck, 1981) felt that this apparent success rate was probably partly due to the fact that some patients underwent spontaneous remission. Heyck watched 30 patients closely during several bouts, and he found that in approximately 50% of the patients methysergide was consistently effective; by 'effective' he meant immediate and complete relief from attacks.

Large series have been reported on by Graham (1964) who treated 500 cases (90 with cluster headache) and by Friedman and Elkind (1963), who treated 367 patients (54 with cluster headache). According to Graham, a beneficial effect of methysergide may be expected in 50–70% of cases, depending somewhat on the criteria of effectiveness. In summing up their own therapeutic results (Lance *et al.*, 1963) and those of others, Curran *et al.* (1967) found an average improvement rate of 72.5% in a total of 451 patients. Lovshin (1963a,b) has produced evidence to the effect that the beneficial influence of methysergide declines when given in successive bouts, in contradistinction to Heyck's findings. Whereas methysergide in these studies was given prophylactically to 'episodic' cases, Kudrow (1980) studied its effect in chronic cases ($n = 15$) and found that it was effective in only 20% of the cases. In a more recent prospective study, Krabbe (1989b) treated 42 cluster headache patients (including 16 episodic cases) for up to 6 months with a dose escalating from 1 to 9–12 mg if necessary to obtain effect and a later dosage reduction if there were no breakthrough attacks. Only 25–30% of patients showed a good treatment response.

Methysergide was used extensively after its introduction as a prophylactic drug and sometimes in large dosages. Graham *et al.* (1966, 1967) then discovered a tendency to fibrosis formation in the wake of methysergide therapy. Fibrosis can develop in the heart valves and the lungs, but first and foremost it developed retroperitoneally during which process the ureters could be constricted, with subsequent hydronephrosis and uremia. Particular techniques were developed to demonstrate these neoformations, which partly could be successfully removed surgically (Graham *et al.*, 1967). Athough such severe complications are relatively rare, this development has naturally led to some caution in the use of methysergide.

As safeguards during methysergide therapy, the following are recommended. The dosage should be as low as possible, is never to exceed 6 mg day^{-1}, and should preferably not exceed 3–4 mg per 24 h (Table 2.18). The therapy should be interrupted every 4–5 months for 1–2 months. The fibrotic tendency seems to be reversible and, with the above precautions, the chances of fibrosis development should be minimized. Since the duration of a bout is usually short, these precautions cause no big problems as far as the episodic

form of cluster headache is concerned. Other adverse effects are less important: gastrointestinal symptoms, paraesthesiae, numbness, lightheadedness, a
feeling of unreality, and cold extremities (Curran *et al.*, 1967).

Used within a limited time-span, with the mentioned dosage, and under
strict control, methysergide is still a treatment alternative in cluster headache.

Corticosteroids

Horton (1952) mentioned that only two out of four cluster headache patients
responded favourably to cortisone. Graham (1975) stated that 'ergotamine,
methysergide, cyproheptadine, pizotifen, indomethacin all have useful roles
as prophylactic agents. When these fail, short courses of steroids are frequently
successful'. We tried prednisone in an open, prospective study on five patients
having the episodic form and on one having the chronic form (Sjaastad and
Dale, 1974). The dosage was initially 60–80 mg day^{-1} and was then gradually
tapered off. Three patients responded favourably (two episodic and one
chronic), with a transient improvement. Jammes (1975) observed an effect of
prednisone in 17 of 19 patients, while placebo resulted in no improvement. He
used single doses of 30 mg.

Couch and Ziegler (1978) carried out a retrospective study of 19 patients,
with peak dosages of prednisone ranging from 10 to 80 mg day^{-1}. The peak
dosage was maintained for 3–10 days, after which the prednisone dosage was
tapered off. Absolute relief was obtained in 58% of the cases, whereas a relief of
>50% was obtained in 73%. These authors felt that a dosage of at least
40 mg day^{-1} was necessary to counteract the tendency to attack. The response
rate was as good in the chronic as in the episodic form, according to their
estimation. Recurrence of symptoms occurred in 9 of 11 patients followed-up,
when the dose was lowered to 10–20 mg day^{-1}. Recurrence thus seemed to be
related to the level of the actual dose of prednisone. With such short courses
(i.e. for <30 days) there were no general signs of overdosage of cortisone.

It is interesting to consider Horton's original somewhat poor results in the
light of Couch and Ziegler's findings. Horton used a cortisone dosage of
100 mg day^{-1}, corresponding to approximately 20 mg day^{-1} prednisone.
Breakthrough attacks start to appear at this dosage level, when prednisone is
tapered off. The dosage administered by Horton thus seems to have been
inadequate in many cases.

Kudrow (1980) used prednisone at an initial dosage of 40 mg day^{-1}, gradually tapering off the dosage over the course of 3 weeks. He treated 77 cases of
episodic cluster headache that were unresponsive to methysergide and found
'marked relief' in 77% and 'partial relief' in 12% of cases. A 'marked relief'
response was obtained in 40% of 15 chronic cases, as against a 'partial relief' in
33%. In a separate study Kudrow studied 77 patients with episodic cluster
headache and found prednisone to be superior to methysergide (88% vs. 65%
improvement, respectively).

We have recently used 60–90 mg day^{-1} prednisone as an initial dosage, with gradual tapering off, so that the total length of the course was 3–4 weeks (Table 2.18). The outcome has been most satisfactory. For the breakthrough attacks that particularly appear at the lower dose levels, oxygen or ergotamine was used.

Prednisone is probably a first-line drug in episodic cluster headache, particularly in those patients who, on the basis of previous experience, are expected to have no more than 3–5 weeks of the bout left at the time of the initiation of the drug therapy. However, as with indomethacin in chronic paroxysmal hemicrania, the process is only curbed, not extinguished. As soon as the dosage is reduced or the drug discontinued, attacks may break through again. Due consideration will have to be taken of the possible adverse effects of prednisone; the use of prednisone may in cases of gastric trouble be permissible when combined with histamine H_2 blocking agent therapy.

Pizotifen

Pizotifen, an antiserotonin agent, also has a place in the arsenal of prophylactic drugs used against cluster headache. To the best of my knowledge, only one placebo-controlled trial has been done (Ekbom, 1969), each patient serving as his own control. Twenty-eight patients were treated with a mean treatment duration of 5 weeks, using a mean daily dosage of 2.4 mg (range 1–4 mg day^{-1}). Of the patients, 57% experienced 'excellent' or 'good' results. The recommended dosage of pizotifen is 1.5–4.0 mg per 24 h (Table 2.18). The adverse effects of pizotifen are well known (see e.g. Sjaastad and Stensrud, 1969), i.e. increased appetite, weight gain, drowsiness and, in some cases, paraesthesiae. Pizotifen does not seem to possess the propensity for fibrosis formation as possessed by another antiserotonin agent: methysergide. Therefore, pizotifen probably does not have to be given in relatively short periods followed by drug-free intermissions.

In my experience, the effectiveness of pizotifen seems to be somewhat inferior to that of methysergide. In *severe* cases, therefore, one should probably resort to using one of the more potent drugs.

Lithium

Lithium prophylaxis was probably first used for cluster headache in South Africa in 1968 by McGregor (McGregor, personal communication, June 1988) and by Graham in 1973–1974 (Graham, 1974, 1975). Ekbom (1974) also tried lithium. The reason for the introduction of lithium was partly the behaviour of cluster headache patients during attack (described by Graham (1975) as 'maniac-like'). Partly, it was because the cyclic nature of cluster headache called to mind the cyclic changes of manic–depressive psychosis. Lithium soon proved to be an efficacious agent in cluster headache, but Ekbom (1974c) initially found it to be helpful particularly in the chronic variety. This seemed somewhat surprising since it was the *cyclic* nature of cluster headache that was the underlying reason for its original use. This early trend later changed clearly, and it became evident that lithium is of benefit also in the episodic form. Open, non-controlled studies have been performed, but then the severity of the cluster headache attack is such that it does not seem unreasonable to adhere to such a design (e.g. Damasio and Lyon, 1980). Naturally, the evaluation of studies conducted on 'episodic' cases is more difficult than that of studies conducted on 'chronic' cases.

There have been multiple studies of the use of lithium in cluster headache in recent years (e.g. Ekbom, 1977; Kudrow, 1977, 1980; Mathew, 1978; Scuk-Kuberska and Klimek, 1979; Klimek *et al.*, 1979; Manzoni *et al.*, 1983a). Generally, the trials published have been small. One exception is the trial done by Manzoni *et al.* (1983a). As a routine dosage of lithium carbonate, Manzoni *et al.* recommend 300 mg three times daily, but occasionally the total daily dosage was 600 or 1200 mg (Table 2.18). Treatment was only interrupted after 1 week or more of freedom from headache. In this study, the results were evaluated using a headache index ratio, comparing a pretreatment period (chronic cases, 1-month observation; episodic cases, 1-week observation) with an equal length of time within the treatment period. A total of 90 patients were studied (68 'episodic cases'; 22 'chronic' cases, with 16 in the primary and 6 in the secondary chronic group). The chronic cases were followed for 22 months on average. The patients in the episodic group were followed for one ($n = 50$) to three periods. Plasma and erythrocyte lithium levels were estimated weekly during the first month and monthly thereafter. In episodic cluster headache, there was a mean improvement of 68%, approximately three-quarters of patients showing an improvement of >60% (Table 2.19). The mean weekly headache index dropped form 30.3 to 0.6. Plasma lithium levels varied from 0.3 to 0.8 meqv l^{-1}, whereas the erythrocyte levels varied from 0.10 to 0.35. Krabbe (1986) has recommended serum lithium levels of 0.6–1.2 mmol l^{-1}.

Lithium does not seem to shorten bouts, and does not prevent or even delay the next one. In 14 patients treated during two bouts, the average improvement in the second bout was 61% vs. 80% in the first bout. In six patients treated for a third bout, an average improvement of 42% was obtained. In four patients with the episodic form, treatment was continued for 1 year. There were no signs of relapse as long as the treatment continued, but attacks reappeared within 1–3 weeks of discontinuation of the drug. *Chronic* medication can thus possibly influence future cluster episodes, i.e. it can delay or even subdue them. More long-term studies are necessary to substantiate this view.

Manzoni *et al.* (1983a) have clearly shown that lithium not only improves the chronic form of cluster headache (see Chronic Cluster Headache), but also the episodic form, although the responsiveness may be slightly less marked in the latter variety. Other groups have made similar observations. Mathew (1978) treated 14 patients having the episodic form and 17 having the chronic form,

Table 2.19   Effect of short-term lithium therapy of
episodic cluster headache (68 cases)[a]

	No. of patients
Improvement (%)	
>90	26
60–90	26
<60	16
Mean improvement 68.3%	
Adverse side effects	
Severe, requiring discontinuation	0
Mild, allowing continuation	18
Tremor	6
Increased thirst	5
Insomnia	4
Diarrhoea	3
Lethargy	2
Diffuse headache	1
Goitre	1

[a]From Manzoni *et al.* (1983a). Courtesy of *Cephalalgia*.

and found lithium to be equally potent in the two types: an improvement exceeding 90% was observed in 55% of the cases in the study groups, 20% showing no improvement. Klimek *et al.* (1979) found a tendency towards better results in the episodic than in the chronic group. Kudrow (1980), who found good response among both chronic and episodic cases, found a higher degree of improvement among the chronic cases.

Lithium is not an inert 'drug'. Euthyroid goitre developed in one case studied by Manzoni *et al.* and it disappeared after discontinuation of lithium. Tremor and other adverse effects were rarely observed (see Table 2.19). Kudrow (1980) noted occasional episodes of decreased concentration and mental confusion. This is consistent with our own experience. Mathew (1978) also observed nausea, diarrhoea, abdominal discomfort, and lethargy. Patients having *known* renal, thyroid, or cardiovascular dysfunction should not be given this therapy. There are even some hints in the literature to the effect that lithium may create headache (Brainin and Eisenstädter, 1985; Alvarez-Cermeno *et al.*, 1989).

There is little doubt that lithium is effective in cluster headache, and that its effect is durable, although it may decline somewhat over time. The effect sets in almost as rapidly as that of steroids, and more rapidly than that of methysergide. The health hazards connected with lithium are hardly greater than those connected with methysergide or steroids. Graham (personal communication, 1983) is of the opinion that lithium is one of the most potent drugs in the episodic form of cluster headache—it may even be the drug of choice.

Lithium is effective in patients that have previously been treated with other drugs, e.g. methysergide, ergotamine and cortisone (Damasio and Lyon, 1980; Kudrow, 1980).

The mechanism of action of lithium is unknown. According to Okayasu *et al.* (1984), lithium has no appreciable influence on cerebral haemodynamics in cluster headache. Lithium treated patients seem to have an increase of δ sleep, as well as a decrease of rapid eye movement (REM) sleep and an increased latency to the first REM phase.

The effect of lithium on the relatively low erythrocyte choline content in cluster headache (de Belleroche *et al.*, 1984a,b, 1986) may be interesting in this context (see Choline). Choline is a component of acetylcholine, and low levels of acetylcholine in critical organs may conceivably also be present in cluster headache patients. Lithium also influences the prostaglandin cascade, which may be of importance in this context. However, lithium has many known—and probably also unknown—effects, and its beneficial effect in cluster headache may be due to an unknown effect.

Calcium entry blocking agents

Meyer *et al.* (1985) demonstrated that cerebrovascular resistance is significantly lowered during treatment with various calcium antagonists. If the underlying pathology in cluster headache is 'vascular', calcium antagonists could, theoretically, exert a beneficial influence.

Verapamil. Gabai and Spierings (1989) treated 48 patients (33 with the episodic and 15 with the chronic form) with verapamil (isoptin) in an open study. The average dose in the episodic group was 354 mg per day (range 240–600 mg) and in the chronic group 572 mg (range 120–1200). A total of 69% of the patients improved (73% in the episodic group), and the mean interval before relief was 1.7 weeks (range 1–6 weeks) in the episodic vs. 5 weeks (range 1–20 weeks) in the chronic group.

These results appear promising. The fact that patients in the episodic group with a bout as advanced as 32 weeks were included, may have influenced the results to some extent.

Nimodipine. de Carolis *et al.* (1988) studied the effect of nimodipine in cluster headache in an open trial ($n = 13$). de Carolis *et al.* found nimodipine to have almost the same level of therapeutic efficacy as prednisone, i.e. 54% and 57%, respectively. When tried in successive bouts ($n = 2$), the number of treatment failures seemed to accumulate with nimodipine (see also de Carolis *et al.*, 1987).

The size of these series makes it desirable that further studies be undertaken.

Comparison of various prophylactic drugs

The relative virtue of lithium, prednisone, methysergide and ergotamine, and various combinations of these drugs must be clarified. Kudrow (1980) compared various treatment regimes in cyclic and chronic cases in an open study. Prednisone was found to be superior to methysergide in the episodic type (88% vs. 65%). Lithium (87% improved) proved to be superior to both prednisone (73%) and methysergide (20%) in the chronic form ($n = 15$).

THERAPY FOR THE SOLITARY ATTACK

If attacks are long-lasting, it may be worthwhile to try to counteract the single attack. If, however, the attack is relatively short-lasting (i.e. 20–25 min) and the therapeutic remedy can be administered only after approximately 5 min and it does not take effect for another 10–20 min, depending upon the mode of administration, then little can be expected to be achieved by giving the remedy. In some patients having relatively mild attacks as well as in mild attacks in patients who are usually subject to severe attacks, the usual analgesics may be of some benefit. Analgesics are, however, usually too weak to have any effect in cluster headache. In general, there are at present only three ways of treating a solitary attack, i.e. by ergotamine, dihydroergotamine or oxygen.

Ergotamine

In addition to being used prophylactically, ergotamine may also be administered *after* a single attack has started. If the attack is of some length, and if the drug is administered at the very beginning of the attack, ergotamine may give good relief. The mode of administration of ergotamine is crucial in such situations (Ekbom *et al.*, 1983). If the attack is relatively long-lasting, orally or rectally administered ergotamine may be useful.

Parenteral administration may, however, seem to be the route of choice in many cases. We have taught many of our patients to self-administer ergotamine by subcutaneous injections at the beginning of an attack; relief may then be obtained within 10 min or even less (as against 20 min or more with oral dosing). A standard dosage of ergotamine may be used (i.e. 0.25–1 mg subcutaneously; the dosage should preferably not exceed 0.5 mg). This dosage may be repeated once (or twice) daily (Table 2.18).

Horton *et al.* (1948) treated 14 cluster headache patients with ergotamine tartrate ('Cafergot'); 10 patients experienced excellent results and three good results. Ryan (1950) found excellent or good effect of orally administered ergotamine in 42 of 46 patients, provided that the drug was administered at the onset of attack. Friedman and Mikropoulos (1958) gave ergot derivatives to a total of 35 patients, and found some degree of alleviation in 85% of the cases. They felt that suppositories gave better and more rapid effect than tablets. Kudrow (1980) found a response rate of approximately 80% in a series of 100 patients, the routes of administration being inhalation or sublingual application.

If the attacks appear at set times, it is preferable that the drug be administered an hour or two in advance of the expected attack (see Prophylaxis). It should be emphasized that the mode of administration of ergotamine may be of decisive importance for therapeutic success. In patients where only doubtful results have been obtained, injections ought to be tried before the use of ergotamine is given up. Ergotamine may be given for the entire cluster period, provided this is of the usual length (i.e. 6–12 weeks), because it will be washed out in the remission period. A clear drawback to this type of therapy is that ergotamine for parenteral use has in recent years ceased to be commercially available.

Dihydroergotamine

The first effective drug in the treatment of cluster headache was dihydroergotamine (Horton *et al.*, 1945). The toxic effects of this drug are, according to Horton (1961), only one-third of those of ergotamine tartrate. He claimed that this is the drug of choice for intravenous use. Ryan (1963) stated that 1 ml (=1 mg) of dihydroergotamine given intravenously can abort an attack within 60–90 s.

Andersson and Jespersen (1986) conducted a double-blind randomized trial with dihydroergotamine (1 mg dosage) and placebo nasal spray. Twenty-five patients participated in the trial, three of whom became headache-free after a few days. In the remainder, 133 attacks were treated with placebo and 137 with dihydroergotamine. Whilst dihydroergotamine seemingly had no effect on the duration of attacks, the intensity of attacks seemed to be modified.

Oxygen therapy

Horton was the first to use 100% oxygen therapy in the treatment of the solitary attack of cluster headache (Horton, 1952, 1956a, 1961). In a few cases he found that oxygen inhalation alleviated the pain if the attack was relatively mild and if oxygen was taken during the early part of attack. Friedman and Mikropoulos (1958) stated that a number of their patients occasionally responded quite favourably to oxygen inhalation, although in general oxygen did not prove to be as effective as ergotamine. Nelson (1970) maintained that oxygen by mask is fairly effective if given early, whereas during the peak of the attack it is of little use. Peters (1953) found 100% oxygen (and dihydroergotamine given intravenously) to abort attacks provoked by nitroglycerin or histamine.

Oxygen therapy in cluster headache has been studied in greater detail by Kudrow (1981). Fifty-two patients (33 cases of episodic cluster headache and 19 cases of chronic cluster headache) were treated with 100% oxygen ($7 \, l \, min^{-1}$) by face mask; in each patient, 10 spontaneous attacks were treated. The treatment was continued for 15 min, the patients keeping a record of the timing. Success was defined as at least 7 of the 10 attacks being almost or nearly terminated within 15 min. In those on prophylactic medication, 'breakthrough attacks' were treated. According to these criteria, 75% of patients benefited from this therapy. The response rate was somewhat better among the episodic cases than among the chronic cases. The response rates among patients receiving and patients not receiving prophylactic medication were of the same level of magnitude. Of the patients that responded to treatment, 62% experienced cessation of the attack within 7 min and 93% within 10 min. Oxygen treatment has also been compared with oral ergotamine medication in a randomized cross-over trial (Kudrow, 1981): a somewhat higher response rate was observed with oxygen (82%) than with ergotamine (70%), and the response was slighly more rapid with oxygen.

The results of oxygen therapy in other centres in recent years may seem to have been somewhat less favourable than Kudrow's results (e.g. Graham, personal communication; Sjaastad, unpublished results). Oxygen therapy is, however, without complication and should, therefore, if at all possible be tried as a first line therapeutic approach for a single attack. Oxygen therapy is inconvenient in terms of the problem of transporting the oxygen tank. However, oxygen tanks can be used at home (even at the bedside) as well as in the work place. There is no definite information at hand to show whether, and to what extent, oxygen loses its potency over time.

Hyperbaric oxygen (2.0 ATA (atmospheres absolute)) has been tried in a single patient, who was refractory to all treatment modalities, including oxygen delivered by nasal catheter. The treatment was tried during two attacks, apparently with optimal effect (Weiss *et al.*, 1989). The effect may well have been a real one. However, the timing of the events during this experiment was not clearly stated: the usual duration of attack in this patient was 45 min. While the time between initiation of treatment and effect was approximately 20 min, it was not stated how much time elapsed before treatment could be started. Specific details of the second attack are not given, and this was the last attack of a bout. Taking into consideration that the last attacks of a bout may be of shorter duration than usual, the possibility cannot be rejected that the observed recoveries were spontaneous and not caused by oxygen.

These findings, therefore, must be substantiated in a larger trial, a conclusion also reached by the authors.

Fogen (1985) compared the effects of oxygen ($6\,l\,min^{-1}$) and air, both administered by face mask, in a double-blind, crossover study in 19 cluster headache patients. The patients rated the relief experienced using a 0–3 scale (3 = complete relief) in up to six attacks. In the oxygen group, the average relief score was 1.93 ± 0.22 (SEM), as against 0.77 ± 0.23 in the air group, the difference being highly statistically significant. The clinical observations concerning oxygen therapy thus have a scientific foundation, the improvement not being due to psychological factors, the attention, the mask, etc.

Drummond and Anthony (1985) found that oxygen inhalation reduced supraorbital and temporal artery pulsations during provoked attacks. The reductions on the symptomatic side during attack were significantly larger than those observed in the remission and in controls.

OTHER DRUGS USED IN THE PAST OR *SUB JUDICE*

β-Receptor blocking agents

Damasio and Lyon (1980) have stated that propranolol is occasionally effective in preventing recurrence of cluster periods, but is not definitely effective in counteracting a current cluster of attacks. To my knowledge no data have been presented that substantiate this contention. Kunkel (1981) claimed that propranolol (120–240 mg day^{-1}) 'may benefit some patients'.

Maxwell (1982) made an interesting observation in one out of eight patients treated with radiofrequency trigeminal gangliorhizolysis. The continuous succession of pain attacks was interrupted in this patient. Weaker attacks started to appear in clusters and propranolol appeared to be effective against *these* attacks, whereas it had been ineffective prior to the gangliolysis.

Cyproheptadine

Damasio and Lyon (1980) maintain that cyproheptadine occasionally may be instrumental in preventing (or delaying?) future cluster episodes. No controlled studies have been conducted, as far as prevention is concerned, and as far as I am aware, there have been no studies that prove the effect of cyproheptadine in a current cluster episode.

Sumatriptan

The new serotonin agonist, sumatriptan (agonist for a 5-HT$_1$-like receptor subtype), has also been tested in an open study (Krabbe, 1989a) in a total of 13 attacks in six patients. Subcutaneous injection of 3–6 mg led to a marked relief of nine attacks in four patients. The future position of sumatriptan cannot be assessed on the basis of the present results. However, the drug seems quite promising.

Lisuride

Raffaelli *et al.* (1983) claim that lisuride in dosages ranging from 0.05 to 0.4 mg day^{-1} had an alleviating effect in 10 cases of cluster headache, of which five were episodic cases. The study was an open one; no quantification of attack frequency was attempted. The cluster headache was partly combined with common migraine and temporal arteritis. Since the claim that lisuride is beneficial in cluster headache has not been substantiated by any data, any possible beneficial effect of this drug in cluster headache remains *sub judice*.

Budipine

Krüger *et al.* (1988) treated 23 episodic and 2 chronic cluster headache patients with budipine (butyldiphenylpiperidine), in an open fashion. All episodic patients were enrolled in the early phase of the cluster period. In only one patient was 'slight' relief obtained. On doses from 30 to 60 mg day^{-1}, the other patients experienced 'complete' or 'substantial' relief. The effect appeared within a mean of 4 days, and adverse effects were few. More recently, Krüger (1989) has conducted a double-blind, randomized placebo-controlled pilot trial with budipine ($n = 14$; 11 with the episodic form). Budipine seemed to be active as early as the second week of treatment. If these findings are reproduced, budipine will be another valuable drug for cluster headache treatment.

Sodium valproate

Cluster headache has been considered a disorder with a disrupted circadian rhythm. Since sodium valproate has been shown to modify circadian periods, it was tried therapeutically in cluster headache (Hering and Kuritzky, 1989). Fifteen patients (episodic type, $n = 13$; chronic type, $n = 2$) were treated with sodium valproate in dosages ranging from 600–2000 mg day^{-1} in a non-controlled, open fashion. Nine patients responded fully, while in two patients there was a partial response. There was poor correlation between plasma sodium valproate levels and the efficacy of therapy. With three exceptions, treatment was started early in the cluster period, and the effect generally appeared within a week. There was mild nausea in three patients. These results may seem promising, but they need to be corroborated by further studies.

Chlorpromazine

Caviness and O'Brien (1980) tried chlorpromazine in an open study in doses of 75–700 mg day^{-1}. The clientele consisted of 13 cluster headache patients, two of whom were chronic cases. In 12 patients, headache reportedly ceased completely within 2 weeks. In nine patients, chlorpromazine was discontinued within 2–3 weeks after the cessation of attacks, without further symptoms. Other drugs were given together with chlorpromazine for the first week, when 6 of the 13 patients underwent remission. However, Caviness and O'Brien suspected that spontaneous remissions may have occurred making the assessment difficult. This is quite possible because in a number of cases attacks did *not* recur after drug discontinuation. The authors, nevertheless, felt that chlorpromazine is apparently more effective than lithium and cortisone in cluster headache prophylaxis. This investigation clearly needs further corroboration before its conclusion can be accepted.

Indomethacin

Indomethacin is the drug of choice in chronic paroxysmal hemicrania, where the effect is *absolute*. The drug is generally not clearly effective in regular cluster headache patients (Sjaastad and Dale, 1974). As a matter of fact, the condition of some of our patients deteriorated during such therapy. This may or may not be a consequence of the property of indomethacin to generate headache *de novo*. It is, however, possible that some selected patients with cluster headache (or perhaps a cluster headache-like picture) show a moderate, positive response to indomethacin (Sicuteri *et al.*, 1965; Graham, 1975; Mathew, 1981; Kunkel, 1981; Sjaastad and Hørven, 1982).

Histamine desensitization

Horton (1941) introduced this treatment and recommended it as the treatment of choice for cluster headache: 'Histamine treatment is as specific for this syndrome as insulin is in the treatment of diabetes mellitus'. The idea behind this treatment was based on Horton's observations during the attack: the patient had a higher temperature in the temporal area on the symptomatic than on the opposite side; and sometimes a redness of the skin was also observed. Horton speculated that these changes were caused by an 'anaphylactoid reaction' towards histamine 'at the cellular level'. To enhance the patients' tolerance towards the endogenous histamine he tried to desensitize them by giving increasing dosages of histamine subcutaneously. He recommended that the therapeutic procedure be conducted as follows: a solution of histamine diphosphate was used (0.225 mg histamine diphosphate per ml). The initial dose was 0.05 ml subcutaneously. This dosage was then increased to 0.05 ml twice daily, given about 8–12 h apart. Each dose was then slowly increased by 0.05 ml until the ultimate dosage of 0.5 ml was reached. At times, the final dose was 0.75 ml or even 1.0 ml, depending upon the tolerance of the individual.

This ultimate dosage could then be continued for weeks or 'indefinitely', in the latter case as one injection per day for some time, and later to be given as 2–3 injections per week (Robinson, 1958). Horton (1956a,b) stressed that each patient must have a 'tailor made' dose schedule. If the patient under desensitization experienced headache, facial flush, or throbbing, he might be undergoing 'sensitization' instead of desensitization. In such cases the next dosage was reduced by half, and was subsequently built up again to just below the level at which the patient had started to react.

Horton (1956a,b) claimed that attacks were aborted within 10–20 days. Of his patients 90–95% responded favourably to this treatment. He also claimed that the recurrence rate was only approximately 36% the first year. The latter prognostic figure may seem to be somewhat better than the general prognosis in cluster headache.

Time and again, Horton (e.g. 1956b) reverted to the considerable problems related to treating patients who had been treated one or more times previously with histamine desensitization, in comparison with the ease with which the first episode can be treated. Under such circumstances, the histamine dose must be decreased consistently; if it is kept at the same level in successive therapeutic series the drug may have an adverse instead of a beneficial effect.

Various clinical investigators have found histamine desensitization useful. Thus, Blumenthal (1950) who used the intravenous route for histamine desen-

Table 2.20   Results of histamine desensitization[a]

Total No. patients	No. of patients whom desensitization was tried in	Results of desensitization		
		Positive	Negative	Equivocal[b]
20	15	6	5	4

[a]From Robinson (1958). Courtesy of *Medicine* (*Baltimore*).
[b]Either hard to evaluate or sometimes positive and sometimes negative.

sitization, treated 20 patients and obtained great relief 'within several days'. Robinson (1958), who was fully aware of the intermittent long-term course of cluster headache, also reported positive results of desensitization, although at a somewhat lower level (Table 2.20). In the hands of others, this therapy has not worked as well, be it because of the inherent difficulties with this treatment (it must be tailor-made for each patient) or for other reasons (e.g. that it really is ineffective). Thus, Kunkle *et al.* (1954) found that histamine desensitization was of no avail in the 11 (out of 30) of his patients in whom it was tried. Others have also found that the treatment is of no particular value (e.g. Gardner *et al.*, 1947; Symonds, 1956; Friedman and Mikropoulos, 1958). As negative results accumulated, the method became discredited. It is only fair to say that, at the present time, the method has lost its reputation completely, and this treatment is no longer popular. The story of histamine desensitization contains some almost tragic elements. It is a story of a waste of energy and work. The reasons for the discrepancy between Horton's results and the more recent ones are probably manifold: Even in 1952, i.e. many years after the cluster phenomenon as such had been mentioned in the literature, Horton did not specifically mention the temporal accumulation of attacks. Although in later years he was aware of the fluctuating course of the disorder, he obviously did not fully appreciate the fact that there *usually* is a regular clustering of attacks. For this reason, he has apparently, to a not inconsiderable extent, confounded a spontaneous recovery with a drug-induced improvement. It is remarkable, however, that investigators who were fully aware of the cluster phenomenon have partly reported beneficial results from histamine desensitization (e.g. Robinson, 1958) (see Table 2.20). Stern (1969), from his study on a small series of patients, advocated the use of histamine desensitization.

Horton (1941) also treated a wide variety of headaches of various types (e.g. migraine, 'psychogenic headache' and hypertension) with the same desensitization procedure. In all groups, there was a remarkably similar trend towards improvement. Horton's conclusion is worthy of note:

> In view of the diverse characteristics of the clinical conditions typified by these groups, this observation suggests either that histamine therapy had uniformly beneficial effects on each type, which is hardly credible, or that it had no effect on any group included in this total sample. Lacking a control group of untreated or placebo treated patients, the spontaneous remission rate is conjectural, but *at all* events the improvement noted does not exceed a

reasonable expectation of spontaneous relief, especially as it is likely that most patients consulted the clinic at the peak of their symptoms.

I am of the opinion that a placebo effect is not commonplace in cluster headache. However, in this situation with a slow and gradual onset of the possible effect, and with the uncertainty as to the natural course of a given bout, it would have been highly desirable to include a control group.

Histamine H₁ and H₂ receptor antagonists

Histamine has various actions in man. Its effect on the vasculature results in dilatation of blood vessels and pooling of blood, with a secondary fall in blood pressure. Histamine causes contraction of the smooth muscles of the respiratory system and gastrointestinal tract. Histamine can also cause symptoms resembling those resulting from anaphylactic reactions. These actions, termed H_1 receptor actions by Ash and Schild (1966), are antagonized by the so-called conventional or anti-allergic antihistamine preparations. The latter have, therefore, become known as histamine H_1 receptor antagonists.

Other actions of histamine are not antagonized by the conventional antihistamine preparations. These include the effect on heart rate and the stimulation of gastric acid secretion. The histamine H_2 receptor antagonists counteract these effects. Experimental studies in the cat, dog and monkey have shown that both histamine H_2 and H_1 receptor sites are present in the carotid vasculature. Stimulation of these receptor sites produces vasodilatation (Saxena, 1975).

The concept that cluster headache might be a 'vascular' headache requires further investigation; it would, therefore, appear that further consideration should be given to the possible pathogenetic role of a vasoactive substance such as histamine. The therapeutic potential of both histamine H_1 and H_2 receptor blocking agents has, therefore, been tested.

Histamine H_1 receptor blocking agents. Histamine H_1 blocking agents have been used in cluster headache. One open, uncontrolled study was carried out on 16 patients, in whom 'the headaches occurred sufficiently often to make a therapeutic test possible' (Tucker and O'Neil, 1952). The study was apparently carried out over at least 2 months and with a dosage of 100 mg day^{-1} benadryl. Benadryl was considered ineffective in only 3 of the 14 patients that could be evaluated properly. It was inactive or only marginally effective in migraine and 'atypical headache'. Other H_1 receptor blocking agents were not found as effective as benadryl. The details of the study were not given, and the diagnostic criteria were not specified. The results of this study clearly conflict with those of other studies: Horton (1941, 1956a), McElin and Horton (1945), Emblem (personal communication), Kunkle *et al.* (1952, 1954) and Eadie and Sutherland (1966) found no convincing, beneficial results with histamine H_1

antagonists. Friedman and Mikropoulos (1958) found negative results in 50% of their patients, and slight or doubtful improvement in the rest.

Histamine H_2 receptor blocking agents. In the early 1970s, a new type of antihistaminic was introduced, the so-called histamine H_2 receptor antagonists (Black *et al.*, 1972). These substances are potent inhibitors of nocturnal (Milton-Thompson *et al.*, 1974) and stimulated gastric acid secretion (Mainardi *et al.*, 1974). Cimetidine was the first drug to gain wide acceptance as a histamine H_2 receptor antagonist for clinical use.

The first study done on cluster headache prophylaxis using the histamine H_2 receptor antagonist cimetidine was done by our group (Veger *et al.*, 1976). The series studied consisted of 16 patients and the design was that of a double-blind, crossover study. Patients were randomly allocated to treatment according to one of four treatment schedules. In these schedules the drug was changed every week or every other week. Cimetidine 400 mg or placebo was taken 4 times daily. As regards the mean number of headache attacks per week, 9 of the 16 patients completing the trial improved on cimetidine medication and 6 deteriorated, whereas 1 remained unchanged. The mean number of attacks per week on placebo was 6.5 as against 6.1 on cimetidine (Russell *et al.*, 1977). When the mean numbers of weekly attacks on placebo and cimetidine were used as figures for comparison, cimetidine was not superior to placebo ($p > 0.5$, Student's *t*-test). In those patients who experienced improvement on cimetidine, the improvement was usually only moderate. We found no statistically significant difference between cimetidine and placebo treatment with regard to the intensity or duration of headache attacks.

A controlled trial of cimetidine in cluster headache has also been carried out by Anthony *et al.* (1978) with a negative result. The study included 20 patients, and the dosage was 400 mg, 4 times daily. Cuypers *et al.* (1979) also obtained a negative result with cimetidine.

If cimetidine does have a therapeutic effect in cluster headache, the results described above would suggest that it is minimal. These results, therefore, seem to exclude the possibility that H_2 receptors *per se* play a fundamental role in the pathogenesis of cluster headache.

A combination of histamine H_1 and H_2 receptor blocking agents. The possibility remained that separate H_1 and H_2 receptor blockades are not sufficient, but that a combination of H_1 and H_2 receptor blockade could influence cluster headache attacks. Anthony *et al.* (1978) undertook a study to investigate this possibility. In their study, cimetidine (400 mg, 4 times daily) was combined with 16 mg day^{-1} of the histamine H_1 receptor blocking agent chlorpheniramine, and compared with placebo in 20 patients. A similar study was carried out by Russell (1978) in a double-blind fashion. No significant difference was found between the two treatment modalities in either of the two studies. Cuypers *et al.* (1979) obtained somewhat better results.

The failure of a combination of histamine H_1 and H_2 antagonists as a treatment for cluster headache casts further doubt on the possible role of histamine in the pathogenesis of cluster headache. It does not, however, exclude such a role: it has been postulated that H_1 receptor antagonist drugs, in ordinary doses, probably do not counteract the so-called 'induced' or 'nascent' histamine (Schayer, 1962; Kahlson and Rosengren, 1971) if such a histamine form really exists. It is also possible that there exist as yet undiscovered histamine receptor sites, which are not blocked by either histamine H_1 or H_2 receptor antagonists. Admittedly, however, the theory of histamine mediation of cluster headache has certainly lost a lot of ground in recent years.

Histaminase

One, rather strong piece of evidence indicating that Horton has misinterpreted his therapeutic results on cluster headache is his therapeutic trials concerning histaminase (Horton, 1941). He treated nine cluster headache patients with histaminase, given by mouth. In eight patients 'excellent results from the use of this drug' were obtained, periods without recurrence lasting from 1 to 10 months. No further details concerning doses, duration of treatment, etc., were given. Histaminase *by mouth* must *a priori* be considered absolutely inactive.

Cocaine

Barré (1982) observed that cocaine hydrochloride may abort an attack of cluster headache. During the application of the drug, the patient must be in a supine position, with the head hyperextended and turned towards the painful side and must remain in this position for 30 s. A 5–10% solution of cocaine was used and a dosage of 25–35 mg was instilled in the nasal cavity on the symptomatic side. Barré contended that an improvement of 65–100% was obtained in more than 55% of the attacks in 11 patients (with one exception), and the improvement might occur within 15 s to 3 min. When not resorting to this treatment more than twice in 5 h, the systemic effects of the treatment were reportedly negligible. Barré, therefore, considered that this approach is a valuable supplementary, therapeutic measure. According to Barré, this therapeutic success implies that 'the origin of much of the pain of cluster headache may be found in the pterygomaxillary fossa region'.

This therapeutic approach was tried decades ago in 'atypical facial neuralgia'. It was totally written off in that context by, for example, Glaser (1928, 1940: see Sluder's Sphenopalatine Ganglion Headache and Atypical Facial Neuralgia). As previously stated, a complete failure on the part of atypical facial neuralgia to respond to this treatment does not imply that there may not be other headaches that may really respond. I have no personal experience of the use of cocaine in cluster headache. Until corroborated by other groups, this treatment cannot be advocated.

Topical application of a local anaesthetic agent (4% lidocaine hydrochloride) over the sphenopalatine fossa on the symptomatic side seemed to bring about relief in spontaneously occurring as well as induced attacks (Kittrelle *et al.*, 1985). More studies ought to be done to corroborate this observation.

Somatostatin

Somatostatin blocks the release of substance P from both central and peripheral nerve endings. Somatostatin also has other biological effects, such as inhibition of noradrenaline and acetylcholine release. Due to the first-mentioned property, somatostatin has been tried in cluster headache.

Sicuteri *et al.* (1984) treated a total of 72 attacks in eight male patients and compared the effect of somatostatin (intravenous infusion of 25 μg min^{-1} for 20 min) to that of ergotamine (250 μg intramuscularly) and placebo in a double-blind fashion. Somatostatin was significantly better than placebo and seemed to give a pain relief equal to that produced by ergotamine.

Since somatostatin had to be administered intravenously during the first study, Geppetti *et al.* (1985) tried to give it subcutaneously. They provided some evidence that the drug could be measured in relatively high concentrations in the plasma for some minutes after subcutaneous administration. They claim that it was active during the attack, although not at quite the same level as ergotamine (30 attacks in five patients).

Testosterone

Klimek (1985b) treated 15 cluster headache patients (12 with the episodic form) with daily intramuscular injections of 25 mg testosterone proprionate for 7–10 days, and thereater with 10 mg per day for a similar time period. In 10 episodic cases the attacks stopped completely. In the chronic cases no beneficial effect of testosterone was found. Whether and to what extent spontaneous recovery interfered with the result is an open question in a study like this.

Antiandrogenic drugs: cyproterone acetate

Due to the male preponderance of cluster headache, Sicuteri (1988) tried a synthetic steroid with antiandrogenic properties in 40 cluster headache patients. This treatment with only a few exceptions gave rise to a slight to marked improvement which was particularly apparent in patients resistant to lithium.

DRUG TREATMENT: GENERAL CONSIDERATIONS

Drug treatment of both the chronic and the episodic forms of cluster headache has been upgraded appreciably during the last few decades, mainly due to the increased number of available active drugs. However, the situation is still far from ideal. For an acute attack of the episodic type, oxygen and ergotamine afford major benefit to the patient. However, even when a positive response is obtained, with this approach the patient must suffer part, or even the major part of an attack, and in a number of patients this treatment has little or no effect. In addition, even in those patients whom this treatment usually helps, occasional attacks are not alleviated. If the attack frequency during a bout is high, prophylaxis with ergotamine, lithium, methysergide, prednisone, or pizotifen is preferred; the latter drug is probably only beneficial in relatively weak attacks. Calcium antagonists may also be of considerable benefit. During relatively short-lasting bouts, there do not seem to be any great health risks attached to the prophylactic use of methysergide, prednisone, lithium or ergotamine treatment.

In individual difficult-to-treat patients a thorough trial of the various treatment modilities should be made. Furthermore, a combination therapy, with two or even three drugs, may also be an avenue worth pursuing. An example of such a combination therapy is the treatment of breakthrough attacks with ergotamine or oxygen, when the patient is on continuous prednisone medication. The toxicity of such treatment combinations must be carefully worked out, e.g. with combinations like methysergide and ergotamine.

At present, lithium seems to be emerging as the solitary drug of choice, even in the episodic form of cluster headache. Lithium is probably one of the least noxious of the major drugs suitable for the relatively short-lasting bouts. With prednisone treatment, courses of 3–4 weeks duration are usually used. Prednisone should preferably be used during the period at the top of curve. The long-term effects of lithium will have to be looked into more closely. The tachyphylactic aspects of the various drug therapy strategies have not been worked out for cluster headache.

Kudrow (1980) gives priorities to various therapeutic regimes based on age groups and partly also on the frequency of attacks. It may be difficult to adhere strictly to such rules because the attack frequency during a single bout may be steadily changing. To base the therapeutic approach on the frequency of attacks may, at least in a number of cases, lead to some confusion.

One other future line of approach may be worthwhile pursuing. It is an interesting development that in recent years anti-inflammatory agents have gained popularity for use in both migraine, episodic cluster headache, and chronic paroxysmal hemicrania. This may point to a similarity between these headaches, as far as pathogenesis is concerned (Sjaastad, 1985b; Sjaastad and Bjerve, 1986). Prednisone is a major drug in cluster headache, whereas indomethacin does not help the ordinary cluster headache patient appreciably; in chronic paroxysmal hemicrania the utility of these drugs seems largely to be the other way around. The special effect of indomethacin was only discovered after a thorough search among anti-inflammatory agents.

We have also *partly* studied the effect of such agents in cluster headache, i.e. indomethacin (13 cases), butazolidine (five cases), and ketoprofen (19.583 Rhone Poulenc) (four cases), without any notable positive findings (Sjaastad and Dale, 1974). Admittedly, the number of cases studied was rather small. It is also a question of trying out *more* drugs. Further therapeutic trials should be carried out with such drugs. A last reservation about the results obtained with non-steroidal anti-inflammatory drugs (NSAIDs) in migraine is that the dosage may have been (far?) too low. Be that as it may, the selection process has, so far, given rise to a far better pharmacological, therapeutic agent for chronic paroxysmal hemicrania than for migraine or cluster headache. A thorough search should, therefore, be made among the NSAIDs for better therapeutic alternatives for the two other headache types (Sjaastad, 1985b). Only minor differences in the molecular structure and pharmacological effects of a drug may give rise to great differences in response. A new view on the dosage question may be necessary for many of the synthetic anti-inflammatory agents. The importance of dosage in this context is illustrated by the recent development of another antiphlogistic drug, naproxen. This drug was originally tried in migraine by our group (Lindegaard *et al.*, 1980). The dosage used was that recommended in those days, i.e. 500 mg day^{-1}. The results were only marginal as far as the migraine prophylactic effect was concerned. Later, the optimal dosage of naproxen was felt to be higher. With this new dosage (i.e. 1100 mg day^{-1}), Welch (1986) and Ziegler and Ellis (1985) both found promising results in migraine prophylaxis. Similarly, the optimal dosage of ibuprofen has also been increased considerably in recent years.

SURGICAL TREATMENT

Episodic cluster headache is, in principle, a medical disorder. In general, therefore, surgery should not be used for episodic cluster headache. Exceptions may be those patients that, as far as the temporal pattern is concerned, approach the chronic form and those patients that have exceptionally frequent, long-lasting and/or severe attacks which are entirely unresponsive or only respond to a small extent to medical therapy. For more details on surgical approaches, see Chronic Cluster Headache.

VARIOUS TESTS AND EXAMINATIONS CARRIED OUT IN CLUSTER HEADACHE.

In studies of cluster headache it may be important whether spontaneous or provoked attacks are studied, whether and when any drugs have been given and whether the study, if carried out during the bout, stems from the early or late phase of the bout.

HISTAMINE METABOLISM

Histamine cephalalgia was originally considered to be a vascular disorder, and Horton thought that histamine (one of the early known vasoactive substances) might be a pathogenic agent in this disorder. A natural approach to cluster headache pathogenesis would, therefore, be the study of a possible implication of histamine by biochemical methods. Horton (personal communication) assayed some blood samples from cluster headache patients for histamine. It was, however, not until many years after the discovery of cluster headache, i.e. the early 1960s, that the role of histamine could be extensively studied with modern techniques (Beall and Van Arsdel, 1960; Sjaastad and Sjaastad, 1964). Not all parameters of histamine metabolism could be readily studied at the time, but some catabolic products could. Thus, free, unconverted histamine and its catabolic product, conjugated histamine (which is partly or entirely identical with N-acetylhistamine) (Tabor and Mosettig, 1949; Urbach, 1949) could be quantified. The following metabolites could also be measured: 1.4 methylhistamine and 1.4 and 1.5 methylimidazoleacetic acid (Tham, 1965; Granerus and Magnusson, 1965; Granerus, 1968). The catabolic pattern (see Figures 4.10 and 4.11) could be studied after oral or parenteral administration of radioactive histamine by means of the isotope dilution technique of Schayer (Schayer and Cooper, 1956) as well as by two-dimensional paper chromatography combined with autoradiography.

The *total turnover of histamine* in the body is probably best studied by assessing histamine and its catabolites in the urine. Since only 1–5% of endogenous histamine is excreted unconverted in the urine (Schayer and Cooper, 1956; Kobayashi and Freeman, 1961), a total picture of histamine catabolism cannot be obtained by studying this parameter only; it would be a prerequisite to know the catabolic pattern of histamine in each condition and disorder to be studied. Even a small change in catabolic pattern and in the total inactivation of histamine could theoretically result in considerable changes in the urinary excretion of the free fraction. Urinary 1.4 methylimidazoleacetic acid (1.4MeImAA) is probably the best solitary indicator of the total turnover of histamine in the body. The immediate, momentary status of histamine in the body could be assessed by estimating the unconverted histamine fraction in whole blood, but preferably it should be measured in the plasma because the whole-blood histamine level mostly reflects the basophilic blood cell content of histamine.

Urinary excretion of histamine and metabolites

The urinary excretion of histamine itself in cluster headache was first studied by our group (Sjaastad and Sjaastad, 1964, 1970, 1977b). As far as urinary free histamine (=histamine) excretion in cluster headache is concerned, two methods have routinely been used, i.e. Duñer and Pernow's (1956, 1958) method and Wetterquist and White's (1970) method. Wetterquist and White's

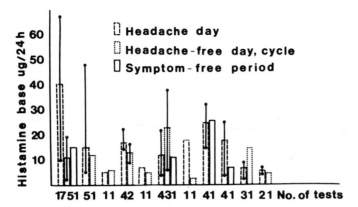

Figure 2.12 Episodic cluster headache: urinary excretion of histamine on days with paroxysms, days without headache during cycle and symptom-free days between two bouts (cycles) in 11 patients. Vertical bars represent the individual range of excretion. (From Sjaastad and Sjaastad (1977b). Courtesy of the *Journal of Neurology*.)

(1970) method uses Dowex-50 for the adsorption of histamine instead of Amberlite IRC-50, which is used in Duner and Pernow's method. The final assay with both methods is a biological one. Some modifications were introduced to secure isotonic or close to isotonic eluates (Sjaastad, 1967). The specificity of biological methods for histamine estimation is a crucial question (see e.g. Lindell and Westling, 1966; Sjaastad, 1975a).

Twenty-two patients (18 males and 4 females) were studied. Two types of controls were used: the patients partly served as their own controls, the attack status being compared with that of the free interval. The histamine excretion in cluster headache patients was also compared to that in an adult control material; the unweighted control urinary excretion of histamine base was 12.6 ± 6.3 (mean ± SD) and 2–31 (range) μg per 24 h (Sjaastad, 1966a). The corresponding values for conjugated histamine were 30.0 ± 23.6 and 1–99 μg per 24 h. It should be emphasized that no correction has been made for the loss during recovery (the mean recoveries for histamine and N-acetylhistamine were 72% and 74%, respectively).

The values for free histamine in cluster headache were: 20.5 ± 20.1 and 10.3 ± 6.4 μg base per 24 h during attack and the free interval, respectively ($p < 0.05$) (Sjaastad and Sjaastad, 1977b). In 11 patients, the urinary excretion of histamine could be estimated in various phases of the headache (Figure 2.12). A comparison of three entirely different methods has also been carried out to ensure that the histamine-like activity in urine measured by the two ion-exchange methods really corresponds to histamine (Døhlen *et al.*, 1973). The methods compared were the so-called specific isotopic method (Snyder *et al.*, 1966), a specially developed (Døhlen *et al.*, 1973) bi-dimensional paper-chromatography method with isotope marking combined with autoradiography (see also Figure 4.12), and Duner and Pernow's (1956, 1958) ion-exchange method. A certain difference between the three methods was found as far as

Table 2.21   Migraine: mean 24 h urinary excretion of free histamine
(unweighted values)[a]

	Histamine excretion	No. of examinations	No. with increased excretion
Attacks	15.4	31	5
Free intervals	23.9	24	7

[a]Control levels: 12.6 ± 0.9 µg of histamine base (range 2–31 µg) per 24 h. From
Sjaastad and Sjaastad (1977b). Courtesy of the *Journal of Neurology*.

the *levels* of histamine were concerned, but the *ratio* between the results
obtained with the various methods was rather stable.

The mean urinary excretion of histamine in migraine was found to be well
within control limits (Table 2.21). The mean excretion was even *lower* during
attacks than during attack-free periods. Still, in some cases increased excretion
was observed, both during and outside attacks.

The underlying mechanism for the observed rise in mean urinary histamine
during attacks of cluster headache may be increased formation, liberation, or
altered catabolism. Patients with cluster headache were shown to be capable of
conjugating histamine both during and outside attacks. The excretion of
conjugated histamine was, moreover, invariably within normal limits and was
found to be of the same order of magnitude whether the excretion of free
histamine was increased or not (the average increase of free histamine in the
'increased' histamine vs. the 'normal' group was 3.3-fold). Thus, the conjugated histamine/free histamine ratio proved to be much lower in the group
with 'increased' than in the group with 'normal' histamine excretion (Table
2.22). If the gastrointestinal lumen were the source of the extra histamine, the
increment in conjugated histamine output would have been far out of proportion to that of histamine, thus rendering a markedly increased conjugated/
free histamine ratio. If histamine is administered into the intestinal tract of
man, or formed within it, histamine is readily conjugated intraluminally or,
possibly, also upon absorption. This results in a conjugated/free histamine ratio
of >17 (up to more than 200) (Sjaastad, 1966b; Døhlen *et al.*, 1973). In the
'increased' histamine excretion group, the conjugated/free histamine ratio was
of the same order of magnitude, i.e. less than 1.0 (Table 2.22), as when
histamine formation takes place in the tissues, following oral or parenteral
L-histidine administration.

In other words these observations clearly infer the origin of the excess
urinary histamine which is occasionally found in cluster headache: it does not
stem from the lumen of the gastrointestinal tract. It is not known whether
histamine originating within the *wall* of the gastrointestinal tract of man results
in increased conjugated histamine excretion. Thus the possibility that the extra
histamine on days with increased excretion stems from the gastric mucosa

Table 2.22 Episodic cluster headache: inter-relationship of free and conjugated histamine excretion[a]

	Total material				Increased free histamine excretion				Normal free histamine excretion			
	No. of examinations/patients	Free histamine	Conjugated histamine	Ratio of conjugated/free histamine	No. of examinations/patients	Free histamine	Conjugated histamine	Ratio of conjugated/free histamine	No. of examinations/patients	Free histamine	Conjugated histamine	Ratio of conjugated/free histamine
Weighted values	18	35.2	41.7	1.18	8	55.8	46.5	0.83	10	16.7	38.0	2.28
Unweighted values	8	40.8	42.9	1.05	5	56.4	45.8	0.81	3	14.7	38.0	2.59

Control limits

Free histamine
  Weighted values 2–31; mean 14.0 μg per 24 h
  Unweighted values 2–31; mean 12.6 μg per 24 h
Conjugated histamine
  Weighted values 1–130; mean 28.0 μg per 24 h
  Unweighted values 1–99; mean 30.0 μg per 24 h
Mean unweighted *control* conjugated/free histamine ratio 2.38

[a] From Sjaastad and Sjaastad (1977b). Courtesy of the *Journal of Neurology*.
[b] From Sjaastad (1966a). All values in μg per 24 h.

Table 2.23 Episodic cluster headache: histaminuria secondary to intravenous L-histidine loading (7.5 g)[a]

	Mean (and range) (μg base per h)		
	Pre-test	0–4 h	4–8 h
Cluster headache	0.6 (0.1–1.3)	3.3 (1.8–6.7)	1.4 (0.6–2.6)
Controls	0.5 (0.3–0.7)	6.8 (3.7–9.8)	0.7 (0.5–0.8)

[a]Data from Sjaastad and Sjaastad (1977b). Courtesy of the *Journal of Neurology*.

cannot be *definitely excluded*—although this is highly unlikely because of the high metabolic activity of the liver. Furthermore, histamine formation as a consequence of oral and parenteral L-histidine administration are of the same level of magnitude (Sjaastad, 1966c; Døhlen *et al.*, 1973). These observations strongly indicate that extragastrointestinal tissues are of importance in this type of histamine formation. The question of *where* the extra histamine during an attack stems from is of particular interest because of the alleged liability to ulcer formation in cluster headache patients.

The urinary excretion of the main metabolite, 1.4 methylimidazoleacetic acid (1.4MeImAA), was estimated on attack days ($n = 3$) (partly the selected days for study of attacks coincided with days of increased free histamine excretion, i.e. 38 and 54 μg per 24 h, respectively). The 1.4MeImAA excretion was entirely within control limits, i.e. mean 5.6 mg per 24 h, range 7.0–3.1 mg per 24 h versus controls: mean 3.2 mg per 24 h, range 8.0–1.3 mg per 24 h. Granerus (1968) found a slightly more limited excretion range of 1.4MeImAA in controls, i.e. 2.5–5.9 mg per 24 h (mean 3.7), on a 'mixed' diet. It is remarkable that the one patient who showed the highest 1.4MeImAA excretion had a low normal excretion of histamine, i.e. 11 μg per 24 h. Conversely, a clearly increased urinary histamine excretion was combined with the lowest 1.4MeImAA excretion. The 1.5MeImAA variety was not found in the patients' urine samples. Thus, even these limited data indicate that there is no invariably increased urinary excretion of 1.4 and 1.5MeImAA during the cycle of cluster headache.

The possibility remained that the histamine metabolic abnormality might be centred on the attacks, and that an increased excretion of histamine during the few hours of abnormality might be swamped in 24 h samples. This was looked into by collecting urine in four portions per 24 h in eight patients during attack days and during attack-free days (0–4, 4–8, 8–12, and 12–24 h portions). There did not seem to be any consistent tendency for increments in urinary histamine excretion in connection with attacks (Sjaastad and Sjaastad, 1977b).

The *formation* of histamine has also been assessed during attacks of cluster headache (Sjaastad and Sjaastad, 1977b). After L-histidine administration, there was no increase in urinary histamine in excess of that observed in controls (Table 2.23). This investigation did thus not render any evidence for an increased histamine formation under such circumstances. Histamine *liberation* could not be clinically measured in a satisfactory way at the time of these studies; no attempt was, therefore, made to assess histamine liberation.

Since urinary excretion of histamine is only occasionally increased during attacks, and since the elevation is so moderate, our findings indicate that the urinary excretion of histamine is more likely to be a consequence of than the cause of an attack of cluster headache. In keeping with this assumption, the urinary excretion of the main metabolite, MeImAA, was within the control range. Thus on the basis of these investigations there is little evidence for a fundamental, causal role of histamine in cluster headache pathogenesis.

Catabolism of 'extrinsic' histamine

Some of the metabolites (see Figure 4.10), e.g. imidazole acetic acid (ImAA), could not be assessed with the previously mentioned methods. In order to obtain a still more complete picture of histamine metabolism in cluster headache and a more firm basis for assessing whether catabolic changes could be responsible for the histaminuria in cluster headache, isotope studies were conducted. The catabolic pattern was studied after subcutaneous as well as oral [^{14}C] histamine administration during attacks and compared to the findings in control individuals (see also Chronic Paroxysmal Hemicrania). The following two methods were used to identify the urinary metabolites (Sjaastad and Sjaastad, 1974, 1977a):

Autoradiography: urine specimens (100–400 μl) were spotted on each of 3–4 bi-dimensional paper chromatograms. On some chromatograms, internal standards, i.e. histamine diphosphate, N-acetylhistamine, 1.4 methylimidazoleacetic acid (1.4MeImAA), 1.4 methylhistamine, and imidazoleacetic acid (ImAA) were also spotted for the identification of the radioactive histamine and its metabolites. Reference ImAA-riboside (ImAA-R) (see Figure 4.12) was not available. However, by doing chromatography prior to and after the splitting of the bondage of ImAA-R, the ImAA-riboside could easily be located. Three different developing systems were used for the descending chromatography. Kodak X-ray films were exposed to the chromatograms for 6–8 weeks. For identification of the metabolites, the chromatograms with the reference substances were stained with either ninhydrin or iodine in ethanol (1% w/v). Sections of the chromatograms, corresponding to the shadows on the X-ray films, were cut out on the unstained chromatograms. The sections cut out were either mounted on counting plates and counted in a Beckman flow-counter (Low-beta II) with a background activity of 4–6 cpm and a counting efficiency of about 37%, or put into counting vials with Instagel after which the radioactivity was counted (Packard Tri-Carb spectrometer). In this way, histamine itself and the three main metabolites (i.e. MeImAA, ImAA and ImAA-riboside) and methylhistamine as well as minor fractions such as N-acetylhistamine could be identified (Sjaastad and Sjaastad, 1974, 1977b).

Schayer's isotope dilution technique for [^{14}C]histamine and its metabolites: outlines of this method have been published (Schayer and Cooper, 1956; Nilsson *et al.*, 1959; Eliassen, 1969; Sjaastad and Sjaastad, 1974). The main features of the technique are as follows: to set amounts of urine containing the radioactive metabolites, carrier non-isotopic histamine, 1.4MeImAA, ImAA, or N-acetylhistamine was added, after which the respective substance was extracted. It was then treated with activated charcoal and crystallized as the pipsyl or picrate derivative. Each sample was redissolved, retreated with activated charcoal, and recrystallized until constant radioactivity was obtained. This was taken to indicate that satisfactory purification of the substance had been obtained. After each crystallization, the crystals were placed on plates of 2.5 cm diameter and counted using the Beckman flowcounter, at infinite thickness. The conversion factor between histamine counted at zero thickness and histamine picrate (counted at 'infinite' thickness) was 35.2; the corresponding figure for pipsyl histamine was 36.1 (mean values).

Total ImAA was determined, the riboside being converted to the free acid by acid hydrolysis (170° for 5 h in sealed tubes). Care was taken that sufficient acid was added to keep the final pH below 1.5 during this procedure; this secures a *complete* conversion of the ImAA-R (Eliassen, 1969). Conjugated histamine was determined as the increment in [^{14}C]histamine after acid hydrolysis. 1.4Methylhistamine was not available to use as carrier in this study. It was, therefore, only measured by paper chromatography (see previously). The histamine/methylhistamine complex may be determined by autoradiography, and histamine may be estimated by means of the Schayer technique. The methylhistamine fraction *per se* may then be estimated roughly by comparing the results of these two techniques. In addition, the total radioactivity excreted in the urine and faeces was determined in successive portions. The exhaled CO_2 radioactivity was also estimated by using a technique based on fractional exhalation sampling (Sjaastad and Sjaastad, 1974).

The total catabolic pattern was studied in three patients with the cluster headache syndrome in the drug-free state, after oral or subcutaneous application of radioactive histamine (total number of tests = 5). The catabolic pattern was similar in reference individuals and in cluster headache patients during attack periods, both with regard to the total urinary radioactivity excretion, the CO_2 exhalation, the faecal excretion (Tables 2.24 to 2.26), as well as with regard to the excretion pattern of urinary [^{14}C] histamine and its metabolites (Tables 2.27 and 2.28) (Sjaastad and Sjaastad, 1977a). In one patient with chronic paroxysmal hemicrania, a striking abnormality of ImAA-riboside excretion was seen (Table 2.28) (see Chronic Paroxysmal Hemicrania).

Beall and Van Arsdel (1960) also studied the catabolic pattern of intravenously administered [^{14}C]histamine in three patients with cluster headache and found no deviation from normal. The chromatographic system used by Beall and Van Arsdel does not separate the two main histamine catabolites in man, i.e. ImAA and 1.4MeImAA (Kobayashi and Freeman, 1961). Beall and

Table 2.24 Cluster headache syndrome: excretion of urinary radioactivity as a function of time after oral [^{14}C] histamine loading (per cent of dosage administered)[a]

Test No.	Time after loading (h)				Later excretion	Total excretion
	0–6	6–24	24–48	48–72		
1[b]	40	23	11	—	—	74
2	48	31	3	0.4	0.2	83
3	50	20	2	0.5	0.1	73
4	17	14	4	—	—	35
5	56	28	3	0.6	—	88
Healthy controls[c]	33–44	27–33	3–5	0.3–0.5	0.2–0.5	68–80

[a]From Sjaastad and Sjaastad (1977a). Courtesy of the *Journal of Neurology*.
[b]Patient with chronic paroxysmal hemicrania, symptom-free 5 days after discontinuation of indomethacin.
[c]From Sjaastad and Sjaastad (1974).

Table 2.25 Cluster headache syndrome: total excretion of radioactivity as a percentage of given oral [^{14}C]histamine[a]

Test no.	[^{14}C]Histamine excretion (%)			
	Urine	Faeces	CO_2	Total
1[b]	74	1	22	97
2	83	2	32	117
3	73	11	1	85
4	35	37	15	87
5	88	24	—	—
Healthy controls[c]	68–80	13–19	2–18	91–109

[a]From Sjaastad and Sjaastad (1977a). Courtesy of the *Journal of Neurology*.
[b]Patient with chronic paroxysmal hemicrania, symptom-free for 5 days after discontinuation of indomethacin. Tests carried out on days with paroxysms, except for test No. 1.
[c]From Sjaastad and Sjaastad (1974).

Table 2.26 Episodic cluster headache: total excretion of radioactivity after oral [^{14}C]histamine loading[a]

	Mean [^{14}C]histamine excretion (%)			
	Urine	Faeces	CO_2	Total
Cluster headache[a] ($n = 3$)	72	13	18	103
Controls[b] ($n = 5$)	74	16	9	99

[a]Data from Sjaastad and Sjaastad (1977a). Courtesy of the *Journal of Neurology*.
[b]Data from Sjaastad and Sjaastad (1974).

Table 2.27 Cluster headache syndrome: relative urinary excretion of [14C]histamine metabolites ([14C]histamine given orally) as a percentage of the sum of the three major metabolites[a]

Test no.	Time after loading (h)								
	0–6			6–24			0–24		
	ImAA-R	ImAA	MeImAA	ImAA-R	ImAA	MeImAA	ImAA-R	ImAA	MeImAA
1[b]	27	12	61	50	5	45	34	10	56
2	38	9	53	56	4	40	43	8	49
Healthy controls[c]	34–50	6–13	41–57	55–75	3–7	23–42	43–60	4–11	34–48

[a]Measured by autoradiography. Data from Sjaastad and Sjaastad (1977a). Courtesy of the *Journal of Neurology*.
[b]Test No. 1 was carried out during a symptom-free period, 5 days after discontinuation of indomethacin. Patient with chronic paroxysmal hemicrania.
[c]From Sjaastad and Sjaastad (1974).

Table 2.28 Episodic cluster headache and chronic paroxysmal hemicrania: fate of subcutaneously administered [^{14}C]histamine determined using the autoradiography and isotope dilution technique (percentages of the sum of the three actual metabolites)[a]

Test No.[b]	0–6				6–24				0–24			
	ImAA-R	ImAA	Sum ImAA-R/ImAA	MeImAA	ImAA-R	ImAA	Sum ImAA-R/ImAA	MeImAA	ImAA-R	ImAA	Sum ImAA-R/ImAA	MeImAA
1	27	14	41	59	48	7	55	45	33	12	45	55
2	28	10	38	62	–	–	–	–	–	–	–	–
3	21	29	50	50	–	–	–	–	–	–	–	–
4	2	54[c]	56	44	11	30	41	59[d]	6	47	53	47

Time after loading (h)

[a]Data from Sjaastad and Sjaastad (1977a). Courtesy of the *Journal of Neurology*.
[b](1) Patient with ordinary cluster headache and (2) patient with chronic paroxysmal hemicrania, both having attacks. (3 and 4) Tests were carried out on the other patient with chronic paroxysmal hemicrania; (3) test done 12 days after discontinuing indomethacin treatment when the attack pattern was just starting, but with only very moderate pain; (4) test was done on a day of heavy paroxysms.
[c]Calculated: Total ImAA − ImAA-R = ImAA.
[d]Determined by means of the isotope dilution technique.

Van Arsdel's observations do thus not allow any definite conclusions to be drawn with regard to the relative importance of the two main metabolites or, in other words, of the catabolic pattern of histamine in cluster headache. They also studied the elimination of total radioactivity via the urine after intravenous administration of labelled histamine and found, as we did later, no deviation from normal. It was, however, not specifically mentioned whether these studies were conducted during a bout (cycle) or between two bouts.

In conclusion, there is evidence for increased urinary histamine excretion in some patients having cluster headache. This histamine in all probability stems from the tissues and not from the gastrointestinal lumen, and probably not from the gastrointestinal wall. The increased excretion hardly has any causal relationship with the headache. The excess urinary histamine is most probably secondary to the disease process (and/or possibly to the 'stress' accompanying the attack).

Histamine and serotonin in blood

At a later stage, *whole* blood histamine levels and what they termed 'plasma' serotonin levels were measured by Anthony and Lance (1971a,b) during 13 attacks in 20 cluster headache patients. In a proportion of their cases, precipitated attacks were studied. They used Shore *et al.*'s (1959) fluorometric method for histamine estimations and Crawford and Rudd's (1962) fluorometric method for serotonin estimations. The mean whole blood histamine levels were 0.045, 0.053 and 0.049 μg ml^{-1} (histamine base values (?)) before, during and after the headache attack, respectively. The corresponding values for 'plasma' serotonin were: 0.48, 0.57 and 0.59 μg per 10^9 platelets, respectively. Whereas the statistical analyses (non-parametric tests) for histamine showed a significant increase during attacks, the one for serotonin did not reach significance ($p = 20$–30%). This apparently was so in spite of the fact that the mean increment (from 'before' to 'during') was of approximately the same order of magnitude, i.e. approximately 18% for both histamine and serotonin. The trend for both variables was the same. No such increase in whole blood histamine was found in migraine (Lance, 1982). Conversely, there was a clear change as far as the platelet-rich 'plasma' serotonin level during migraine attacks was concerned.

Anthony and Lance felt that their findings gave credence to Horton's hypothesis that attacks of cluster headache are due to a 'release' of histamine. They maintained that the fact that pizotifen (a serotonin (and histamine) antagonist) prevents nitroglycerin from provoking cluster headache attacks (Ekbom, 1969) strengthens this view. The mean histamine level in cluster headache patients during attacks (i.e. 0.053 μg ml^{-1}) was in fact lower than the levels observed in some control individuals (i.e. range 0.048–0.075 μg ml^{-1}). As far as I am concerned, this strongly indicates that the histamine in the whole blood *as such* does not play a causal role in the pathogenesis of this headache (see also On the Significance of Blood Histamine Levels).

On the significance of blood histamine levels

Histaminology is a whole, separate world in science. Admittedly, it is next to impossible for the ordinary clinical investigators working in the headache field to appreciate the intricacies of histamine research and the signficance and impact of various findings. Anthony and Lance's (1971a,b) own interpretation of their blood histamine findings was somewhat more optimistic than our interpretation of our own findings. The former optimistic attitude seems to have stirred the minds of many clinicians in this field. Much over-simplified reasoning has followed in the wake of the histamine investigations. Such a development may hamper rather than promote progress. I have attempted to clarify the enormous methodological difficulties and some of the fallacies of interpretation, particularly with regard to the headache field, and the reader is referred to this review for details (Sjaastad, 1975a).

It is well established that patients with chronic myelogenous leukemia have enormously high blood histamine levels, ranging up to 27 μg ml^{-1} (i.e. $\geq$500 times higher than the levels observed by Lance and Anthony's study (1971a,b)). In other words, the histamine quantities circulating in the blood in these patients correspond to many times the lethal dose of histamine in man. Nevertheless, such patients do not have symptoms that can be clearly ascribed to toxic effects of histamine. Thus, an increment in *whole blood histamine* during cluster headache attacks does not allow any conclusion as to a relationship between this finding and the clinical symptoms of cluster headache. Whole blood histamine mainly reflects the number of circulating basophilic leucocytes (Lindell and Westling, 1966).

What really matters as far as blood histamine and symptom production is concerned is probably the level of *plasma histamine*, which is most likely the biologically active form of histamine, the cell bound form being inactive. The study of plasma levels of histamine in cluster headache patients between and during attacks should thus provide important information. The determination of plasma histamine levels is, however, a most intricate task, the plasma levels of histamine being seemingly infinitesimal. The problem is, however, not so much that such small quantities cannot be measured, but that disintegration of histamine containing blood corpuscles may take place during the *in vitro* preparation of the blood aliquot; in this way it is next to impossible to judge whether or not an increase in plasma histamine really is present *in vivo*. It should be mentioned that an attempt at measuring plasma histamine in migraine has been made (Heatley *et al.*, 1982).

The clinical studies done with histamine H$_1$ and H$_2$ receptor blocking agents (Russell, 1978) to some extent substantiate our findings (or, to put it more exactly, our interpretation of them) that no clear-cut abnormalities of histamine metabolism are present in cluster headache. As stated elsewhere, however, these findings do not *rule out* an involvement of histamine in cluster headache pathogenesis. As we postulated in 1975 (see Figure 2.13), it is most likely that

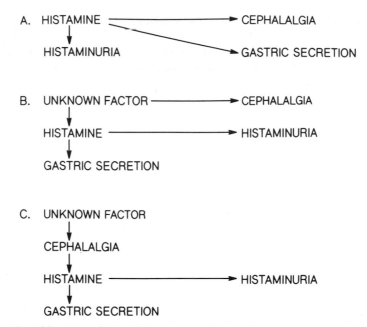

Figure 2.13 Possible interrelationship between histamine turnover, headache and gastric secretion in cluster headache. Possibility A: histamine is the causative agent for headache and gastric secretion. Possibility B: increased histamine turnover as a phenomenon independent of the headache. Possibility C: increased histamine turnover as a secondary phenomenon.

the minor histamine abnormalities observed during attacks of cluster headache are either associated with or are secondary phenomena in the disease process (possibilities B and C in Figure 2.13).

The interrelationship of histamine, the headache and the gastric acidity is another controversial matter. Various theoretical models can be conjectured (Figure 2.13). It should also be emphasized in this context (see also Gastroduodenal Ulcer and Gastric Ulcer) that it does not seem to have been proven that increased gastric acidity is an invariable accompaniment of cluster headache. However, increased gastric acid production has been demonstrated in some cases, even in connection with solitary attacks (Alford and Whitehouse, 1945; Graham *et al.*, 1970). The model which I favour is possibility C (see Figure 2.13) (provided that gastric secretion really *is* a feature of the cluster headache attack).

An *in vitro* study of the possible histamine involvement in cluster headache was carried out by Hardebo *et al.* (1980). There seemed to be no major difference between controls ($n = 5$) and episodic cluster headache patients ($n = 6$) in the ability of the superficial temporal artery to dilate in response to histamine exposure. On the other hand, vessels from chronic cluster headache patients seemed to react more strongly than those from controls. The responses to a number of vasoactive agents, such as noradrenaline, serotonin, acetylcholine,

VIP (vasoactive intestinal polypeptide) and prostaglandin $F_2\gamma$ also were of the same magnitude in headache patients and controls. If there is a histamine mediated dilatation of the temporal artery on the symptomatic side during attack, this would seem to be due to increased quantities of histamine rather than to a super-sensitivity reaction.

MAST CELLS IN THE SKIN

The main source of histamine in the human body is the mast cells and these have been the aim of various studies on cluster headache. Appenzeller *et al.* (1978, 1981a) detected an increased number of mast cells in the skin in the painful temporal area in cluster headache patients. Seemingly, more degranulating mast cells were observed in patients ($n = 6$) than in controls ($n = 3$). These findings were made in the cluster period as well as in the quiescent phase, and the findings did not predominate on the symptomatic side. The mast cells were detected perivascularly, in close proximity to cutaneous nerves in the patients, but only perivascularly (and not in the vicinity of nerves) in the controls (Appenzeller *et al.*, 1981). Because of this close proximity, Appenzeller *et al.* wondered whether antidromic impulses in sensory axons might cause a release reaction, mediators being liberated from an increased number of mast cells. They hypothesized that the unilaterality of the pain might be caused by periodic, unilateral axonal reflexes.

The Lodz group has also been involved in such studies (Prusinski and Liberski, 1979; Liberski, 1980; Liberski and Prusinksi, 1982; Liberski and Mirecka, 1984). They found a clearly increased number of mast cells in the skin biopsies from the painful area (30 ± 11.4) when compared to controls (9 ± 5.7; $p < 0.05$) (Prusinski and Liberski, 1979). Later (Liberski and Prusinski, 1982), their material was extended to 23 patients. The difference found between skin samples from control individuals ($n = 6$) and from the painful side in cluster headache patients was as in the previous series. However, the mean number of mast cells on the symptomatic and non-symptomatic sides was of the same order of magnitude, i.e. 35 and 31, respectively. In Liberski and Mirecka's (1984) study, biopsies from cluster headache patients in the drug-free state ($n = 13$) were obtained a few hours after attack and were compared with biopsies obtained from patients with diagnoses other than headache ($n = 10$). An electron-microscopic pattern of 'piece-meal' degranulation or dissolution was found, with perigranular membrane fusion and localized, reduced granule electron density. This dissolution pattern was not observed in the controls.

Dimitriadou *et al.* (1989) removed the temporal artery (on the symptomatic side?) in 20 cluster headache patients (four with the episodic form, all in the bout), and compared the findings with those in eight controls. The adventitia of the artery frequently contained mast cells localized in the vicinity of the autonomic nerve fibres. Whereas the mast cells from controls contained a great number of granules evenly distributed in the cytoplasma, the mast cells from cluster headache patients showed degranulation in 17 of 20 cases.

Cuypers *et al.* (1980), however, who partly studied patients 2–4 days after attack, did not find such changes. This time delay can hardly explain the discrepancy between the results of the latter group and those of the former groups, since Appenzeller also studied cases in the quiescent phase.

Another study may also have a bearing on the mast cell investigations. Nasal smears were prepared from 10 cluster headache patients during spontaneously occurring headache attacks and during the pain-free period. Ten suitable controls were also studied. The smears were stained with Giemsa and hematoxylineosin. There were no appreciable differences between patients and controls either in the 'total number of cells' or in the relative number of basophils. This study thus does not provide any evidence that chemotactic factors influence the basophils in the nasal mucosa during the attack. The concentration of histamine storing cells in these areas *may* thus only concern the mastocytes (Selmaj and Pruszcynski, 1984).

The mast cell studies are interesting, but it is uncertain what inferences can be drawn from them. The total turnover of histamine in some cluster headache patients may be increased (Sjaastad and Sjaastad, 1977b). The possibility exists that there is a causal relationship between the above-mentioned findings and the increased histamine turnover. However, the mast cell study findings do not prove that the histamine changes are primary; they may well be secondary. In addition, there *may* even be simple explanations for these findings, such as e.g. rubbing of the skin during attacks.

HISTOLOGICAL EXAMINATION OF THE SUPERFICIAL TEMPORAL ARTERY

Temporal artery biopsies were taken from the affected side in 15 patients with cluster headache (eight with the chronic form and seven with the episodic form; all except one were taken within a bout) and in five controls (Krabbe and Rank, 1985). The biopsies were investigated with light and electron microscopy, and the diagnostic work was carried out blindly. Most of the specimens from both patients and controls showed adventitial and intimal fibrosis. There were no signs of inflammation or of atheroma formation. The vasa vasorum appeared in equal numbers in the three groups. Mast cells appeared in normal quantities and appeared to be of normal shape. Electron microscopy did not reveal any further information. The not infrequent involvement of the temporal artery during attacks of cluster headache thus does not seem to have left any scars. There is, however, no specific information on whether or not the patients studied clinically had shown any temporal vessel dilatation during attack.

HISTAMINE SKIN TEST

The triple response has been studied by Giacovazzo *et al.* (1985) in cluster headache ($n = 20$), as well as in migraine patients ($n = 20$) and healthy volunteers ($n = 20$). Histamine was deposited in a scratch on the forearm, and three parameters were followed, i.e. latency before erythema development, the diameter of hyperaemia, and the extinction time. It did not seem to matter which forearm was used for the test. The latency time was significantly shorter in cluster headache patients than in controls. The last two parameters mentioned showed significantly increased values in cluster headache patients.

This test has also been used by the Lodz group (Bogucki and Prusinski, 1985). The histamine (200 ng histamine diphosphate) was injected intradermally at the point of maximum pain in the frontotemporal area. In principle, the response to histamine on the headache side and the non-symptomatic sides was compared. No difference was found. The response seems, at least to a certain extent, to depend upon the histamine salt used, histamine itself having a slight local irritant effect. Therefore, further work remains to be done before the value of this test is clear.

KININS

Because of the putative vascular nature of cluster headache, kinins might be of importance in the syndrome. Blood is a predilection site for kinin formation, and kinins play a role in pain generation and exert a marked effect on smooth muscles and the vasculature. In some preliminary studies, we have measured blood kinin parameters (Sjaastad, 1970; Sjaastad, unpublished observations), that is the levels of kinins, kallikrein, total kininogen, and kininase, during the various phases of migraine attack and in cluster headache (multiple tests in six patients). We also determined the urinary excretion of kinins. The interrelationship of these factors is evident from Figure 2.14. The following technique was used for the *blood kinin* level determination: 2 ml of arm-vein blood were withdrawn after minimal stasis and passed through a siliconated canule directly into 10 ml of ice-cooled absolute alcohol. After evaporation, the residue was dissolved and tested on rat uterus. *Kininase* was determined as described by Rugstad (1966). *Kininogen* was determined by means of the trypsin method (Dinitz *et al.*, 1961), as described by Ofstad (1970). The other methods are largely the same as described by Ofstad.

Increased amounts of kinins were found in brachial vein blood (i.e. amounts above the control levels of 4–5 ng ml^{-1}) during some attacks of cluster head-

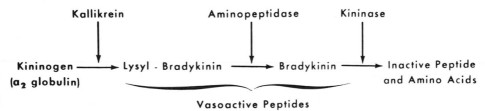

Figure 2.14   Schematic representation of the kininogen–kallikrein–kinin–kininase system. (From Sjaastad (1970). Courtesy of Danmarks apotegerforening.)

ache in five of the six patients studied. A corresponding decrease seemed to occur in total blood kininogen, whereas no definite changes were noted in the other parameters. No definitely pathological findings were made in the urine.

This study was a preliminary one, and it was done with the relatively crude and unrefined methods of the time. Double siliconation of the sampling equipment was done so that glass activation, etc., was hindered. Nevertheless, one crucial issue in this context is whether the kininogen transformation really takes place in the circulating blood or whether it is formed during the sampling procedure. These results should, therefore, be viewed as those of a pilot study. More investigations are clearly needed in this field in order to assess the possible role of kinins in cluster headache. Even if the findings described above were to be verified, the same reasoning as for the significance of the histamine findings would be appropriate.

PROSTAGLANDINS

Prostaglandins are potent vasoactive substances which may possibly be involved in the mechanism of pain, for which reason a study of prostaglandins in cluster headache was carried out (Bennett *et al.*, 1974). In accordance with the hypothesis proposed by Sandler (1972), femoral arterial blood samples were used. Blood was taken from four control subjects and from 13 patients suffering from either migraine or cluster headache during and sometimes several days after an attack. Plasma prostaglandin-like activity was extracted and assayed against PGE_2 on rat fundus preparations.

Blood levels in controls varied from undetectable amounts to 0.28 ng ml^{-1} prostaglandin-like activity, assayed as PGE_2. The average total prostaglandin-like activity in the various groups was as follows: controls, 0.13 ± 0.3; migraine patients during an attack 0.47 ± 0.23; migraine patients outside an attack 0.45 ± 0.21; and cluster headache patients during an attack 0.45 ± 0.21 ng ml^{-1} PGE_2.

Patients with headache tended to have higher levels than healthy controls, but the differences were not significant, largely due to the wide spread of values in the control group. Prostaglandin-like activity varied between different samples taken from the same patient, but the levels did not seem to correlate well with the degree of pain. It is, however, still possible that circulating prostaglandins may contribute to the pain in a variety of ways, for example by interactions with other vaso-neuro-active substances (by altering the sensitivity to other pain-producing stimuli). Such a sensitization could be long-lasting and for this reason blood prostaglandin levels might not correlate with pain at the time of sampling.

This study did not provide any evidence for any special link between cluster headache and prostaglandins. The equal levels of prostaglandins in migraine and cluster headache patients during attacks suggest that the findings are non-specific and are probably secondary to the disease process. These studies were carried out with the crude and inadequate techniques for prostaglandin estimation in use at the time. The results obtained should, therefore, be viewed in this light.

CORTISOL

A chronobiological study of plasma cortisol was carried out by Chazot *et al.* (1984) in 11 cluster headache patients, who were in the cluster cycle, and eight control individuals. There was a tendency to lower amplitude and mesor in the cluster headache patients as a whole, i.e. 4.3 and 6.7 mg per 100 ml, respectively. The corresponding values in the controls being 6.3 and 9.1 mg per 100 ml, respectively. Cortisol acrophase was advanced, particularly in three cases in whom there was also a marked reduction in mesor melatonin. These findings contrast with those of Facchinetti *et al.* (1986), who found higher values (partly significantly so) in cluster headache patients ($n = 9$) than in controls ($n = 7$) (Figure 2.15). These patients were studied during the third and fourth weeks of a bout, and none had received drugs for the week prior to study. Waldenlind (1987) found that the 24 h mean serum cortisol values are generally higher *during* a bout than outside bouts (Figure 2.16). Facchinetti *et al.* (1986) contend that stress associated with experiencing a bout is the mechanism underlying the elevation of cortisol levels. These findings also lend some support to the view that cluster headache is a dyschronic disorder with disruption of chronobiological rhythms.

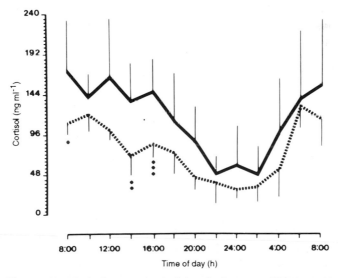

Figure 2.15 Chronogram of plasma cortisol levels (mean ± SD) in episodic cluster headache patients (————) and controls (– – – –). Student's *t*-test: *$p < 0.05$; **$p < 0.02$; ***$p < 0.01$. (From Facchinetti *et al.* (1986). Courtesy of *Cephalalgia*.)

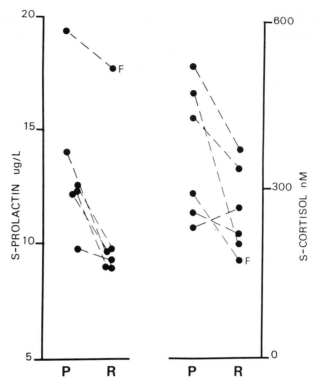

Figure 2.16 A comparison of 24-h mean prolactin and cortisol levels in episodic cluster headache patients (n = 6; one female). Patients did not get any headache attacks during the study even though they were in an active period. P, active period; R, remission; F, female patient. (From Waldenlind (1987). Courtesy of E. Waldenlind.)

Nappi *et al.* (1987) found a parallel phase delay of cortisol and adrenocortico-trophic hormone (ACTH) of approximately 2 h in patients as compared with controls.

The hypothalamopituitary axis seems to function normally in cluster headache, as evidenced by a normal response to the dexamethasone suppression test (Devoize *et al.*, 1986; Frediani *et al.*, 1988). The ACTH response to dexamethasone was also normal (Frediani *et al.*, 1988).

MELATONIN

Melatonin (*N*-acetyl-5-methoxyserotonin) is a good indicator of pineal gland cyclic activity. The plasma level of melatonin exhibits a clear nocturnal climax and, in addition, shows seasonal variations (melatonin secretion is known to peak during the dark season). Melatonin is converted from serotonin by acetylation and methylation. *N*-Acetyltransferase seems to be the enzyme that to a large extent regulates the rhythmical formation of melatonin. This conversion takes place in the pineal gland. However, the regulation of the enzyme activity responsible for the melatonin oscillations is rather compli-cated. This regulation seems to be steered by the suprachiasmatic nucleus, which is innervated by retinohypothalamic fibres. The message from the hypothalamus passes through sympathetic neurons via the superior cervical ganglion to the pineal gland. This system will accordingly be extremely sensitive to the light–dark cycle.

Chazot *et al.* (1984) studied the diurnal variation in the serum concentration of melatonin. They used a radioimmunological method for the assay of melatonin and found relatively low nocturnal plasma levels in the attack-free period of bouts in cluster headache patients, and in one patient the melatonin oscillations were eliminated. The mesor was 34.4 and 17.6 pg ml^{-1} in controls ($n = 8$) and patients ($n = 11$), respectively, whereas the corresponding values for the acrophase were 58.7 and 18.7 pg ml^{-1}. There was a slightly advanced acrophase in the patient group. Lithium may normalize these changes (Chazot *et al.*, 1987). The three patients with the lowest melatonin plasma levels had the largest shift in cortisol acrophase (see Cortisol).

Waldenlind *et al.* (1984a) studied the diurnal variation in the serum concen-tration of melatonin in 24 patients having episodic cluster headache, four patients with chronic cluster headache, and nine healthy individuals. Blood samples were drawn eight times per 24 h (every 2 h during the night). Melatonin concentration in serum was measured by means of the radio-immunoassay technique. Patients only studied during an active period exhibited lower values during the night than those only studied during a remission, but the findings did not differ significantly. However, in eight patients studied both during and between bouts, significantly lower nocturnal melatonin levels were found during than outside the bout. Nocturnal urinary excretion of melatonin was of the same order of magnitude in patients and controls. The studies of the individual patients were carried out within the same season, so that the influence of seasonal variation should have been obviated. These observations indicate that, due to existing interindividual differences, comparative intraindividual studies ought to be carried out in order to obtain meaningful data.

The dysfunction leading to the plasma melatonin changes in cluster head-ache could be anywhere along the axis through which the pineal gland receives its regulating signals or in the gland itself. The dysfunction could even be in the metabolism of melatonin. Due to the retinal connections with the suprachias-matic nucleus, light/dark fluctuations will exert their influence on this struc-ture. Hormones *not* connected with the pineal gland, e.g. cortisol, also show abnormalities. If the cortisol changes in cluster headache are reproducible, there might be a common denominator for the aberrations concerning cortisol and melatonin. The dysfunction could be in the hypothalamus (suprachiasma-tic nucleus or neighbouring structures), because not only melatonin-regulating, but also steroid-regulating rhythms seem to stem from these structures. These findings are clearly of great importance in the understanding of possible 'central' mechanisms in cluster headache.

TESTOSTERONE

Approximately 83% of cluster headache cases are males (Table 1.6). Male patients have a leonine appearance; moreover, some of the few female cases have been claimed to have a particularly masculine physiognomy ('female lions') (Graham *et al.*, 1970; Graham, 1975). Another natural approach to cluster headache pathogenesis would, therefore, be to study male sex hormones. Kudrow (1976) studied serum testosterone in two small, separate groups of male cluster headache patients; both groups were studied in both the active phase and the remission period. The clinical analyses of the two series were carried out in two different laboratories. Decreased serum testosterone levels were found in both series during the active phase of cluster headache, both when compared to the findings in controls and when compared to the remission periods. Even the remission levels were lower than the control levels in the first series (Table 2.29).

Nelson (1978), in essence, compared testosterone levels in cluster headache and migraine patients in the headache-free stage. The control range for testosterone was given as 300–850 ng dl^{-1}. In females, the control range was 10–65 ng dl^{-1}. The mean blood level in cluster headache patients was 460.4 ng dl^{-1}, as against 431.5 ng dl^{-1} in migraine patients (Table 2.29). There was no significant difference between the groups. Five out of 27 cluster headache patients showed decreased testosterone levels (19%), as against seven of 26 migraine patients (27%). Some cluster headache patients were studied during attacks (four altogether), and on no occasion was a decreased testosterone level observed. The levels in four female patients studied in the interparoxysmal period of the bout were at or above the upper normal limit. Kudrow's original findings were, therefore, not entirely reproduced in this study. In a more recent study, Kudrow (1980) used the patient as his own control and compared testosterone levels in five patients in the active phase and the remission. The mean plasma testosterone levels in the active phase and in the remission were still significantly different (Table 2.29).

Romiti *et al.* (1983) compared plasma testosterone levels prior to and during the attack, as well as in the remission phase in cluster headache patients ($n = 29$, chronic and episodic cases) with those in a control group of 29 patients having various types of headache. The mean testosterone level in the control group was not significantly higher than that in the cluster headache group during remission. In 11 male patients with episodic cluster headache there was a significant mean decrease in the testosterone level during attacks as compared with the level between attacks. No such difference was observed in the chronic cluster headache patients, nor was there any difference between headache and headache-free periods in the control group.

Klimek (1982b) studied plasma testosterone levels in the drug-free state in 23 male cluster headache patients (during the interparoxysmal periods of a bout) and compared them with those of 10 patients with trigeminal neuralgia, 14 with

Table 2.29 Blood testosterone values in cluster headache and other headaches

Authors	Cluster headache				Migraine		Various painful conditions		Units
	Remission	Bout, inter-paroxysmally	During attack	Controls	Attack-free	Attack	Trigeminal neuralgia	Radicular pain	
Kudrow (1976b) (A)	401 ± 79	238 ± 144		530 ± 181					ng/100 ml
Kudrow (1976b) (B)	675 ± 160	425 ± 38		796 ± 277					ng/100 ml
Kudrow (1980)	634 ± 191	479 ± 106		—					Probably ng/100 ml
Nelson (1978)	460 ± 155	—	631	300–850[a]	432 ± 177	490			ng/100 ml
Klimek (1982b)	—	240 ± 112	—	385 ± 128[b]			175 ± 71[c]	162 ± 99[c]	ng/ml
Romiti et al. (1983)	651	580	438	400–900[d]					ng/100 ml
Facchinetti et al. (1986)		4.4 ± 1.1[e]		6.6 ± 0.8[e]					ng/ml

[a] Range, healthy individuals.
[b] Blood donors.
[c] Not age-matched with cluster headache patients (mean age: cluster headache, 34; radicular pain, 41; trigeminal neuralgia, 63 years).
[d] Patients with various headaches.
[e] Mesor (mean integrated 24-h values).

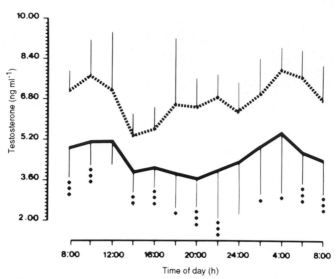

Figure 2.17 Chronogram of testosterone plasma levels (mean ± SD) in episodic cluster headache patients (———) and controls (– – – –). Student's *t*-test: *$p < 0.05$; **$p < 0.02$; ***$p < 0.01$. (From Facchinetti *et al.* (1986). Courtesy of *Cephalalgia*.)

radicular pain, and 14 blood donors, all males. The lowest mean plasma levels were found in patients suffering from radicular pain (162 ng ml^{-1}) and trigeminal neuralgia (175 ng ml^{-1}). In the latter group of patients, the mean age (63 years) was rather higher than that of the cluster headache patients (34 years). In the cluster headache and blood donor groups (mean age 30 years), the mean plasma levels were 240 and 385 ng ml^{-1}, respectively. The fact that the mean ages of the various groups were dissimilar probably influenced the results to some extent, since testosterone production gradually reduces with increasing age. There was a marked difference in the mean ages of the cluster headache (34 years) and trigeminal neuralgia (63 years) groups. However, the mean ages of the cluster headache (34 years) and radicular pain (41 years) group were such that the difference in age do not necessarily invalidate the results. The mean testosterone level found in the radicular pain group was the lowest one obtained in the entire study. The observed lowering may thus be secondary to the pain as such. In fact, Fanciullacci *et al.* (1987) have found significantly higher testosterone levels in patients than in controls.

Like other hormones, the plasma level of testosterone shows a fluctuating curve. The above-described studies on testosterone levels in cluster headache patients were 'point observations'. Facchinetti *et al.* (1986) compared the 24 h variation of testosterone in patients (in the bout) and controls and found that the mean serum testosterone levels in cluster headache patients were significantly reduced most of the time (Figure 2.17). As mentioned elsewhere (see Cortisol), Facchinetti *et al.* found the mean plasma cortisol level in cluster headache patients to be elevated (Figure 2.15). Cortisol has a lowering effect on plasma testosterone. Facchinetti *et al.*, therefore, ascribed the lowering of plasma testosterone in cluster headache to the co-existent, elevated cortisol levels. Increased cortisol levels may have contributed to the low plasma testosterone levels in cluster headache, but this may only be part of the explanation for the testosterone findings. It cannot be concluded at present that theses changes indicate a *primary* hypothalamic dysfunction, as was originally suggested.

It would also have been of interest to have analysed the free and protein bound fractions of testosterone in cluster headache patients (Fanciullacci *et al.*, 1987). This was actually studied by Murialdo *et al.* (1989), who used a 'simulatory computerized method based on the mass action law'. Total, free, and carrier-bound testosterone levels were found to be significantly diminished in the chronic variety only.

LUTEINIZING HORMONE

The lowered testosterone level could be due to a pituitary failure. Pituitary luteinizing hormone (LH) release is characterized by pulses, appearing at approximately 1-h intervals, depending on the parallel pulsatile release of the hypothalamic LH–releasing hormone (LH–RH) into the hypophyseal portal circulation. It was accordingly natural to estimate the level of LH in cluster headache patients. Kudrow (1980) found that, in each of four patients, the plasma LH value was lower in the cluster phase than during remission, the average values being 9.7 and 15.3 MIU ml^{-1}, respectively. Facchinetti *et al.* (1986) studied morning LH levels in nine males with episodic cluster headache and in seven age- and sex-matched controls. The average plasma values in the patient and control groups were 7.3 and 7.4 MIU ml^{-1}, respectively. Similar results were obtained by Polleri *et al.* (1983b) and later also by Fanciullacci *et al.* (1987). These studies do not allow the conclusion to be drawn that the level of LH is different in patients and controls; there is thus no proof of a pituitary failure in this respect.

Micieli *et al.* (1987) studied the LH 'pulsatility' in cluster headache and found signs of a disordered secretion. The hypothalamic pathways regulating the LH release seem to be subject to a cyclic vulnerability in cluster headache. Murialdo *et al.* (1987, 1989) found that the LH peak values after intravenous administration of LH–RH were decreased in chronic cluster headache, but not in episodic cluster headache, be it inside or outside the bout. Basal and peak (LH–RH induced) follicle stimulating hormone serum levels were found to be significantly elevated in both episodic and chronic cases.

PROLACTIN

A study of the level of prolactin circadian secretion may give important information about various conditions (Polleri *et al.*, 1983). Polleri *et al.* (1982) studied the diurnal variation in prolactin blood levels in nine cluster headache patients (four with the episodic variety), seven patients with 'atypical facial pain', and 10 healthy controls. Blood samples were obtained every 2 h by means of an indwelling catheter, so that sleep was not disturbed. A double antibody radioimmunoassay technique was employed. No significant difference was found between the three groups as regards the arithmetic mean levels of prolactin. However, when the periodicity was scrutinized, the usual pattern of a nocturnal peak and a diurnal trough was not present in cluster headache but persisted in atypical facial pain. The pain attacks *per se* thus seem to be the synchronizing event which leads to an increase in prolactin levels.

Boiardi *et al*. (1983) found basal serum prolactin values to be of approximately the same magnitude in 10 male cluster headache patients and 10 age- and sex-matched controls. The prolactin response to stimuli such as insulin and L-dopa were also of the same order of magnitude.

Thyrotropin releasing hormone (TRH) is a tripeptide which stimulates the production and release of thyroid stimulating hormone (TSH) from the thyreotropic cells in the anterior portion of the pituitary gland. Its role in the release of prolactin has not been defined. TRH production and release at the hypothalamic level are regulated by facilitating monoaminergic noradrenergic and serotoninergic fibres.

Bussone *et al*. (1988) studied 10 cluster headache cases in and outside the bout, and seven controls were studied with regard to blood levels of TSH and prolactin. No significant difference was found between the three groups with regard to the basal serum levels for TSH and prolactin. Even after TRH stimulation the mean levels were not significantly different with regard to TSH and prolactin in the three groups. However, the *maximum* TSH values were significantly lower after TRH stimulation in cluster headache patients in the active period than in the remission period ($p < 0.001$) and than in controls ($p < 0.05$). There thus seems to be a somewhat blunted TSH response on TRH stimulation, whereas the prolactin response was within control limits. The blunted TSH response has recently been verified in a large clinical series (32 patients in the cluster period; 16 in remission) (Bussone *et al*., 1989).

Ferrari *et al*. (1983) found that, in the single patient, the chrono-organization of prolactin secretion could be intact. In the cluster headache group as a whole, however, there was a lack of statistically significant circadian rhythm of prolactin secretion. Although there was a marked individual variability in rhythmometric changes in the cluster headache patients as a whole, there seemed to be a more evident dysrhythmic condition in the chronic than in the episodic form.

Klimek (1985) studied in the plasma levels of prolactin in nine cluster headache patients (six males and three females), 10 migraine patients (three males and seven females) and two control groups, i.e. patients suffering from constant radicular pain (nine patients; six males and three females) and 10 healthy individuals (five males and five females). The patients in both headache groups were studied interparoxysmally, but prior to treatment. The serum concentration of prolactin was determined by radioimmunoassay; it was assessed in the basal state (samples taken at the same time of the day), as well as every 30 min up to 2 h after the administration of metoclopramide (10 mg intramuscularly), a D_2-type dopamine receptor blocking agent. Metoclopramide serves as a prolactin releaser from the pituitary gland due to dopamine antagonistic activity.

The mean basal prolactin level in cluster headache patients was 10.6 ± 2.95 ng ml^{-1}. A maximum level (77.13 ± 40.37 ng ml^{-1}) was attained 30 min after metoclopramide administration. The corresponding values in the migraine group were 8.29 ± 2.66 and 127.28 ± 44.5 ng ml^{-1}, respectively. In the two control groups, the corresponding values were: healthy group 9.80 ± 4.38 and 101.3 ± 64.96 ng ml^{-1}; and radicular pain 11.09 ± 3.33 and 139.29 ± 67.90 ng ml^{-1}, respectively.

The basal level of prolactin was thus within the control range in the cluster headache group. The increase following stimulation was seven-fold in the cluster headache group, which is considerably less than in the other groups. The peak levels in the cluster headache group differed significantly from that in healthy controls ($p < 0.05$).

Waldenlind and Gustafsson (1987) studied the circadian rhythmicity of serum prolactin in cluster headache patients (27 episodic cases; 4 chronic cases) and healthy controls ($n = 14$), and 16 patients were studied both during and between bouts. The 24 h average serum prolactin levels were lower during remission and during the bout than in healthy controls, but not significantly so. Prolactin levels frequently increased during attacks (Figures 2.16 and 2.18).

The significance of the changes in prolactin serum level rhythmicity in cluster headache is not obvious. Until proven otherwise, it is not unreasonable to consider the changes to be secondary to the disease process.

GROWTH HORMONE

Patients with cluster headache may have a rugged, leonine appearance (Graham, 1972, 1975). Serum growth hormone was, therefore, studied by Klimek (1985) in nine cluster headache patients (six males and three females), 10 migraine patients (three males and seven females), nine patients with constant radicular pain (six males and three females) and 10 healthy individuals (five males and five females), the last two groups serving as controls. The groups were not quite age-matched. The cluster headache and migraine patients were studied interparoxysmally and prior to starting treatment.

Serum levels were measured prior to and subsequent to (i.e. every 30 min up to 2 h) administration of a D_2-type dopamine receptor antagonist (metoclopramide, 10 mg intramuscularly, given at the same time of day). Growth hormone was assessed by radioimmunoassay.

The mean basal growth hormone level was 0.46 ± 0.49 ng ml^{-1} in the cluster headache group. Metoclopramide administration caused an increase in growth

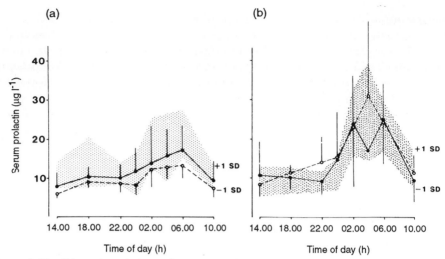

Figure 2.18 Diurnal variation of serum prolactin levels in males and females with episodic cluster headache. (a) Males: (●) cluster period, $n = 13$; (○) remission period, $n = 17$; (□) controls, $n = 6$. (b) Females: (●) cluster period, $n = 5$; (○) remission period, $n = 8$; (□) controls, $n = 8$. For the female patients the data at 24.00 and 04.00 h are from one patient only. (From Waldenlind and Gustafsson (1987). Courtesy of E. Waldenlind and *Cephalalgia*.)

hormone with a maximum level of 4.95 ± 2.41 ng ml^{-1} appearing after 1 h. The corresponding values in the migraine group were: 5.22 ± 3.17 and 17.46 ± 20.8 ng ml^{-1}, respectively.

In the radicular pain group the corresponding values were 1.0 ± 0.39 and 1.95 ± 1.34 ng ml^{-1} (at 30 min) and in the second control group these values were 2.09 ± 1.30 and 6.96 ± 4.54 ng ml^{-1}, respectively. Thus, the mean basal growth hormone value in cluster headache was within control limits.

According to Klimek, an increase of 2–3 times in growth hormone level following stimulation is to be considered normal. The increase in percentage was more marked in the cluster headache group than in any of the other groups, but the post-stimulation values were also within the control range.

Boiardi *et al.* (1983) found normal basal serum growth hormone levels in 10 male cluster headache patients when compared to 10 age- and sex-matched healthy individuals. Furthermore, the growth hormone responses to such stimuli as insulin (0.1 IU kg^{-1} intravenously), L-dopa (500 mg orally), and thyrotropin releasing hormone (TRH) (400 μg intravenously) were within normal limits. An abnormal growth hormone response to TRH is encountered in connection with deficient control of the whole hypothalamic–pituitary regulation. The normal response suggests that this regulation is intact in cluster headache. Depressed patients behave differently on this test. These results may, to some extent, detract attention from the 'central' hypothesis in cluster headache (see Pathogenesis)

β-ENDORPHIN, β-LIPOTROPIN, ADRENOCORTICOTROPHIC HORMONE AND METENCEPHALIN

β-Lipotropin (β-LPH), β-endorphin (β-EP) and adrenocorticotrophic hormone (ACTH) seem to derive from a common pituitary precursor, proopiomelanocortin. Their rhythmic secretion seems to depend on the activity of the corticotropin releasing factor (CRF). This factor is under neural control.

Interesting findings concerning β-EP have been made in migraine, where lowered levels have been found in the blood (Baldi *et al.*, 1982) and cerebrospinal fluid. Anselmi *et al.* (1980) found a lowered level of encephalin in the cerebrospinal fluid of migraine patients. Studies of such parameters were, therefore, also indicated in cluster headache.

Appenzeller *et al.* (1981) found elevated serum β-EP levels during the attack, which they interpreted as a secondary phenomenon. In the cluster phase ($n = 7$), plasma β-EP was found to be within normal levels (6.9 ± 1.1 fmol ml^{-1} (mean $\pm$ SE) in patients and 6.7 ± 0.9 in controls) in another study (Nappi *et al.*, 1985b; see also Nappi *et al.*, 1985c). β-LPH and ACTH levels were also studied in the same patients and were found to be within control limits. Hardebo *et al.* (1985) found that serum β-EP levels were of the same order of magnitude in cluster headache and control patients (neurological patients with minor symptoms). 'A tendency to lower levels' of cerebrospinal fluid β-EP between and during attacks was observed in patients as compared with controls.

Central opioid activity can also be evaluated in another way: opioids exert a tonic inhibition on luteinizing hormone–releasing hormone (LH–RH) neurons at the hypothalamic level. Naloxone is an antagonist of opioid activity at the receptor level. Naloxone administration will, therefore, lead to an annulment of the inhibition of the LH–RH neurons and subsequent release of LH into the blood.

A naloxone challenge test (4 mg intravenously as a bolus) was given to 10 cluster headache patients and 12 healthy controls and the additional secretion of LH was measured (Facchinetti *et al.*, 1988; see also Facchinetti *et al.*, 1987). In the control group, a value of 497.5 ± 85.5 (mean $\pm$ SE) mIU ml^{-1} over 120 min was found as compared with 450.5 ± 70.4 mIU ml^{-1} in cluster headache patients and 357.8 ± 78.9 mIU ml^{-1} in classical migraine. These values are not significantly different. In non-classicial migraine (155.3 ± 71.7 mIU ml^{-1}, $p < 0.05$, vs. controls) and migraine with interval headache (104.1 ± 53.7 mIU ml^{-1}, $p < 0.01$ vs. controls), significantly reduced levels were found. In none of the patient categories did the LH response to LH–RH stimulation ($10\,\mu$g intravenously) differ from that in controls, indicating that there is no pituitary dysfunction responsible for the alterations in response. There thus appears to be a tendency towards normal naloxone effect on the LH–RHLH axis in the headache categories where normal β-EP levels have been demonstrated in blood and cerebrospinal fluid and impaired reaction in those categories showing reduced cerebrospinal fluid β-EP levels, such as in migraine.

Nappi *et al*. (1985a) also studied the rhythmicity of the blood levels of β-EP and β-LPH in patients in the third and fourth weeks of a cluster period. Whereas controls showed a significant secretory rhythmicity of β-EP and β-LPH with almost simultaneous acrophases, no such rhythmicity was detected in a group of seven cluster headache patients. A higher mesor was found in the patient group than in controls.

The cerebrospinal fluid content of metencephalin was found to be below the assay sensitivity (<0.6 pmol ml^{-1}) in five cluster headache sufferers, as compared to a mean level of around 25 pmol ml^{-1} in four controls (Anselmi *et al*., 1980). Hardebo *et al*. (1985) found the following levels in cerebrospinal fluid: outside attacks 55, during attacks 83 and in controls 176 fmol ml^{-1}. The plasma metencephalin levels (mean 32 fmol ml^{-1}) in cluster headache patients were considerably lower than the cerebrospinal levels. Since the blood–brain barrier seemed to be intact even during attacks (as indicated by the normal cerebrospinal fluid/plasma albumin ratio), the lowered mean cerebrospinal fluid metencephalin level could reflect a true deficiency in the central nervous system. The reduced cerebrospinal fluid metencephalin levels indicate an increased turnover or a deficiency in central encephalinergic neurons. Chinese acupuncture (Hardebo *et al*., 1989) caused the lowered cerebrospinal metencephalin level to increase, whereas β-EP levels were not influenced by this procedure. The disentanglement of the abnormal levels and rhythmic patterns of β-EP, β-LPH, melatonin and cortisol may render new insight into the basic mechanisms of cluster headache.

PLASMA NORADRENALINE DURING ATTACKS

Brachial arterial and internal jugular vein noradrenaline concentration was assessed during the remission ($n = 6$) and during spontaneous ($n = 3$) and provoked attacks ($n = 6$) (Igarashi *et al*., 1987). During the remission, the mean noradrenaline concentration in brachial artery and jugular vein blood was 149.8 and 143.8 pg ml^{-1}, respectively. After nitroglycerin administration, there was a rapid and rather marked increase in blood noradrenaline concentration (89% for the arterial sample and 130% for the venous sample). The noradrenaline levels returned to the basal level after approximately 30 min, and the headache appeared after a mean of 37 min. There was a second rise in noradrenaline blood levels in connection with the attack and another drop at the end of the attack. During spontaneous attacks, there was an increase in blood levels of noradrenaline during the attack and in a parallel fashion in arterial and venous blood.

The minor differences between spontaneously occurring and nitroglycerin induced attacks as regards blood noradrenaline levels are interesting. In spontaneously occurring attacks the noradrenaline increase did not precede the pain and there was no preferential increase in the internal jugular vein noradrenaline concentration. To me, these findings do not suggest a *primary* role of noradrenaline in cluster headache attacks.

GASTRIN

In earlier days, the stomach played a central role in the thinking about cluster headache pathogenesis (e.g. Graham *et al.*, 1970). Nattero *et al.* (1985) have examined the serum gastrin levels in cluster headache patients ($n = 8$) both during attacks and interparoxysmally. They used a radioimmunoassay method. The mean level during attack was 101.4 pg ml^{-1}, against 52.1 pg ml^{-1} in the interparoxysmal period. In only one of the patients was no difference found between attack periods and attack-free periods. Later on (Nattero *et al.*, 1987a), a control group was added, and the following values were found: cluster headache ($n = 25$) 50.6 pg ml^{-1}, versus controls ($n = 20$) 27.5 pg ml^{-1}. These values differed significantly.

Nattero *et al.* found a mean serum gastrin level of 37.4 ± 28.8 pg ml^{-1} in migraine patients during the pain-free interval ($n = 62$) and 28 ± 14.5 pg ml^{-1} in the control group ($n = 40$). There was a statistically significant difference between the serum gastrin levels of migraine patients during and between attacks (69.9 ± 56.6 ($n = 23$) and 52.3 ± 40.0 pg ml^{-1}, respectively). On this occasion the blood samples were drawn in the morning. These findings seem to make the findings regarding serum gastrin levels in cluster headache patients unspecific.

Results diametrically opposite to these were found by Klimek (1982) who estimated the serum gastrin concentration in migraine ($n = 23$, females) and cluster headache ($n = 23$, males) patients and control individuals ($n = 26$, 10 females and 16 males). Blood samples were taken in the morning after overnight fasting, outside of attack, and prior to the start of treatment. The method used was a radioimmunological one, and the individual results were based on three parallel assays. No appreciable difference was found between male and female controls, for which reason the two subgroups were treated as one. The average gastrin level in the migraine group was 35.7 ± 15.9, in cluster headache 39.8 ± 21.3 and in the controls 55.3 ± 16.1 pg ml^{-1}. While the mean gastrin levels in cluster headache and migraine patients were not significantly different, the mean values for these groups both differed significantly from the mean level for the controls ($p < 0.01$ and <0.001, respectively).

The variation in these results is marked, and more questions are raised than are solved by these investigations. One wonders what the influence of drugs might have been, and what the impact of the difference between the assay techniques used might have been. Likewise, the composition of the sample (relative content of 'big gastrin', 'little gastrin', and 'mini gastrin') might have influenced the outcome of the test.

INFLAMMATION—POSSIBLE ROLE IN THE PATHOGENESIS

Viral disease has been mentioned as a cause of the exacerbations of cluster headache. Graham (1975) observed that bouts started in the wake of a herpes simplex virus flare-up. More recently, Hardebo (1986) has also described this. Graham speculated that the demonstration of herpes simplex virus in the Gasserian ganglion at autopsy (Baringer and Swoveland, 1973) may have a bearing on cluster headache pathogenesis: activation of vira in cranial nerves may sensitize these patients to various stimuli, e.g. vasodilating ones.

Hardebo and Ryberg (1988) have looked more closely into the aspect of inflammation. Cerebrospinal fluid was obtained at various phases of the bout, and the findings were compared with those in controls. Three of 33 cerebrospinal fluid samples showed a cell count exceeding 5 cells, and seven samples had a cell count exceeding 3. Thirteen of 33 cerebrospinal fluid samples from 19 cluster headache patients showed increased levels of total protein. The cerebrospinal fluid/serum albumin ratio was increased in nine of 28 samples. The cerebrospinal fluid IgG/albumin index was elevated in only two of 28 samples.

No absolute values were given for these variables. Be that as it may, most patients did not show pathological findings. On the other hand, the cerebrospinal fluid was collected at some distance from the region where the crucial events probably take place. These findings for cerebrospinal fluid may, therefore, only vaguely reflect what goes on at the base of the brain. These findings may have some significance for cluster headache pathogenesis.

IMMUNOLOGICAL STUDIES

Klimek (1985c) determined the total complement level and the levels of C_3, C_4, IgG, IgA and IgM in 39 cluster headache patients and 70 controls. Cluster headache patients were found to have significantly reduced mean C_3 and IgA fractions.

Visintini *et al.* (1986) studied serum immunoglobulins, complement components and immune complexes in 47 patients with cluster headache, 32 patients with common and 12 with classical migraine, as well as in 93 age- and sex-matched controls. The cluster headache patients were studied in the various phases of the headache. Serum IgG, IgA and IgM concentrations in the headache groups did not differ from those in controls. Similarly, C1q, C_3 and C_4 levels were within the normal range in all the headache groups, as was the alternative pathway protein, factor B. In addition, no conversion products of C_3 or factor B were detected. A search with three different assays was made for immune complexes of various sizes, from the small IgG complexes to the larger IgM complement-fixing aggregates. No definite differences between the headache and control groups were detected.

There were no differences in the levels of these compounds between the remissions and bouts in the cluster headache patients or for any of the other parameters mentioned. Consequently, this study does not provide any evidence to implicate activity of the complement system in cluster headache pathogenesis.

PLATELET STUDIES

Electron microscopy

Experiment on animals have shown that serotonin is embodied within the *very dense* bodies of the platelets, and reserpine causes a virtual disappearance of the *dense* bodies (osmophilic granula) (Pletscher *et al.*, 1971). The serotonin storing organelles of animal platelets can be easily seen using electron microscopy of ultrathin sections. Experiments by Anthony *et al.* (1969) indicated that the mechanism behind serotonin depletion during migraine attacks may be similar to that operative in reserpine depletion. In other words, blood serotonin fluctuation during migraine attacks could be a reflection of the change in the number, shape or structure of the dense bodies. Because migraine and cluster headache bear many similarities, and because a 'general factor' (see Pathogenesis), in addition to a local one, has been suspected to also be present in cluster headache, platelets from cluster headache patients have been studied alongside platelets from migraine patients.

The ultrastructure of platelets has been studied (Grammeltvedt *et al.*, 1975) during and between attacks of classic migraine ($n = 5$) and cluster headache ($n = 6$), the patients being their own controls. Four controls were also investigated. Venous blood samples were drawn 2–4 h after the onset of attacks of migraine, and from the later part of cluster headache attacks, since these generally were short-lasting. The patients were drug free. Blood was drawn directly into 2.5% glutaraldehyde in 0.1 M phosphate buffer. After fixation, the platelet pellet was post-fixed in osmium tetroxide. The final sections were examined using an electron microscope. The total number of platelets was counted. About 100 sectioned platelets, selected at random, were studied on micrographs, and the dense bodies were counted. The various subcellular platelet structures were also studied. Platelet adhesiveness was estimated, according to the Hellem II method (Hellem, 1971).

The mean number of dense bodies per 100 sectioned platelets from the four healthy individuals was 27 (range 20–35) (Table 2.30). No significant difference was found between the number of dense bodies in platelets obtained during and between attacks in either migraine or in cluster headache. There was no significant difference between cluster headache and migraine patients as to the number of dense bodies present during and between attacks, whereas the mean number of dense bodies in both groups outside attacks was somewhat lower than in the control group.

No systematic attack-induced alterations could be observed in cluster headache with regard to the various subcellular platelet structures, such as α-granules, mitochondria, the vacuole system, glycogen granules, or the surface connecting system. Platelet counts during and between attacks of cluster headache did not differ greatly (mean 296 000 and 289 000, respectively). The mean platelet adhesiveness during and between cluster headache attacks was

Table 2.30 Number of very dense bodies per 100
sectioned platelets in samples taken from episodic
cluster headache and migraine patients[a]

	No. dense bodies	
	Mean	Range
Controls	27.1	20–35
Migraine		
Attack-free interval	21.8	12–39
During attack	20.2	13–38
Cluster headache		
Attack-free interval	21.3	14–31
During attack	20.0	11–38

[a]From Grammeltvedt *et al*. (1975). Courtesy of *Headache*.

86% (7 patients, 12 tests) and 83% (5 patients, 6 tests), respectively, the
corresponding values in migraine being 88% and 90%, respectively.

There was no marked tendency to attack-induced reduction in the number of
dense bodies in either migraine or cluster headache patients. This was a rather
surprising observation. It should be emphasized, however, that the serotonin/
dense body interrelationship was less well known in man than in animals at
that time. In any event, electron microscopy ought to be sensitive enough to
detect the expected changes in the number of dense bodies.

Platelet counts

In cluster headache, the mean platelet count during attack was 296 000 (range
191 000–362 000; 12 tests in 8 patients). In the interparoxysmal period, the mean
platelet count was 289 000 (range 200 000–475 000; 17 tests in 9 patients). The
mean platelet count in migraine was lower (221 000) during than between
attacks (270 000) (Grammeltvedt *et al*., 1975).

Waldenlind *et al*. (1984) found a similar number of platelets outside pain
attacks in cluster headache patients ($n = 33$, 165 700 ± 34 600 platelets per μl)
migraine patients ($n = 34$, 173 300 ± 38 700) and healthy controls ($n = 128$;
169 400 ± 56 900). No statistically significant difference was found when comparing the two headache disorders by sex. The groups were age matched, and
no drugs had been administered for ≥3 days previously.

In vivo **activation**

The platelet contains three types of storage granules each having different
contents; the lysosomes, with the acid hydrolases; the α granules, with e.g.
coagulation factors, β-thromboglobulin (β-TG) and platelet factor 4 (PF 4); and
dense granules, with e.g. ATP, ADP and serotonin. Weak agonists, such as

ADP and adrenaline elicit α-granule and dense granule secretion, but no acid hydrolase secretion. Strong agonists, such as thrombin and collagen, provoke secretion from all three types of storage granule (e.g. Holmsen, 1986).

D'Andrea *et al.* (1986) studied platelet activation in a total of 17 cluster headache patients, nine during remission and eight during a bout, that is during attacks as well as in the interparoxysmal period. The specific protein, β-TG, was increased in the plasma during remission (71.2 ± 30.1 ng ml^{-1} $\pm$ SD) (as compared with that in controls (32.6 ± 5.9; $p < 0.005$, Student's t-test for unpaired data). The same trend was observed for PF 4, i.e. 14.6 ± 8.5 and 6.0 ± 1.3 ng ml^{-1}, respectively. During the interparoxysmal period of a bout the mean value for β-TG was 63.8 and for PF 4 16.6 ng ml^{-1}.

During attacks, average β-TG and PF 4 levels were reduced to normal levels, i.e. 34 and 6μg ml^{-1}, respectively. β-TG and PF 4 are both markers of *in vivo* platelet activation. Thus, platelet activation seems to take place in cluster headache, the activation being most marked outside attacks. The factors causing activation and the reasons for the discrepancy between attack and attack-free periods remain unknown.

Monoamine oxidase

A number of biologically active monoamines are oxidatively deaminated by monoamine oxidase (MAO). There are two types of MAO: MAO$_A$ and MAO$_B$. The human platelet contains only MAO$_B$, which has a wide range of substrates, e.g. telemethylhistamine and phenylethylamine. Histamine has been invoked in cluster headache pathogenesis (see Histamine Metabolism).

Bussone *et al.* (1977) found a low platelet content of MAO in a group of cluster headache patients.

Glover *et al.* (1981) compared the platelet MAO contents in various groups of headache sufferers of both sexes (a total of 111 patients) with those of sex-matched control groups. All patients were studied in the headache-free interval. The MAO assay was carried out in duplicate and blindly with [^{14}C] tyramine as substrate and the activity expressed as nanomoles of tyramine oxidized per milligram of protein in 30 min. A group of 41 male cluster headache patients was studied together with 30 male controls. Of the cluster headache patients 39 were in a bout, but did not have a pain attack at the time of testing. Fifteen of these patients returned for retesting in the remission period.

There were no significant differences in MAO levels between any of the female groups or between these and controls. The mean values $\pm$ SEM were: female controls 16.7 ± 1.5; classical migraine 15.3 ± 1.4; common migraine 16.6 ± 0.9; and tension headache 15.9 ± 1.6. In males, however, the following values were obtained: male controls 16.3 ± 1.3; classical migraine 10.9 ± 0.9; common migraine 13.9 ± 1.1; tension headache 10.7 ± 1.1; and cluster headache 9.0 ± 1.3. The average values in males having classical migraine and tension headache were significantly lower ($p < 0.01$) than the average values in controls, and the values for cluster headache were lowered even more signifi-cantly ($p < 0.002$). The findings were similar inside and outside bouts.

This study attests to the non-specificity of the lowering of the MAO level. The fact that the MAO level is permanently lowered indicates that this phenomenon *per se* does not underlie the attack generation.

The platelet protein concentration was found to be of the same order of magnitude in male patients studied in the pain-free phase (2.4 ± 0.3 mg ml^{-1}) and controls (2.4 ± 0.2 mg ml^{-1}).

In another study by the same group (Littlewood *et al.*, 1984) the low platelet MAO activity in cluster headache was confirmed. The activities of two other enzymes, that is phenolsulphotransferase M and succinate dehydrogenase, were determined in the same platelet samples. Low levels of succinate de-hydrogenase activity were found. This appears to represent a separate phenomenon, since there was no correlation between the activity of this enzyme and that of MAO. The low platelet MAO activity in cluster headache thus does not seem to reflect a generalized platelet enzyme defect.

Waldenlind *et al.* (1984b) and Ekbom (1987) studied the thermolability and kinetics of platelet monoamine oxidase (MAO$_B$). A total of 33 patients with cluster headache (27 in the remission), and 34 migraine patients were com-pared with 128 age- and sex-matched healthy controls. None of the headache patients were studied during ongoing attacks, and none had received any medication the 3 days preceding the blood sampling. In the assay, radio-labelled phenylethylamine in various concentrations was used as the sub-strate. The thermolability was studied by pre-incubating the aliquots at 52°C and 4°C.

The MAO activity (i.e. the initial velocity, V_0) was significantly lower in both headache groups than in controls. It was also significantly lower in cluster headache than in migraine, both when the whole group and both sexes were compared. The maximal enzyme velocity (V_{max}) was significantly lower in male cluster headache patients than in male migraine patients. In both headache groups, V_{max} was lower than in controls. With regard to the Michaelis constant (K_m), cluster headache did not differ from controls. Plate-let MAO from cluster headache patients was more thermostable than MAO from migraineurs.

Smoking seemed to influence the result, heavy smoking being associated with the lowest V_{max} levels.

The difference in MAO activity between the cluster headache and control groups was caused by the difference in V_{max} values. Platelet MAO in cluster headache and migraine may also differ essentially. The possibility that medication—or other external influences unrelated to the basic disturbances in these headaches—influenced the tested variables cannot be rejected at this stage. The significance, if any, of the demonstrated lowered V_{max} values for MAO in cluster headache is doubtful.

CHOLINE, PHOSPHATIDYLCHOLINE AND LEUKOTRIENE B$_4$

The choline levels in erythrocytes are raised in mania, a disorder that, like cluster headache, responds to lithium. Choline levels have been measured (de Belleroche *et al.*, 1984a,b) in erythrocytes and plasma in male patients with the episodic form of cluster headache ($n = 27$) and male controls ($n = 14$). When compared to controls, there were decreased average erythrocyte choline levels both between and during cluster periods, the mean levels being 55.2 and 58.6%, respectively. In the lithium treated group, a drastic elevation of erythrocyte choline levels of up to 500 times the pre-treatment level was found. The effect of lithium on the erythrocyte content of choline lasted 3–4 months on discontinuation of treatment, which indicates that the effect lasts until the erythrocytes have decayed; in other words, the effect of lithium is irreversible. Erythrocyte choline levels were normal in migraine (de Belleroche *et al.*, 1986). It is interesting that Fragoso *et al.* (1988, 1989a,b,c) found the phosphatidylcholine fraction to be reduced in cluster headache in experiments in which polymorphonuclear cells were incubated with radiolabelled arachidonic acid. Whether arachidonic or oleic acid was the substrate, the phosphatidylcholine fraction formed seemed to be smaller in cluster headache than in controls.

The effect of lithium in the blood, as far as choline is concerned, seems to be restricted to the erythrocytes. The plasma levels were 30–40% of the erythrocyte levels in de Belleroche *et al.*'s studies. In lithium treated patients, the erythrocyte transport system for choline is inhibited bi-directionally. The increased erythrocyte choline level during lithium treatment seems to be produced inside the erythrocytes from phosphatidylcholine catabolism through the mediation of a phospholipase.

Erythrocyte choline levels would *a priori* not be believed to change much in the course of a relatively short-lasting attack; this was shown to be the case. The fact that the erythrocyte choline level is low both during and between cluster phases indicates that the low level *per se* does not evoke the attacks. However, combined with another factor (other factors?), this abnormality may possibly be symptom productive. There is another possible mechanism for its action, i.e. that choline combines with acetyl to form the neurotransmitter acetylcholine. Choline may be the rate-limiting factor in this reaction. What is found in erythroyctes may conceivably reflect the situation in neurons. Choline may be a marker in cluster headache. Much work, however, remains to be done to clarify these problems.

In later work in this field, de Belleroche *et al.* (1986) extended their study to include the investigation of membrane-bound lipid fractions such as membrane phosphatidylcholine, total phospholipids and cholesterol in erythrocytes. A significantly increased membrane phosphatidylcholine to cholesterol ratio was found in cluster headache as compared to controls. These findings indicate that the turnover of phosphatidylcholine is reduced. A significant reduction in high-affinity prostaglandin receptor stimulation of lymphocyte adenylate cyclase also suggests abnormal membrane function in cluster headache.

This reduction in response co-existed with a lack of change in the number or affinity of receptors. This might indicate a defective coupling between receptor and adenylate cyclase. In a later study, the polyphosphoinositide system was investigated by de Belleroche *et al.* (1988). This system is a major pathway for mediating the effects of neurotransmitters. Upon receptor activation of this system two second messengers are formed: inositol triphosphate and diacylglycerol.

The receptor-mediated activation of the polyphosphoinositide system in polymorphonuclear leucocytes was studied in patients having common migraine ($n = 12$) or cluster headache ($n = 14$) and in appropriate controls. The polymorphonuclear response to chemotactic factor stimulation was reduced in migraine (mean 42% of controls), while in cluster headache there was a slightly exaggerated response.

Incubation experiments with polymorphonuclear cells from cluster headache patients and controls and radiolabelled arachidonic acid, oleic acid, or serine as substrates have been carried out by Fragoso *et al.* (1989a,b,c). The fraction of phosphatidylserine formed appeared to be slightly increased, whichever substance was used as substrate. Phosphatidylserine is an important activator of protein kinase C, an enzyme contributing to transmembrane signalling. Whether the possible increase in phosphatidylserine in cluster headache is of importance in cluster headache pathogenesis cannot be determined at the present time.

The leukotrienes belong to a group of potent proinflammatory mediators, being converted from arachidonic acid through the action of lipo-oxygenase. There are two major groups of leukotrienes derived from the leukotriene A_4: the peptidylleukotrienes, the well-known slow reacting substance of anaphylaxis (SRS-A); and leukotriene B_4.

Selmaj *et al.* (1986) used *in vitro* experiments to study leukotriene B_4 levels in polymorphonuclear leucocytes from cluster headache ($n = 8$) and migraine ($n = 14$) patients during and between attacks. A control group of eight healthy individuals was included. Attack levels of leukotriene B_4 exceeded the free interval levels ($p < 0.05$), the leukotriene level seemingly being correlated to the interval from attack onset to blood sampling. The values for the two headache groups did not differ significantly from those in the control group. Leukotriene B_4 is apparently present in the blood at an early stage of attack, whereafter the level decreases. There was no difference between attack and attack-free levels in migraine, and these values did not differ significantly from those in controls.

There is certainly much more to be done before all these findings can be understood in terms of cluster headache pathogenesis.

ELECTROENCEPHALOGRAPHIC INVESTIGATIONS

Electroencephalograms (EEGs) have been recorded in the headache-free interval in various studies. It has generally not been mentioned whether the EEGs were recorded in an asymptomatic period between two bouts or in the interparoxysmal stage. In Friedman and Mikropoulos' (1958) series of 50 patients, normal EEGs were invariably obtained. No details were given. Stowell (1970) also generally found normal EEGs in 100 patients. In another study (Sutherland and Eadie, 1972), electroencephalography was performed in eight patients. Normal recordings were obtained in six, with bilateral non-specific changes being present in the other two patients. Heyck (1976) obtained normal EEGs in 14 of 18 cases. In three cases, paroxysmal, bilateral θ waves were observed after hyperventilation, in one case even spontaneously. Heyck, however, also found such manifestations in the free interval in the migraine patient, which points to their non-specificity.

The EEG pattern during attack was thus unknown until it was studied by our group in 1976 (Hasan *et al.*, 1976). In 30 patients (24 males and 6 females) with cluster headache, 98 EEGs were recorded in the interparoxysmal period, and in 15 of these patients (4 females and 11 males) 21 EEGs were recorded during paroxysms. All medication was discontinued >2 days prior to study, and only spontaneously occurring attacks were studied. Photic stimulation and hyperventilation were invariably included. The recordings in the interparoxysmal period were always done post-prandially, in order to obviate the influence of hypoglycaemia.

In the pain-free period, EEG abnormalities were found in one-third of the patients (Table 2.31). Focal θ activity, be it on the symptomatic side, the opposide side, or bitemporally, seemed to be the most frequently occurring abnormality. Half of the female patients showed abnormal standard EEG recordings, the abnormal activity being localized on the symptomatic side. EEG abnormalities in male patients were not as frequent (i.e. in 29% of the patients) and not so well localized to the side of the headache as those in the female patients.

Table 2.31   EEGs recorded during attacks and in the interparoxysmal period in episodic cluster headache patients ($n = 15$)[a]

EEG result	Without attack	During attack
Within normal limits	10	$\left.\begin{array}{c}9\\+3\end{array}\right\} = 12$
Pathological	5	$\left.\begin{array}{c}1\\+2\end{array}\right\} = 3$

[a]From Hasan *et al.* (1976). Courtesy of *Clinical Electroencephalography*.

In 10 of the 15 patients in whom EEGs were recorded both during and outside attack, a normal EEG was obtained outside attack. The EEG deteriorated during attacks in only one case (a slight decrease in frequency was recorded). In three of the five patients who showed a pathological EEG outside attacks, the EEG improved during attack. Thus, more cases improved than deteriorated during attacks, as far as the EEG is concerned (Table 2.31). The EEG was normal in 12 of 15 patients studied during attacks of cluster headache.

Focal EEG abnormalities similar to those recorded in some patients with focal cerebral symptoms during classic migraine attacks were not found during cluster headache attacks. The general lack of attack-induced additional EEG changes is remarkable. It seems to indicate that, if there are cerebral changes during attacks of cluster headache, they are rather discrete, or are located in electroencephalographically 'silent areas'.

SLEEP STAGES AND ATTACKS: A POSSIBLE RELATIONSHIP

An interesting study concerning the temporal relationship between headache and sleep stages was published by Dexter and Weitzman in 1970 (see also Dexter, 1974; Dexter and Riley, 1975). The patients studied suffered from cluster headache ($n = 3$), nocturnal migraine ($n = 3$), or 'psychogenic headache' ($n = 1$). During a total of 45 patient nights, 19 headache attacks occurred. In cluster headache/migraine patients, 11 headache attacks occurred during the rapid eye movement (REM) phase, four within 3 min of a REM phase, whereas two attacks occurred within 10 min of a REM period. By contrast, the patient with 'psychogenic headache' on two occasions woke up and stayed awake for upwards of 20 min before the headache started. Sleep reversal studies carried out in a single case (four nights, three headache attacks) showed that headache attacks were still temporally connected with the REM stage.

Even if nocturnal attacks could be explained as appearing within or in close temporal relationship to a certain sleep phase with a low pain threshold, this is not helpful in explaining attacks that appear during the day. It is interesting in this connection that there seem to be daytime correlates to the REM stage sleep (Othmer et al., 1969). So, notwithstanding the fact that the patient is behaviourally awake, the possibility exists that attacks may be set off during diurnal periods phenomenologically related to REM sleep, periods that may be associated with augmented vulnerability. The autonomic outbursts during the REM stage may, in part, give rise to a symptomatology similar to that observed during a cluster headache attack.

It is noteworthy that the findings were seemingly made as often in migraine as in cluster headache. Migraine and cluster headache are in all probability two distinct disorders. If some particular mechanism is present in two different headaches, we may be faced with a more general principle in headache, and not a principle of particular significance for only one headache type (in this case, cluster headache).

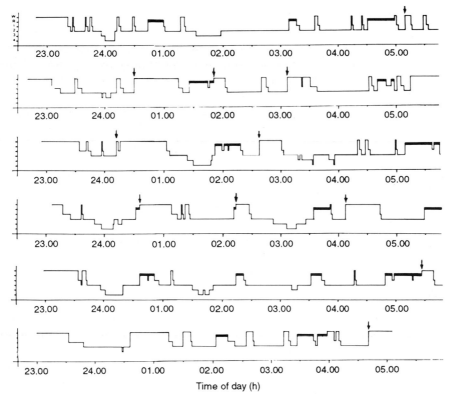

Figure 2.19 Whole night polysomnographic recordings in three patients with episodic cluster headache (total of six nights). Vertical arrows indicate onset of attacks. The heavy horizontal lines indicate REM sleep. (From Kayed and Sjaastad (1985). Courtesy of *Annals of Clinical Research*.)

In a small study of nocturnal cluster headache attacks (Kayed and Sjaastad, 1985), we were only partly able to confirm the above-mentioned findings: three patients were monitored for two nights each, during which time a total of 11 attacks occurred (1 + 1, 3 + 1 and 2 + 3, during the two nights in the three patients, respectively). There was no temporal relationship between attack occurrence and REM sleep in five attacks (Figure 2.19); on two occasions, the attacks started within 10–15 min of the end of a REM phase; only on four occasions did the attack actually start during a REM phase. These observations, although limited in number, may accordingly cast some doubt on the original findings. Results along the same lines have more recently been obtained by Pfaffenrath *et al.* (1986).

Bono *et al.* (1985) have shown that triazolam, a benzodiazepine which acts by delaying the REM cycles, reduced by approximately 60% the occurrence of nocturnal attacks in 20 episodic cluster headache patients having a nocturnal prevalence of attacks. The same investigators also demonstrated that sleep deprivation, a procedure which influences biorhythms, has short-term as well as protracted attack-preventive effects in cluster headache.

SLEEP APNOEA

Kudrow *et al.* (1984) studied the frequency of sleep apnoea in five episodic and five chronic cluster headache patients in a one night polysomnographic study. The occurrence of parasomnias and sleep symptoms were unknown to the investigators at the time of patient selection. A stop in air flow exceeding 10 s was considered to be an episode of apnoea. Sleep apnoea was diagnosed if >5 episodes occurred within 1 h. Six of the 10 patients had sleep apnoea by the above definition; four of the central type, and two of the obstructive type. All five episodic cases displayed sleep apnoea. The apnoeas ranged in number from 19 to 141 per hour. Sleep apnoeas occurred as frequently during the non-REM as in the REM phase. The headache attacks seemed partly to be, and partly not to be, preceded by oxygen desaturation. The minimum haemoglobin saturation in the sleep apnoea patients ranged between 65 and 89%. In the non-sleep-apnoea group, attacks were not preceded by oxygen desaturation.

Mathew and Frost (1984) in a polysomnographic study of three cluster headache patients found that two of the patients showed signs of upper airway obstruction, one having in addition a sleep apnoea/hypersomnia syndrome. Dexter (1984) examined four patients with chronic cluster headache, for a minimum of two nights with and two nights without attacks. Sleep characteristics were normal, and there were no demonstrable, consistent differences between symptomatic and symptom-free nights. Occasional apnoea periods were observed, but in none of the cases was there any night with >50% of the >70 episodes of apnoea per night, required for the sleep apnoea diagnosis.

Oxygen desaturation at the level demonstrated in some cases by Kudrow *et al.* does not *per se* seem to be a prerequisite for the initiation of cluster headache attacks. It is probably not even *one* of two or more factors mandatory for the creation of attacks. The possibility exists that it *facilitates* the creation of (certain?) attacks.

The frequency of sleep apnoea in episodic cluster headache seems to be high. However, sleep apnoea is a frequent disorder, and no decisive conclusion as to its significance in cluster headache can be made on this basis.

These series do not provide sufficient data for conclusive statements to be made. The selection of cases may also have been of crucial significance. To venture a cautious suggestion, it could be that there is a difference between the episodic and the chronic types of cluster headache in this respect. It would be helpful to know the sleep pattern and oxygen saturation of these patients in the remission phase. The results obtained during the symptomatic period must also be compared with findings in control series.

PNEUMOENCEPHALOGRAPHIC AND COMPUTED TOMOGRAPHY FINDINGS

The issue of whether structural cerebral changes are present in cluster headache was studied by our group by means of computed tomography (CT) scans and pneumoencephalography (Russell *et al.*, 1978). Twenty-four male and four female cluster headache patients with a mean age of 43 years (range 17–70 years) were examined by CT scanning (Delta scan 25) during symptomatic cluster periods. Prior to the introduction of CT scanning, 14 of these patients had been examined by pneumoencephalography, the interval between the two investigations varying between 2 and 6 years. The timing of the CT scan examination varied with regard to the interval following the onset of cluster periods (1–20 weeks) and the interval following the most recent headache attack (0–48 h). Three patients were examined by CT scanning on three occasions during the same cluster period; one of these examinations was carried out during a headache attack.

None of the 28 patients examined by CT scanning showed cerebral parenchymal low densitometric areas, similar to those previously described on CT scan examination in 13–59% of patients with grave attacks of migraine (Cala and Mastaglia, 1976; Hungerford *et al.*, 1976; Mathew *et al.*, 1977; Masland *et al.*, 1978). Borderline widening of the ventricles was assessed as being present in three of the pneumoencephalographic examinations, but in only one of the CT scan examinations. One other patient showed slight cortical atrophy on both pneumoencephalography and CT scanning. The inherent difficulties in defining exact upper normal limits of the widths of the various parts of the ventricular system and cortical sulci on both pneumoencephalography and CT scanning may explain the slight discrepancy which was found on comparison of findings obtained with the two methods. The increase in width of ventricles and sulci which was found in a few patients, just exceeded our normal criteria. The significance of these findings is, therefore, uncertain. The borderline abnormalities observed are probably coincidental findings. There is no evidence for a causal relationship between the changes in central and cortical surface topography and the pathological process in cluster headache. If 'central' changes are present in cluster headache, they are likely to be of a *discrete* nature.

To the best of my knowledge no autopsy studies of cluster headache have been published.

CEREBRAL ANGIOGRAPHY

Carotid arteriograms were obtained in the pain-free phase in five cluster headache patients 'with oculosympathetic paralysis' (Nieman and Hurwitz, 1961) and normal results were obtained in all cases.

CEREBROSPINAL FLUID: VARIOUS STUDIES

Intrathecal injection of saline during attack could ease the headache of cluster headache if it were associated with dilated intracranial arteries. Kunkle *et al.* (1952) did not find that their two cases improved with this technique. On the other hand, the pain was rapidly abolished by ergotamine administered intravenously. Thomas and Butler (cited in Kunkle *et al.*, 1952) arrived at the opposite conclusion: in three of their four patients, pain was readily terminated by injection of saline. Kunkle *et al.* concluded that, in some cases of cluster headache, dilated branches of the external carotid artery are the principal contributors to the pain, while in other patients the source of pain seemed to be intracranial arterial branches.

Kunkle (1959) estimated the content of acetylcholine-like activity in the cerebrospinal fluid from 14 cluster headache patients. Patients with several different types of headache ($n = 23$) were also studied, and patients with various neurological disorders served as controls. The acetylcholine assay was carried out with a biological method, using the heart of the clam as the test organ. The method is apparently most sensitive, the detection limit being as low as $0.001\ \mu g\ ml^{-1}$. Various confirmatory tests for acetylcholine were carried out. Acetylcholine-like activity was found in five male headache patients, four of them suffering from cluster headache ($0.004–0.06\ \mu g\ ml^{-1}$), all apparently being in the symptomatic phase.

The parasympathetic barrage theory in cluster headache still has considerable support, and the interesting results described above may provide further evidence for it. These experiments should be repeated.

THERMOGRAPHY

Horton *et al.* (1939) found the 'surface temperature on the side of the head involved' to be increased by 1–3°C above that on the opposite side under standardized conditions during attacks. The exact areas involved were not specified.

Wood and Friedman (1974) found multiple, small, well demarcated spots of coolness (average diameter 0.5 cm) in the medial, supraorbital area on the symptomatic side during remission in two-thirds of cases (1.0–1.5°C colder than the surrounding skin). The mentioned area is supplied by the frontal and supraorbital branches of the ophthalmic artery. In some cases, small islands of coldness were also found in areas supplied by the external carotid artery. In migraine patients, such changes were only rarely found (2.3% of the cases) and in non-headache controls they were found even more rarely (6 out of 3300 thermograms). The findings, therefore, appeared to be *rather* specific. The authors consider the changes to be manifestations of a 'fixed vascular state'.

In the early phase of attack, Lance (1982) found the forehead to be cooler (by 1°C) on the symptomatic than on the non-symptomatic side, but as the pain approached its maximum a hot spot was frequently detected in the medial part of the orbit on the symptomatic side. During spontaneous ($n = 11$) and induced ($n = 22$) attacks, the area of increased 'heat loss' spread from the orbital area to the supra- and infra-orbital areas and the temporal area. Oxygen inhalation annulled the asymmetry in those patients who also experienced pain relief (Drummond and Lance, 1984). There thus seems to be a transition from one state to another in the course of the attack. As mentioned elsewhere, we (Hørven and Sjaastad, 1977) have demonstrated that the corneal temperature on the symptomatic side also increases during attacks. There may be a connection between these findings.

DOPPLER FLOW-VELOCITY STUDIES

Flow acceleration in the supratrochlear arteries during attacks was invariably found by means of the Doppler technique ($n = 6$, four spontaneous and two nitroglycerin provoked attacks) (Schroth *et al.*, 1983). A moderate flow acceleration was found in the external carotid arteries during attacks, when compared with the headache free stage.

The pulsed Doppler spectral analysis system was used to study extracranial flow velocity in cluster headache (Russell and Lindegaard, 1985). The study group consisted of 37 patients (35 males) who were drug free for at least 48 h prior to study. Velocities were determined in the supratrochlear, temporal, external carotid, internal carotid, common carotid, and vertebral arteries during the interparoxysmal period of a bout and in 18 patients also during a spontaneously occurring attack (during which the common carotid and vertebral flow velocities were not measured). Average and maximum velocities did not differ significantly on the two sides, either during the asymptomatic period or during the attack, as for any of the variables tested.

During attack, the flow velocity was significantly increased in one solitary artery, i.e. the supratrochlear artery, on the symptomatic side in comparison with the pre-attack level, whereas a minor increment on the non-symptomatic side did not reach significance. However, an increase in average and maximum flow velocity was lacking in 6 of 18 attacks. This finding in combination with the lack of flow-velocity asymmetry during attack makes it unlikely that vascular changes on the symptomatic side alone underlie the pain generation.

Ocular (corneal indentation pulse) amplitudes (Hørven and Sjaastad, 1977) invariably increase during attack. Interestingly, flow changes in an 'adjacent' area, the supratrochlear artery were present in only two thirds of the cases studied by Dahl *et al.* (1990). One would *a priori* have expected that rather similar findings would have been made in both areas as regards circulatory variables. The variables studied were of course different in these two investigations, and this may explain the discrepancy between the findings. There may, however, be another explanation for the discrepancy observed; i.e. in the corneal indentation pulse studies only severe attacks were studied. Russell and Lindegaard (1985) did not mention the severity of attacks and it is possible that they studied partly weak attacks.

Gawel and Krajewski (1988) studied the flow velocity in intracranial vessels in 42 cluster headache patients (mean age 42 years) and 44 controls (mean age 51 years). Age was shown not to be a determinant for these parameters. Of the patients studied, 32 suffered from the episodic variety; 35 patients had attacks at the time of examination, two of whom were also studied during attack. Twenty-two patients were on medication (verapamil or lithium) but were still having attacks. No major difference in the mean and peak flow velocities was observed between cluster headache patients and controls. However, there was a significantly more marked interhemispheric difference in patients than in controls, both with regard to the middle and posterior cerebral artery flow velocity (symptomatic > non-symptomatic side) and to anterior cerebral artery flow velocity (symptomatic < non-symptomatic side). These differences were more pronounced when analysing data from the cluster period. In patients on medication, the asymmetry in the middle and posterior cerebral artery velocities was annulled, whereas that in the anterior cerebral artery was accentuated.

Dahl *et al*. (1990) studied middle cerebral artery flow velocity by means of the transcranial Doppler technique. The patients ($n = 25$) were studied interparoxysmally in the bout. Fifteen patients were given 1 mg glycerol trinitrate sublingually, and eight of these developed a headache attack. In addition, 10 spontaneously occurring attacks were studied. Single photon emission computerized tomography (SPECT) with ^{133}Xe inhalation was carried out in seven of the patients in whom attacks were provoked, and a repeat study was conducted in the pain-free phase. The patients were drug free for at least 24 h prior to study. For the flow velocity studies, 10 not quite age- or sex-matched control individuals were used; for the SPECT study, there were 25 control individuals.

A significant flow velocity asymmetry was observed during the interparoxysmal period (69 ± 12 and 65 ± 11 cm s^{-1}, on the symptomatic and non-symptomatic sides, respectively). There was no significant difference between findings on the symptomatic side and the control values.

Nitroglycerin ($n = 15$) caused a significant, bilateral reduction in flow velocity, with a predominance on the symptomatic side (from 68 ± 14 to 49 ± 9 cm s^{-1} on this side and from 63 ± 13 to 50 ± 10 cm s^{-1} on the contralateral one, the *fall* in velocity on the symptomatic side being significantly more marked than that on the opposite side). The fall in flow-velocity values in controls, i.e. from 65 ± 10 to 49 ± 10 cm s^{-1}, did not differ significantly from that in patients. During spontaneously occurring attacks, the flow velocity was reduced from 74 ± 10 to 58 ± 10 cm s^{-1} on the symptomatic side and from 71 ± 10 to 59 ± 11 cm s^{-1} on the opposite side, a non-significant side difference. The decrease *per se* was significant bilaterally ($p < 0.05$). In eight provoked attacks the flow velocity dropped significantly ($p < 0.05$) on both sides, i.e. from 66 ± 13 to 49 ± 11 cm s^{-1} on the symptomatic and from 61 ± 12 to 50 ± 11 cm s^{-1} on the contralateral side.

The maximum decrease in velocity in those who developed attacks and in those who did not ($n = 7$) was of the same order of magnitude. In addition, the magnitude of velocity decrease was essentially no different in those with spontaneous and provoked attacks. There were no drastic changes in flow velocity just prior to onset of attack. It is remarkable that the flow velocity during spontaneous and provoked attacks seems to differ (e.g. on the symptomatic side 58 ± 10 and 49 ± 11 cm s^{-1} respectively).

The reproducibility of the method was tested in 20 healthy individuals (two tests done within 1 h by the same examiner), and a correlation coefficient of 0.95 was found. This is essential information, as far as this type of technique is concerned.

The mean hemispheric cerebral blood flow and the regional cerebral blood flow in the middle cerebral artery perfusion area were within control limits. A test of reproducibility showed that this was good. It was not reported whether the experiment was double-blind.

These two studies employing the transcranial Doppler ultrasound technique had some findings in common: there was a interhemispheric flow velocity asymmetry in cluster headache in the headache-free period. Since Dahl *et al.* found regional cerebral blood flow values (F) within normal limits during attack, the reduction in flow velocity (V) indicates that there is a concurrent increase in vessel diameter ($R = $ radius), according to the equation $F = R^2 \times V$.

The bilateral changes during attack to some extent count against the possibility that these changes are the only mechanism underlying the unilateral attack. The observation that there was no difference in flow velocity reduction in those who did and did not develop an attack in the nitroglycerin experiments points in the same direction.

A particularly intriguing observation is that Gawel *et al.* found a discrepancy between the velocity-flow characteristics in the middle and posterior cerebral arteries on the one hand and anterior cerebral artery on the other. *One* aspect that has not been estimated in these works is the pCO_2 levels during attack. Lowering of pCO_2 exerts a marked influence on cerebral vessel diameters. It is known that cluster headache patients not infrequently hyperventilate during attacks (Sulg and Sjaastad, 1983).

No further speculation can be made on the basis of the presently available data.

WASHOUT OF RADIOISOTOPES INTRADERMALLY

An attempt at measuring cutaneous forehead blood flow during and between attacks was done with intradermally injected ^{99m}Tc pertechnetate (Sjaastad *et al.*, 1974). The patients were without any medication, and only spontaneous attacks were investigated. Patients were in the recumbent position, and had rested at least 5 min prior to the test (room temperature approximately 20°C). The nature of this procedure does not allow measurements to be carried out at the beginning of the attack. An injection of 20 uCi in 0.05 ml of isotonic saline was carried out bilaterally, 4 cm above the outer angle of the eye over the course of 1 min. No skin disinfectant was employed. The washout of the isotope was monitored by means of a γ camera, and background corrected semilogarithmic plots of radioactivity versus time were constructed. The time was measured

Table 2.32   Fractional rate of ^{99}Tc pertechnetate removal from the forehead in episodic cluster headache patients ($n = 6$)[a]

	Mean fractional disappearance rate	
	Symptomatic side	Non-symptomatic side
Between attacks[b]	0.184	0.202
During attacks[b]	0.169[c]	0.174

[a] Controls ($n = 22$): 0.197 ± 0.029 (mean of right and left sides). A high value indicates fast removal. From Sjaastad *et al.* (1974). Courtesy of *Headache*.
[b] The patients were injected once or twice; in the latter case, the mean values were used.
[c] Significantly different from control values (Student's *t*-test, unpaired data; $p < 0.05$).

from the plots from 4 min after the injection until half the 4 min counting value was reached. The fractional rate of removal was then calculated. In six patients with cluster headache, one or two injections were made during attacks and during the asymptomatic period; 22 injections were done in a control group (Table 2.32).

The lowest removal rate was found on the symptomatic side during attack. None of the side differences were statistically significant (Student's *t*-test, paired data). However, the disappearance rate on the symptomatic side during headache was significantly lower than the disappearance rate in control subjects (Student's *t*-test, unpaired data; $p < 0.05$). Increased removal, however, was found during attack in two patients. Increased pulsatile (corneal indentation pulse) amplitudes (which were measured during other attacks (Hørven and Sjaastad, 1977)) were thus associated with both increased and decreased rate of removal.

There are clear limitations to this type of study. First of all, the local application of the radioisotope is critical. In some cases, slight oozing of blood from the injection site appeared, and this oozing was of varying magnitude. In addition, such injections will locally disturb the *milieu intérieure*, and so the existing local pathological situation, if any, may be interfered with. The traumatic hyperaemia lasts for approximately 15–20 min (Sejersen, 1971). For technical reasons, the washout curve from 4 min after injection had to be used in our experiments, although ideally the calculation should have started at 15–20 min. There is also the question of whether or not the removal rate of the isotope really reflects the flow. Furthermore, there may be a considerable difference between findings concerning a given parameter in various stages of an attack, such as observed for the pulse frequency (Russell and von der Lippe, 1982; Russell and Storstein, 1983; Russell, 1985) and facial temperature. Waxing and waning of attack severity is also experienced by a number of patients, and this may also affect many pathophysiological parameters. The results of this investigation must, therefore, be viewed with caution.

REGIONAL CEREBRAL BLOOD FLOW

The first cerebral blood flow (CBF) measurements on cluster headache syndrome were carried out by our group (Broch *et al.*, 1970). Internal carotid blood flow was measured bilaterally using the electromagnetic flow method, during and between attacks in one patient. No changes were seen which indicates that there were no changes in the resistance to peripheral flow. It is emphasized, however, that the lumen of the carotids themselves may be changed appreciably without influencing the flow. It was later ascertained that this patient suffered from chronic paroxysmal hemicrania.

CBF was studied in an ordinary cluster headache patient by means of the intracarotid ^{133}Xe method (Norris *et al.*, 1976). The patient developed an attack at the end of a carotid angiography. A blood flow study about 10 min after the onset of attack showed flow values in the upper normal range (mean 73.6 ml/100 g/min). A normal response to low p_aCO_2 was demonstrated. The mean hemispheric flow value at 33 min was still higher, i.e. 83.1 ml/100 g/min, and this value was interpreted by the authors as showing hyperperfusion. Henry *et al.* (1978) also used the intra-arterial ^{133}Xe method. Normal flow values without any focal changes were invariably found during attack ($n = 3$). No attempt was made to correct the flow values according to p_aCO_2 levels. Nelson *et al.* (1980), compared CBF in spontaneously occurring attacks and attacks precipitated by histamine, nitroglycerin or alcohol. CBF increased during attacks induced by nitroglycerin in three of five patients. During the spontaneously occurring attacks, CBF was either reduced (from 8 to 34%, in three of four patients) or slightly increased. Two suggestions seem to emerge from this investigation: (1) no *uniform* pattern of CBF seems to characterize the cluster headache attack; the CBF might increase or diminish during attack; and (2) there may seem to be a difference between spontaneously occurring and induced attacks as far as CBF is concerned.

Krabbe *et al.* (1984) studied the regional cerebral blood flow with single photon emission tomography in both the interparoxysmal period and during attack ($n = 18$). Attacks were provoked by 12 g alcohol (+ occasionally 1 mg nitroglycerin sublingually), only one attack occurring spontaneously. Eight attacks with a severity of 30–100% were provoked. In the interparoxysmal phase, rCBF was invariably within normal limits. In addition, no significant deviations from the baseline were observed during attack. There was, however, a moderate increase in the central, basal region as well as in the right parietotemporal region. The authors interpret this flow increase as possibly being due to pain activation.

At least two studies have shown diametrically opposite findings, i.e. those of Sakai and Meyer (1978, 1979). In both studies, spontaneously occurring attacks were studied using the isotope inhalation method. The mean grey matter blood flow during headache ($n = 5$) was raised to 94.8 as compared with 73.1 ml/100 g/min in the headache-free period ($n = 7$). Evidence has been found with

CBF studies for an asymmetrical adrenoceptor disorder consistent with a sympathetic denervation supersensitivity (Yamamoto and Meyer, 1980).

Dahl *et al.* (1990; in press) studied the middle cerebral artery and hemispheric flow in seven male cluster headache patients in the interparoxysmal period and during provoked attacks (nitroglycerin). No definite changes were observed for any of these variables. The middle cerebral artery flow values in the attack-free period were: symptomatic side 59.9 ± 10.2 and contralateral side 60.2 ± 9.8 ml/100 mg/min. The corresponding values during attacks were: 58.2 ± 7.5 and 58.9 ± 8.8 ml/100 mg/min, respectively.

Whether methodological problems or diagnostic problems underlie this discrepancy between results is uncertain. The available evidence suggests that CBF during *provoked* attacks seems to be more or less within normal limits, possibly with the exception of the basal, central area. Unfortunately, it has *not* been demonstrated beyond doubt that drug-provoked attacks are identical to spontaneously occurring ones. Therefore, it is required that CBF studies be carried out during an adequate number of spontaneously occurring attacks if definite conclusions are to be made. The balance of evidence seems to point to a more or less normal CBF in spontaneously occurring attacks.

The available evidence may, however, be interpreted in various ways. Recently, Meyer (1987) has stated that: 'in cluster headache, there are some inconsistencies in reports of cephalic blood flow, although virtually all investigators agree that vascular responsiveness is abnormal'.

ELECTROCARDIOGRAPHIC RHYTHM DISTURBANCES DURING ATTACKS: BLOOD PRESSURE AND CARDIOVASCULAR REFLEXES

Horton (1961) noted that the pulse rate in a few cases slowed down from 70 to 45–50 beats/min during attacks. Bruyn *et al.* (1976) found a marked bradycardia in one case.

Hørven and Sjaastad (1977) studied the pulse rate during corneal indentation pulse amplitude recordings in 18 patients with spontaneous attacks in the drug-free state, the measurements generally being made during the pain maximum or late phase of the attack. In most cluster headache patients, slight bradycardia was demonstrated during pain attacks. The average free interval pulse rate was 72.9 beats/min, as against 67.9 beats/min during the attack (no significant difference) (Table 2.33).

Russell and co-workers have made a thorough study of heart rate during attacks (Russell and von der Lippe, 1982; Russell and Storstein, 1983). At the onset of attacks there was a mean *increase* in heart rate, followed by a relative *decrease* during attacks (Figure 2.20). Attacks with onset during sleep started with a heart rate of approximately 18 beats/min lower than those starting when the patient was awake.

These findings suggest an instability in the central regulation of autonomic influences to the heart during attacks. This concept is, to some extent, supported by observations made in patients in whom autonomic impulses via

Table 2.33 Pulse rate in episodic cluster headache patients[a]

	Between pain attacks	During pain attacks	t[b]
Cluster headache ($n = 18$)	72.9	67.9	1.826
Atypical cluster headache ($n = 6$)	69.3	65.0	0.884
Migraine ($n = 22$)	71.0	76.2	1.017
Classic migraine ($n = 5$)	87.8[c]	71.1	3.356[d]

[a] From Hørven and Sjaastad (1977). Courtesy of *Acta Ophthalmologica (Copenhagen)*.
[b] Statistical method of paired comparison.
[c] During scintillation phase.
[d] The pulse rate during the scintillation phase was significantly ($p < 0.05$) increased when compared to the pulse rate during the pain phase.

the parasympathetic and sympathetic nervous system do not reach the heart. In such a situation, variations in heart rate are greatly reduced. In cardiac transplant recipients, donor heart rates are faster than normal and similar to 'intrinsic' heart rates which are obtained by combined vagal and adrenergic blockade (Jose and Collison, 1970; Stinson *et al.*, 1972). Respiratory influences on the donor heart rate are absent, and there is a reduced or absent heart-rate response to various pharmacological and physiological manoeuvres (Cannom *et al.*, 1973).

The initial rapid and transient increase in heart rate at the onset of attack may reflect the beginning of the disturbance leading to the attack. At present, it is

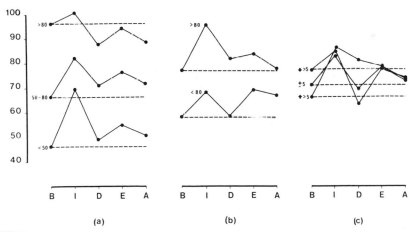

Figure 2.20 Cluster headache, episodic form. Patterns of heart rate change which accompanied attacks, grouped according to: (a) the heart rate before attacks; (b) the initial heart rate (at the onset of attacks); and (c) the change in heart rate during attacks when the latter was compared with the heart rate before attacks (increase >5 beats/min, ±5 beats/min or decrease >5 beats/min). B, Before; I, initial; D, during; E, end; A, after attack. (From Russell (1981). Courtesy of *Cephalalgia*.)

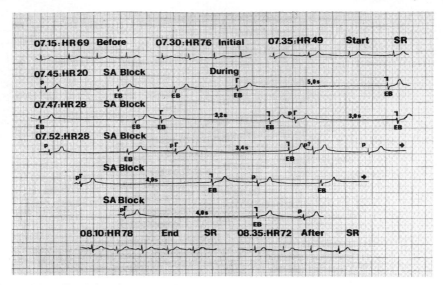

Figure 2.21 Episodic cluster headache: electrocardiogram during an attack, showing bradycardia and sinoatrial (SA) block with nodal or ventricular escape beats (EB). SR, Sinus rhythm; E, end; B, before. (From Russell and Storstein (1983). Courtesy of *Cephalalgia*.)

impossible to explain its cause adequately, but it could be due to an increase in sympathetic activity, a decrease in parasympathetic activity, or a combination of both. It could also be due to a supersensitivity to sympathetic stimuli. The relative decrease in heart rate during the attack suggests a further change in autonomic function as the attack progresses. This finding could be due to a decrease in sympathetic activity, an increase in parasympathetic activity, or a combination of both. A decrease in heart rate does not exclude the possibility of simultaneous parasympathetic and sympathetic stimulation, since it has been shown that moderate vagal stimulation may mask the effects of strong sympathetic stimulation (Levy and Zieske, 1969). The increased variations in heart rate during attacks may also suggest a disturbance in autonomic function to the heart which affects both the parasympathetic and sympathetic nervous systems. On the other hand, it cannot be excluded that turning the activity of only one system 'on' and 'off' may have some rather drastic effects on pulse rate.

Specific electrocardiographic rhythm disturbances, such as sinoatrial block (Figure 2.21), atrioventricular block (Figure 2.22) and atrial fibrillation (Figure 2.23), accompanied attacks of cluster headache in 19% of the cases studied by Russell and Storstein (1983). These rhythm disturbances may also be due to a central disturbance in autonomic function. It is well known that several other conditions which affect the central nervous system may induce electrocardiographic changes and arrhythmia (e.g. Vaisrub, 1975). The pattern of heart-rate change in association with attacks of cluster headache may suggest a 'central'

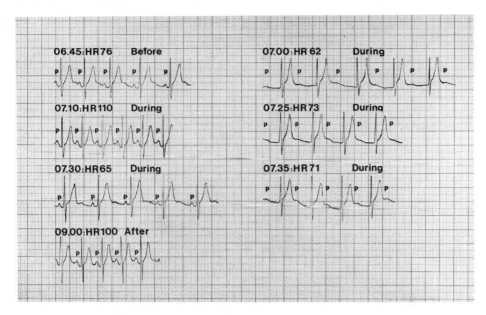

Figure 2.22 Episodic cluster headache: electrocardiogram showing the development of first-degree atrioventricular block during an attack. (From Russell and Storstein (1983). Courtesy of *Cephalalgia*.)

disturbance in autonomic function. More refined underlying mechanisms cannot be defined at the present stage of knowledge. Two things should be borne in mind when discussing the significance of the cardiac rhythm disturbances during attack. First, the intricacies of the autonomic regulatory system for the various autonomically functioning organs are becoming more and more evident. This is also true for the autonomic regulation of the heart. Second, it is not unreasonable to believe that the same type of dysregulation as demonstrated in other organs, e.g. in the sweat glands during cluster headache attack, also takes place in the heart.

Russell and von der Lippe (1982) found that the blood pressure increased slightly, but significantly during attacks in 11 patients with spontaneous attacks (systolic from 127 to 135 mmHg; diastolic from 85 to 94 mmHg). Sacquegna *et al.* (1985) also found an increase in blood pressure in three nitroglycerin induced attacks.

Boiardi *et al.* (1988a) found significant differences between cluster headache patients and controls as regards various tests of cardiovascular reflexes, such as the deep-breathing test, the lying-to-standing test, as well as the Valsalva manoeuvre. Firenze *et al.* (1989) made analogous findings for the first two of these variables. However, no significant difference was found for the Valsalva manoeuvre.

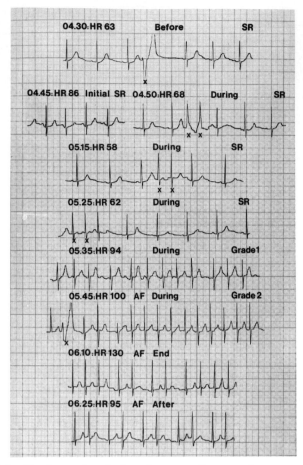

Figure 2.23   Episodic cluster headache: electrocardiogram showing atrial fibrillation (AF), developing during attack and continuing after the attack. SR, Sinus rhythm; ×, supraventricular and ventricular extrasystoles. (From Russell and Storstein (1983). Courtesy of *Cephalalgia*.)

ELECTRONYSTAGMOGRAPHY

Impairment of equilibrium and phonophobia are well recognized features of migraine (Bickerstaff, 1961). For this reason an unselected group of migraine patients (common migraine, $n = 50$; classic migraine, $n = 44$) was investigated by means of electronystagmography and, for comparison, eight cluster headache patients were included (Schlake *et al.*, 1989). All patients were free of medication at the time of investigation. None of the cluster headache patients showed any abnormality. A total of four migraine patients showed various abnormalities, such as spontaneous nystagmus to the one side and spontaneous upbeat nystagmus, which could be suppressed by fixation, indicating a disturbance of central vestibular functions. It is concluded that vestibular dysfunctions, in particular those of central origin, are uncommon in migraine and also in cluster headache. These data contrast with those obtained in previous studies (Raffaelli *et al.*, 1985).

HLA HISTOCOMPATIBILITY ANTIGEN SYSTEM

It is theoretically possible that a disorder like cluster headache can only arise when a combination of two factors is present: a *local* one determining the site of the lesion, and a *general* one allowing the disorder to express itself in that area. The presence of one factor alone makes it permissible to develop the disorder, but the very presence of the other factor would be mandatory for the disorder to become clinically manifest.

In a search for the general factor, the histocompatibility complex has been studied in episodic cluster headache (Kudrow, 1978; Cuypers and Altenkirch, 1979). No definite deviations from normal were found in these studies. Giacovazzo *et al.* (1984), however, have claimed that there are more cluster headache patients than controls that lack human leukocyte antigen B14 (HLA-B14). Another interesting aspect was that patients lacking HLA-B14 seemed to be the best responders to lithium.

Cuypers and Altenkirch (1979) examined five cases of chronic cluster headache, in whom the HLA-A$_1$ antigen was invariably found. The number of cases studied in the latter respect is as yet too limited to allow any definite conclusions to be drawn. This finding may, if reproduced, open up new perspectives in this field. Until proven otherwise, the possibility seems to exist that the chronic form of cluster headache differs fundamentally from the episodic one in this respect.

ORBITAL PHLEBOGRAPHY

Milstein and Morretin (1971) discovered that a patient with sphenoid fissure syndrome (Tolosa–Hunt syndrome) showed pathological changes in the superior ophthalmic vein, a finding corroborated by others (e.g. Muhletaler and Gerlock, 1979; Hoes *et al.*, 1981).

In a series of healthy individuals ($n = 23$), only one positive finding was made, whereas 13 of 19 cases of Tolosa–Hunt syndrome (68%) showed a pathological phlebographic pattern. The pathological findings were as follows: narrowing of the superior ophthalmic vein (either along its entire course or in its third segment), partial occlusion of the cavernous sinus, or collateral veins in the vicinity of the superior orbital fissure (Hannerz *et al.*, 1984). A rather high proportion of patients with Tolosa–Hunt syndrome thus have a normal phlebographic pattern. These findings indicate that in Tolosa–Hunt syndrome there may be false-negative phlebograms, but hardly false-positive ones. An

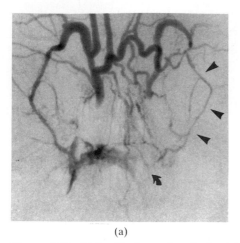 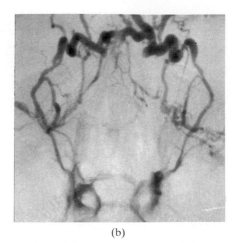

(a)   (b)

Figure 2.24   Episodic cluster headache: (a) narrowing of the entire superior ophthalmic vein on the left side (arrowheads) and partial occlusion of the cavernous sinus (arrow); (b) normal orbital phlebogram for comparison. (From Hannerz *et al.* (1987a). Courtesy of *Cephalalgia*.)

abnormal phlebographic pattern, therefore, seems to have pathological significance. Later, Hannerz *et al.* (1986) also demonstrated that similar phlebographic changes were present in 52% of patients with the characteristic pain of Tolosa–Hunt syndrome, but without the ophthalmoplegia ($n = 96$). Most of these cases, however, had visual disturbances (which also responded to steroids).

Hannerz *et al.* (1987a) then extended their studies to include cluster headache ($n = 13$). The phlebograms were interpreted in a blind manner. In eight of the patients (61%) they found a pathological phlebogram, in five of them on both sides, and in three on the symptomatic side only. In two of the patients with bilateral changes, the abnormality was most marked on the symptomatic side. The changes observed were the same as those that occur in the Tolosa–Hunt syndrome (Figure 2.24). Six patients were studied during and outside attacks. In one patient, a narrowing of a short segment of the supraorbital vein and an irregular calibre of the superior ophthalmic vein were detected during the attack (Figure 2.25). It is thus remarkable that changes typical of the Tolosa–Hunt syndrome also occur in cluster headache and to the same degree and with approximately the same frequency as in the Tolosa–Hunt syndrome (and in Tolosa–Hunt-like syndrome).

The implications of these findings are not obvious: the vascular changes in these headache forms are frequently bilateral, whereas the headache and the clinical deficiency symptoms and signs are unilateral. The subjectivity of the rating of the abnormality is a drawback. On the other hand, the assessment of the phlebograms in Hannerz *et al.*'s studies was done blindly. These findings may, therefore, be of localizing importance in cluster headache. The retro-

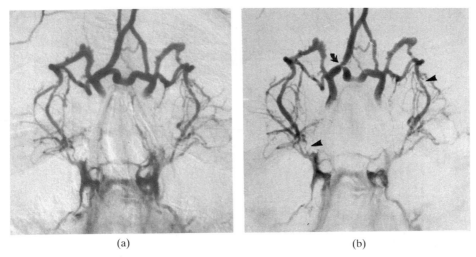

(a)   (b)

Figure 2.25   Episodic cluster headache: orbital phlebography before (a) and during (b) an attack. In (b) a constriction is seen in the supraorbital vein (arrow); caliber variations in the superior ophthalmic veins are shown (arrowheads). (From Hannerz *et al.* (1987a). Courtesy of *Cephalalgia*.)

orbital drainage system—that is, the superior ophthalmic vein and the cavernous sinus—may be affected in all three mentioned disorders and even in chronic paroxysmal hemicrania (see Chronic Paroxysmal Hemicrania) (Sjaastad, 1988b). The *nature* of the involvement in these disorders may be what makes them different, and not the localization (see also Pathogenesis).

CORNEAL INDENTATION PULSE AMPLITUDES: DYNAMIC TONOMETRY

Not only is the *pain* localized in and about the eye in cluster headache, but local phenomena, like conjunctival injection, indicate that pathological processes occur in this area. The eye itself has indeed been proven to be a source of useful information concerning cluster headache attack. A major technique for obtaining such information is dynamic tonometry (Hørven *et al.*, 1971b, 1972; Hørven and Sjaastad, 1977).

The dynamic tonometer (Hørven, 1968) is an improved, standardized, electronic Schiøtz tonometer that records eye tension and corneal indentation pulse (CIP) amplitudes at all tension levels. The output is 1 mV per micrometre of tonometer plunger movement, and the output is linear. An output of 50 mV, therefore, corresponds to 50 μm of plunger deflection, that is one scale reading Schiøtz. The CIP amplitudes recorded by dynamic tonometry reflect the pulse–synchronous alterations in intraocular pressure. This is again dependent on the pulse–synchronous change in intraocular volume (ΔV), caused by the extra amount of blood which enters the eye during systole. An increased pulse rate usually creates a decrease in CIP amplitudes (Hørven and Gjønnæss, 1974).

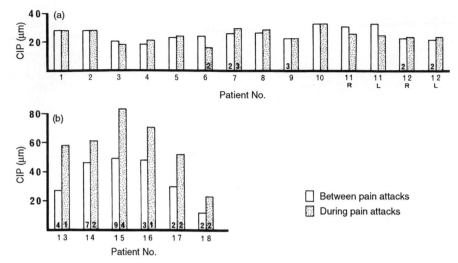

Figure 2.26 Corneal indentation pulse (CIP) amplitudes on the symptomatic side during and between attacks of (a) migraine and (b) episodic cluster headache. R, right side; L, left side. (From Hørven *et al.* (1972). Courtesy of *Neurology* (*Minneapolis*).)

The pulse–synchronous change in intraocular volume (ΔV) may be calculated (in mm^3) from the CIP amplitudes by the use of converting tables based on the data of Langham and Hetland-Eriksen (Hørven, 1970a). Multiplication by the exact pulse rate gives the ΔV per minute. The reproducibility of the method is generally better than ±5%.

A typical registration curve is shown on page 341 under Chronic Paroxysmal Hemicrania (see Figure 4.21). In a preliminary study (Hørven *et al.*, 1971b), 12 migraine and six cluster headache patients were studied during and between attacks (Figure 2.26). In cluster headache, contrary to the case in migraine, there was invariably an increase in CIP amplitudes during attack. In continued investigations (Hørven and Sjaastad, 1977), 18 patients (3 females, 15 males, average age 53.5 years) with typical, episodic cluster headache were examined between and during spontaneously occurring attacks (Table 2.34). This group was compared with two other groups.

1. A group of 22 migraine patients (13 females, 9 males; average age 36.6 years) who were examined during and between pain attacks. Thirteen suffered from classic migraine (five of whom were examined both during scintillation and during a subsequent pain attack) and nine from common migraine ('migraine without aura'). This series was selected because we also wanted to study the 'aura' phase.
2. A group of six patients with 'atypical cluster headache'; two of these cases suffered from what was later recognized as chronic paroxysmal hemicrania. Another case in this group was a female (aged 39 years) with recurring bouts of ipsilateral, retrobulbar neuritis and with a coagulation

Table 2.34 Corneal indentation pulse (CIP) amplitudes (μm) in episodic cluster headache patients[a]

	N	Symptomatic side				Non-symptomatic side			
		Between pain attacks	During pain attacks	t^b	p	Between pain attacks	During pain attacks	t^b	p
Cluster headache	18	23.6	34.8	5.267	<0.001	23.0	28.3	3.290	<0.005
Atypical cluster headache	6	44.2	71.7	4.292	<0.005	40.5	58.5	3.473	<0.02
Migraine	22	26.0	25.1	1.168	—	25.5	24.4	1.098	—
Classic migraine	5	24.8[c]	25.4	0.440	—	24.8[c]	24.8	0.094	—

[a]From Hørven and Sjaastad (1977). Courtesy of *Acta Ophthalmologica* (*Copenhagen*).
[b]Statistical method of paired comparison.
[c]During scintillation phase.

factor (factor XII) deficiency (Sjaastad *et al.*, 1976; Sjaastad *et al.*, 1988b) (see Symptomatic Cluster Headache-like Picture). Two cases demonstrated marked interparoxysmal electroencephalographic changes during bouts and had less clear-cut attacks than is usually seen in cluster headache. These cases were selected as being at variance with ordinary cluster headache prior to CIP amplitude measurements, due to these unusual traits. This group of 'atypical' cases accordingly consisted of various disorders.

No appreciable change in CIP amplitudes was found during *migraine* attacks, be it during the prodromal or the pain phase (Table 2.34). The CIP amplitudes in migraine were of equal size in the two eyes and averaged about 25 μm, which is slightly less than the normal average of 30 ± 10 μm (mean ± SD) (range 13–56 μm (Hørven, 1970b). In the interparoxysmal period in *cluster headache*, the amplitudes were a little lower than those observed in migraine (Tables 2.34 and 2.35). During pain attacks, a statistically significant increase in CIP amplitudes was found, being most pronounced on the symptomatic side. In control individuals, the asymmetry was negligible (Hørven, 1970b).

Attacks also co-existed with increased CIP amplitudes (most pronounced on the symptomatic side) in the *atypical cluster headache* group. However, the CIP amplitudes in cluster headache just barely exceeded the mean control amplitudes. As a matter of fact, the 'atypical cluster headache' patients showed CIP amplitudes which, on average, were about twice as large as those observed in ordinary cluster headache patients (Tables 2.34 and 2.35). The observed cluster headache versus atypical cluster headache (symptomatic side) differences were significant during attacks $p < 0.01$; between attacks $p < 0.01$ (Wilcoxon–White two sample rank test).

Thus, the CIP amplitude pattern seems, to some extent, to distinguish 'atypical cluster headache' patients from ordinary cluster headache patients. The larger CIP amplitudes in most of the atypical cases both between and during attacks suggest either a larger intraocular vascular bed in these patients,

Table 2.35 Corneal indentation pulse amplitudes (μm) in episodic cluster headache, 'atypical cluster headache' and migraine patients, during and between attacks[a]

	N	Between pain attacks				During pain attacks			
		Sympto-matic side	Other side	t^b	p	Sympto-matic side	Other side	t^b	p
Cluster headache	18	23.6	23.0	1.401	NS	34.8	28.3	4.744	<0.001
Atypical cluster headache	6	44.2	40.5	2.412	NS	71.7	58.5	5.518	<0.001
Migraine	22	26.0	25.5	1.308	NS	25.1	24.4	1.061	NS
Classic migraine	5	24.8[c]	24.8[c]	0	NS	25.4	24.8	0.612	NS

NS, not significant.
[a]From Hørven and Sjaastad (1977). Courtesy of *Acta Ophthalmologica* (*Copenhagen*).
[b]Statistical method of paired comparison.
[c]During scintillation phase.

or a true difference in the pathogenesis of these disorders. It is again emphasized, however, that the 'atypical cluster headache' group is heterogeneous; the group even includes some patients with chronic paroxysmal hemicrania. Accordingly, such atypical cases should probably be classified and listed separately from ordinary cluster headache patients, although the link with ordinary cluster headache is appreciable (see So-called Atypical Cluster Headache).

As far as the ΔV per minute is concerned, a statistically significant difference between sides during attacks was found in cluster headache, with larger values on the symptomatic side (mean 220 and 177 mm^3 min^{-1}, respectively) and in atypical cluster headache (mean 453 and 371 mm^3 min^{-1}, respectively). A clear, statistically significant, increment occurred as a consequence of attack on both sides in cluster headache (160 before and 220 mm^3 min^{-1} during attack on the symptomatic side, vs. 157 before and 177 mm^3 min^{-1} during attack on the non-symptomatic side). The increased ΔV per minute during pain attacks in these patients demonstrates that the CIP amplitude increment by far outweighs the bradycardia effect *per se* (Hørven and Sjaastad, 1977). Accordingly, the increment in amplitudes cannot be explained by the bradycardia alone, a factor which should anyway affect the non-symptomatic side to the same degree as the symptomatic side. The asymmetry of the CIP amplitudes seems to be an integral part of the attack, the underlying pathology of which resides within the eye, although it may be influenced by extrinsic forces like the nerve and vascular supply to the eye.

INTRAOCULAR PRESSURE

The intraocular pressure (IOP) (in mmHg) was calculated from the tonometer readings (5.5 g plunger weight) by using Friedenwald's 1955 converting tables

Table 2.36　Intraocular pressure (mmHg) in episodic cluster headache, 'atypical cluster headache' and migraine patients, during and between attacks[a]

		Between pain attacks				During pain attacks			
	N	Symptomatic side	Other side	t^b	p	Symptomatic side	Other side	t^b	p
Cluster headache	18	12.3	12.1	0.756	—	13.7	11.9	3.411	<0.005
Atypical cluster headache	6	12.8	12.8	0	—	15.5	14.1	1.998	—
Migraine	22	14.5	14.5	0.208	—	14.2	14.6	1.128	—
Classic migraine	5	15.0[c]	15.1[c]	0.147[c]	—	14.5	14.9	0.370	—

[a]From Hørven and Sjaastad (1977). Courtesy of *Acta Ophthalmologica (Copenhagen)*.
[b]Statistical method of paired comparison.
[c]During scintillation phase.

(Friedenwald, 1957). The IOP was measured in the same groups of patients used for corneal indentation pulse measurements (see previous section). Between pain attacks, there was no asymmetry in the IOP values in any of the groups, the values in the migraine group being somewhat higher than those in the other groups (Hørven and Sjaastad, 1977). During pain attacks (Table 2.36), a moderate, but invariable and statistically significant increase in IOP was found on the symptomatic side in patients with cluster headache ($p < 0.005$). The average IOP did, however, *not* increase on the non-symptomatic side during attacks. A similar trend was also noted in the 'atypical cluster headache' group but, probably due to the small sample size, no significant difference was obtained. No change in IOP occurred in 22 patients with migraine in either the scintillation or the headache phase.

Barré (1983) has more recently made similar observations to ours in nine cluster headache patients during a total of 15 attacks, induced by nitroglycerin. An asymmetric increase in IOP was observed on 14 occasions (symptomatic side > non-symptomatic side) and a symmetric increase on one, the average increments on the two sides being 48% and 21%, respectively. These increments are somewhat higher than those observed by us. This may have to do with the phase of attack studied or with the fact that Barré studied provoked and not spontaneous attacks.

CORNEAL TEMPERATURE

The corneal temperature was recorded using a specially constructed thermometer probe and a Brush Mark 220 recorder. The temperature tracings can be read to an accuracy of less than 0.1°C (Hørven and Larsen, 1975), and the method gives good reproducibility. Pilot studies of patients with common ('without aura') and classic migraine showed no alteration in corneal temperature during the scintillation and pain phases.

Table 2.37 Corneal temperature (in +°C) during and between attacks in episodic cluster headache patients[a]

Patient No.	Between pain attacks			During pain attacks		
	Symptomatic side	Other side	Difference	Symptomatic side	Other side	Difference
1	33.8	33.7	0.1	34.2	33.7	0.5
2	33.2	33.1	0.1	33.4	32.5	0.9
3	32.5	32.3	0.2	34.9	33.5	1.4
4	32.4	32.6	−0.2	33.9	32.7	1.2
5	32.7	33.0	−0.3	33.6	32.8	0.8
6	34.65	34.8	−0.15	35.3	33.15	0.15
7	32.15	32.1	0.05	32.2	31.4	0.8
Average	33.06	33.09	−0.03	33.93	33.11	0.82
t^b		0.407			5.229	$p < 0.005$

[a]From Hørven and Sjaastad (1977). Courtesy of *Acta Ophthalmologica* (*Copenhagen*).
[b]Statistical method of paired comparison.

In ordinary cluster headache, no side difference was found in the period between pain attacks (Hørven and Sjaastad, 1977), the average corneal temperature being +33.1°C, which is slightly less than the control average of +33.7°C (Hørven, 1975). During pain attacks (Table 2.37), the corneal temperature increased significantly on the symptomatic side as compared with the pre-attack level ($p < 0.005$) and as compared with the non-symptomatic side during attacks ($p < 0.005$). There was no similar increment on the non-symptomatic side. In patients with 'atypical cluster headache' an interparoxysmal difference of +0.6°C was demonstrated, with the higher value on the symptomatic side. This difference increased markedly during pain and had an average value of +1.63°C.

The interpretation of the latter findings is not easy. Theoretically, a rise in corneal temperature could be caused by excessive lacrimation (Mapstone, 1968), or by heat conducted to the cornea from the surrounding tissue, from the ciliary body, or from the posterior part of the eye. That warm tears should affect the registration directly seems rather unlikely, since the contact probe was specially constructed to shield it from the influence of tears. The temperature sensor is located in the very centre of the 3-mm diameter probe tip (Hørven and Larsen, 1975). The possibility that warm tears could conduct heat to the corneal stroma itself was tested in eight healthy subjects with the following results: average corneal temperature before lacrimation, right 34.74°C, left 34.61°C. Following 3 min excessive lacrimation precipitated by mechanical irritation of the nasal mucosa, the mean temperature was: right 34.78°C, left 34.40°C. Accordingly, the effect of lacrimation *per se* on corneal temperature seems to be negligible.

Horton *et al.* (1939) found a ±1–3°C rise in cutaneous temperature on the symptomatic side of the head during attacks in cluster headache patients (see Thermography). However, cold patches have also been found around the eye, even at the beginning of an attack (Lance and Anthony, 1971b; Wood and Friedman, 1974). These cold patches may fade away as a consequence of attack. A mediation of heat from the surroundings to the cornea during attack cannot entirely be ruled out. The most likely explanation for the observed rise in corneal temperature during pain attacks is probably an acute intraocular vasodilatation, which presumably exists (as judged from the dynamic tonometry results). An intraocular vasodilatation might tend to reduce the temperature gradient between the posterior and anterior parts of the eye. Experimentally, a rise in ocular temperature of +2–4°C was found in cats and dogs by compression of the abdominal aorta, thus forcing more preheated blood towards the animal's eye (Colle *et al.*, 1931).

SIGNIFICANCE OF OPHTHALMOLOGIC ABNORMALITIES

What inferences can be made from the results of intraocular pressure (IOP) and corneal indentation pulse (CIP) amplitude measurements? In cluster headache, the CIP amplitudes and ΔV per minute are in fact relatively small prior to attacks. During pain, however, they increase by a mean of somewhat less than 50% on the symptomatic side together with an increase in IOP and corneal temperature. In 'atypical cluster headache', similar, but more pronounced, changes take place during an attack. In most of the latter cases, the CIP amplitudes and ΔV per minute were also relatively large between attacks.

The possibility that the findings can be explained on the basis of methodological errors or by the fact that the patients were examined repeatedly and at different times of the day and at various intervals can probably be rejected. Measurable changes in ocular rigidity did not occur, and the slight bradycardia which was seen during pain attacks can only explain a small fraction of the CIP amplitude increment. It is highly unlikely that voluntary squeezing of extraocular muscles secondary to the pain could explain these findings. First, we did not note any such squeezing during attack when IOP/CIP were measured. Second, the increase in IOP/CIP seems to follow a rather regular curve, values increasing with increasing pain (also observed as far as IOP is concerned by Barré (1983)). The increase is bilateral, and probably almost always less on the non-symptomatic side. To 'squeeze' the extraocular muscles constantly and in such a regular fashion that an IOP of similar magnitude and asymmetry is produced in all attacks is virtually impossible. Last, but not least, in chronic paroxysmal hemicrania—a closely related headache—autonomic phenomena, like lacrimation and sweating (which probably have the same common denominator aetiologically speaking as the IOP/CIP) clearly arise *prior to* the pain. The increase of 50% or more in CIP, as partly observed in cluster headache syndrome and 'atypical cluster headache' patients during pain attacks is, therefore, probably far beyond what can be explained by methodological errors or physiological variations. A statistically significant difference between sides, as present during pain attacks, is never seen under physiological conditions.

There seems to be a certain relationship between amplitude and the state of the intraocular vessels. Even changes in the lumen of the carotid artery, such as in carotid artery occlusive disease or after graded external reduction of the lumen, have a major impact on the CIP amplitudes (reduction in amplitudes) (Hørven et al., 1971; Nornes et al., 1971a,b). If vasospasms occur, like in pre-eclampsia, the amplitudes are small (Hørven and Gjønnæss, 1974). A 50% reduction in amplitude is also observed following retrobulbar injection of adrenaline. However, if vasodilatation prevails, as in Horner's syndrome, an increase in amplitudes is found. Increased amplitudes during attacks may thus indicate that vasodilatation has taken place in the eye. In other words, there seems to be an increment in the pulsatile part of the intraocular vascular bed. These conclusions are drawn mainly by analogy, and for this reason are not necessarily absolutely correct. Deductions as to the total blood flow through the eye can only be made to a limited extent on the basis of such reasoning. The basic abnormality in the vascular system of the eye during attacks of cluster headache does not necessarily have to be a vasodilatation. Hypothetically, vasoconstriction could occur in more distal segments of the intraocular vessels and could be the crucial abnormality. In this case, the increased amplitudes could be a reflection of an effort to overcome an increased resistance to the blood flow through the eye. In our estimation, the latter possibility is unlikely.

The changes observed in CIP amplitudes and ΔV per minute should be viewed as pathophysiological characteristics of these disorders. Dynamic tonometry is, therefore, a practical method which may aid in the diagnosis of patients suffering from cluster headache and 'atypical cluster headache', besides providing an avenue for further insight into these headaches.

Many other autonomic abnormalities occur during an attack of cluster headache, e.g. changes in heart rate, lacrimation, nasal secretion and forehead sweating (see previous sections). It is not unreasonable to assume that there is a *common source* of all these manifestations. These manifestations are widespread and even bilateral. A unilateral defect along the third sympathetic neuron would hardly be sufficient to produce all these manifestations of the attack (see also Pathogenesis). It is also questionable whether all these manifestations are sympathetic in nature. The picture may be very complex, and the possibility also exists that part of the IOP increment could be caused by intraocular extravasation. Neurologically mediated extravasation is known to occur in other intracranial structures and is even beneficially influenced by ergot alkaloids (Markowitz et al., 1988). Oedema formation is observed in extraocular and periocular tissues on rare occasions in cluster headache (see Oedema).

QUANTIFICATION OF SALIVATION

Several investigators have described increased salivation during attack (e.g. Horton, 1952; Graham, personal communication). Some of our patients have told us that they had abundant and thick saliva during attacks.

Salivation has been quantitated by means of a collecting system developed in our laboratory. For details and a validation of the collecting method the reader is referred to Saunte's (1983) work. With this system, the fluid produced can be collected quantitatively from each of the two sides of the mouth floor and expressed in millilitres per minute. The average salivation in the *basal state* (24 tests in 14 patients) was of the same order of magnitude as in a control group of 20 students (i.e. around 0.12 ml min^{-1}). During *the attack* (eight severe and 12 moderate attacks in six patients), only minute quantities of saliva were collected, the quantities being measurable in only three patients. There was no demonstrable asymmetry of saliva production. Increased salivation does thus not seem to be an integral part of the regular cluster headache attack. Naturally, there may be exceptions to this rule.

Pilocarpine administration outside attack (0.1 mg/kg body weight; 24 tests in 14 patients) resulted in drastic bilateral salivation (mean ratio pilocarpine: basal state 13.8 and 13.0 on the symptomatic and non-symptomatic sides, respectively). The pilocarpine stimulated salivation was slightly, but not significantly lower than in controls (Figure 2.27). These observations show that, in general,

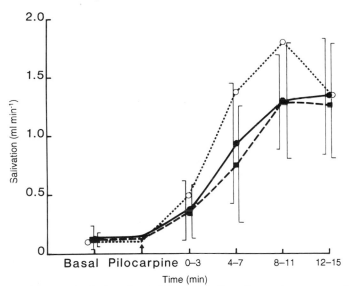

Figure 2.27 Salivation in the basal condition and after pilocarpine provocation (0.1 mg/kg body weight, subcutaneously) in episodic cluster headache patients (14 patients outside attacks) and controls (*n* = 20). Each point represents mean ± 1 SD. (●) Symptomatic side; (■) non-symptomatic side; (○) mean of right and left sides in controls. (From Saunte (1984a). Courtesy of *Cephalalgia*.)

the patterns during attack and as a result of parasympathetic stimulations differ fundamentally as far as salivation is concerned. Although the properties of pilocarpine may seem to be manifold (Newsome and Loewenfeld, 1974; Day, 1979), these results tend to show that the autonomic manifestations of the cluster headache attack are unlikely to be due to an extensive parasympathetic stimulation alone.

QUANTIFICATION OF LACRIMATION

Lacrimation has been quantified in cluster headache in our laboratory by using Schirmer's test tapes (Schirmer, 1909). The average lacrimation during the *basal state* (24 tests in 14 patients) was at approximately the same level (about 18 mm min^{-1}) as in control individuals ($n = 20$), and there was no significant asymmetry (Saunte, 1983, 1984a,b).

A total of eight severe and 12 moderate cluster headache *attacks* were studied in six patients. Lacrimation increasd on the symptomatic side during *all* 'severe attacks' and, on average, increased above the basal secretion by a factor of 2.1. Lacrimation on the non-symptomatic side increased less (by a factor of 1.4), but in six of eight severe attacks the lacrimation also exceeded the basal secretion on this side. The mean symptomatic/non-symptomatic side ratio during eight severe attacks was 2.81, whereas it was 1.90 during the moderate attacks (Table 2.38). *Pilocarpine* administration (0.1 mg/kg body weight; 24 tests in 14 patients) led to a moderate increase in lacrimation which was only slightly asymmetric (slightly greater on the symptomatic side) (Figure 2.28). The increment during pilocarpine stimulation was of the same magnitude in both patients and controls.

The mean *increment* of lacrimation during attack was several times greater on the symptomatic than on the non-symptomatic side. The moderate increase in

Table 2.38 Mean symptomatic/non-symptomatic side ratios of nasal secretion and lacrimation as a function of attack severity in episodic cluster headache patients[a]

	No. tests	Mean attack severity (%)	Mean symptomatic/ non-symptomatic ratio	
			Nasal secretion	Lacrimation
Basal condition	24	0	1.18	1.28
Weak attacks	12	34	1.37	1.90
Severe attacks	8	74	1.80	2.81
Excruciatingly severe attacks[b]	4	90–100	1.94	2.92

[a]From Saunte (1984a). Courtesy of *Cephalalgia*.
[b]These four attacks are also included in the group with 'severe attacks'.

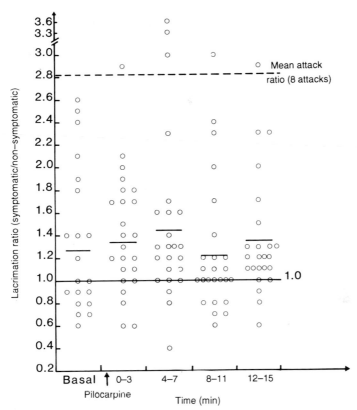

Figure 2.28 Lacrimation in the basal condition and after pilocarpine provocation (0.1 mg/kg body weight, subcutaneously) in episodic cluster headache patients (*n* = 14; outside attack). The horizontal lines indicate the unweighted mean ratio for each time interval. The mean ratio during attacks of headache was 2.8 (six patients; eight attacks). (From Saunte (1984a). Courtesy of *Cephalalgia*.)

attack-related lacrimation on the non-symptomatic side is the main reason why this may not be clinically apparent.

The question then arises whether lacrimation *invariably* increases on the symptomatic side during an attack. This question cannot be answered properly on the basis of our limited data. However, in all of the eight severe attacks studied, lacrimation exceeded the control limits on the symptomatic side (Saunte, 1984a). The techniques used were coarse. If more refined methods had been used, it might have been possible to detect even minor increments, such as on the non-symptomatic side during mild attacks, that the coarse methods could not detect due to a lack of sufficient sensitivity.

QUANTIFICATION OF NASAL SECRETION

Nasal secretion has been quantified by Saunte (1983, 1984a,b), using Schirmer's test tapes (Schirmer, 1909). The strips were inserted to a point approximately

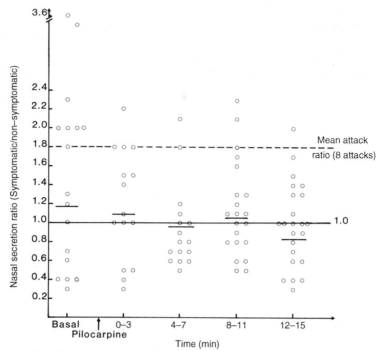

Figure 2.29   Nasal secretion in the basal condition and that produced by pilocarpine (0.1 mg/kg body weight) in episodic cluster headache patients. The mean values for each time interval are marked by a horizontal line and the mean attack ratio is marked by a horizontal broken line, i.e. 1.8 (six patients; eight attacks). (From Saunte (1984a). Courtesy of *Cephalalgia*.)

15 mm above the opening of the nares, and they were made to adhere to the septal mucosa. The secretion measured in this way, therefore, reflects the endogenous secretion from the nasal septal wall. The irritative effect of the strips in this position seems to be very moderate. The secretion under *basal conditions* (24 tests in 14 patients) was slightly higher on the symptomatic than on the non-symptomatic side (Table 2.38). This secretion was of the same magnitude as that in controls ($n = 20$).

Secretion was measured during eight severe and 12 moderate attacks in six patients. During the eight severe attacks, the secretion exceeded the basal one on both sides, but to a higher degree on the symptomatic than on the non-symptomatic side. The mean symptomatic/non-symptomatic side ratio was 1.8 during severe attacks, and 1.37 during moderate attacks (Table 2.38). During *pilocarpine stimulation* (0.1 mg/kg body weight, 24 tests in 14 patients), the secretion approximately doubled and was of the same level of magnitude as that in controls. There was no clear asymmetry (Figure 2.29).

SIGNIFICANCE OF ATTACK-RELATED SALIVATION, RHINORRHOEA AND LACRIMATION

Severe attacks are associated with lacrimation and nasal secretion exceeding normal limits, and the increase is bilateral, although less marked on the non-symptomatic side. In the basal state, there is no clear difference between patients and controls. It should be noted that similar findings, i.e. that the increase is bilateral although most marked on the symptomatic side, have also been made for forehead sweating and corneal indentation pulse (CIP) amplitudes (see appropriate preceding sections and Table 2.39). Intraocular pressure seems to be an exception to this rule, since it has been shown to decrease slightly, if anything, on the non-symptomatic side during attack. The discrepancy between the CIP amplitudes and intraocular pressure in this respect is interesting, but is poorly understood at present. Another remarkable feature is the striking difference between nasal secretion and lacrimation, on the one hand (a clear increment has been found during attack), and salivation (no increase), on the other. This may indicate that the stimuli reaching these autonomically innervated glands during attack are not purely parasympathetic in nature. A sympathetic drive (or, perhaps, supersensitivity phenomena) could possibly explain the lack of salivation and possibly also the lacrimation. It should be emphasized that the situation may be very complicated, since the innervation of the glands involved may be very intricate. The rule of 'one nerve, one transmitter' no longer applies.

Table 2.39 Various 'autonomic' parameters in episodic cluster headache patients[a]

		Between attacks		During attack	
	n	Symptomatic side	Non-symptomatic side[b]	Symptomatic side	Non symptomatic side[b]
CIP[c] amplitude (μm)	18	23.6	23.0	34.8	28.3
ΔV[d] (mm^3 min^{-1})	18	159.9	157.3	219.7	177.1
Sweating (g m^{-2} h^{-1})	8	18	16	98	42
Lacrimation ratio[e]	8		1.28		2.8[f]
Rhinorrhoea ratio[e]	8		1.18		1.8[g]

[a] From Sjaastad *et al.* (1985). Courtesy of *Cephalalgia*.
[b] Note that the values for the non-symptomatic side increase for all variables during attacks.
[c] CIP, corneal indentation pulse.
[d] Pulse–synchronous change in intraocular volume (ΔV); this is caused by the extra amount which enters the eye during the systole.
[e] Symptomatic side; non-symptomatic side.
[f] In six of eight severe attacks, tearing on the non-symptomatic side exceeded the basal lacrimation level. The mean ratio of attack-induced/basal secretion on the non-symptomatic side was 1.4.
[g] Nasal secretion was invariably increased on the non-symptomatic side during eight severe attacks. The mean ratio of attack-induced/basal secretion on the non-symptomatic side was 1.4.

FOREHEAD SWEATING DURING ATTACK

Until we began such studies in 1977 no quantitative estimations of sweating had been carried out in cluster headache and atypical cluster headache (Sjaastad *et al.*, 1978, 1981, 1982; Sjaastad, 1981, 1982a). We monitored sweating in a thermo-room at a temperature of $27 \pm 1°C$ using an Evaporimeter (Nilsson, 1977). Sweating was calculated as grams per square metre per hour $(g\,m^{-2}\,h^{-1})$. Three different sites on the forehead were selected for measurements: directly above the inner canthus (I), above the pupil (II), and above the outer canthus (III), all points approximately 1.5 cm above the superciliary ridge. Much of the time sweating was also measured on two additional spots, that is directly below the eye (IV) and on the upper eyelid (V) (see Figure 2.30). Sweating was also, in the first part of our study, assessed at certain, fixed positions elsewhere on the body, i.e. on the abdomen, thorax, neck and upper extremities. Sweating was always measured bilaterally.

We compared sweating during *spontaneously occurring cluster headache attacks* (31 attacks in 18 patients) with sweating in a control group of healthy individuals (*n* = 25). No drugs had been given on the day of study or on the two

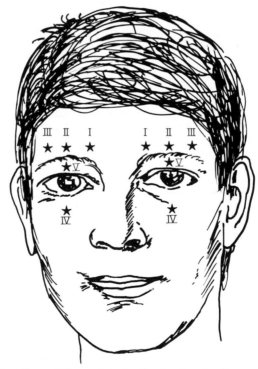

Figure 2.30 The location of the points in the forehead where sweat measurements were routinely carried out. The measurements were always done on the right side first and then on the left side for each of the points I–V. (From Sjaastad *et al.* (1981). Courtesy of *Cephalalgia*.)

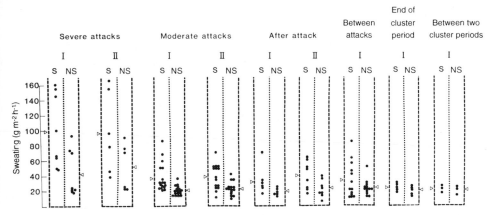

Figure 2.31 Forehead sweating (mean values) during various phases of the cluster cycle in episodic cluster headache patients. The control values were (mean ± SD): position I, 15.3 ± 5.2; position II, 13.7 ± 6.7; position III, 12.6 ± 5.7 g m^{-2} h^{-1}. S, Symptomatic side; N-S, non-symptomatic side. (From Sjaastad *et al.* (1981). Courtesy of *Cephalalgia*.)

preceding days. Most patients also acted as their own controls, in that measurements were also carried out outside attacks, either within the cluster period or between two cycles.

During eight severe attacks (>50% of maximal pain), sweating was *clearly* and *invariably* increased in the central part of the forehead on the symptomatic side, that is site I (symptomatic side 98.9 ± 49.1 (mean ± SD) versus non-symptomatic side 42.4 ± 30.9 g m^{-2} h^{-1}; controls 15.3 ± 5.2 g m^{-2} h^{-1}). The observed asymmetry is statistically significant. Even on the non-symptomatic side, sweating was increased significantly above the interattack level and the level in controls (see also Table 2.39). Sweating decreased *pari passu* with the decrease of pain (Figure 2.31). Sweating on the abdomen, thorax, etc., was invariably normal during attack. A typical example of forehead sweating during a severe attack is shown in Figure 2.32.

Increased forehead sweating during cluster headache attacks is accordingly a much more commonly occurring phenomenon than hirtherto believed. The reason why it had been found so rarely before is that it is mostly subclinical, i.e. <70–80 g m^{-2} h^{-1}.

STIMULATION OF FOREHEAD SWEATING: BODY HEATING AND PILOCARPINE

In order to elucidate the mechanism underlying the attack-related sweating in cluster headache, we have studied sweating provoked by pilocarpine, and sweating as a consequence of increased body temperature, i.e. caused by heating or exercise (Sjaastad, 1981, 1982, 1983; Saunte *et al.*, 1983b). The

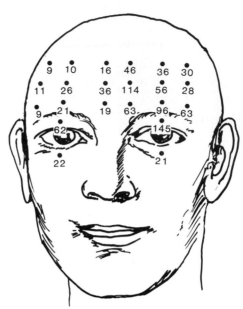

Figure 2.32 Sweat measurements carried out over the entire forehead in a patient (male, 25 years old) with episodic cluster headache during a severe attack on the left side. This patient previously had right-sided attacks. For control values see the legend to Figure 2.31. (From Sjaastad *et al*. (1981). Courtesy of *Cephalalgia*.)

pilocarpine (16 patients, 38 tests), heating (10 patients, 12 tests), and exercise (14 patients, 27 tests) tests were carried out outside of attacks. The control series for these tests consisted of 20, 23 and 15 healthy individuals, respectively, who were not age- and sex-matched with the cluster headache series. It is emphasized, however, that we had previously not found any marked age- or sex-variation as far as *asymmetry* of forehead sweating is concerned. Symmetry of forehead sweating was the parameter which we placed emphasis on, in *this* connection.

During the heating test, the individual was put into a paper bag, covering the body up to the neck; the body was then covered with rubber bags containing hot water. Exercise was carried out on the examination couch, for example by 'bicycling in the air'. Sweating was then measured at its maximum, and preferably when it had exceeded 75 g m^{-2} h^{-1} at one or more points. Pilocarpine was administered subcutaneously in a dosage of 0.1 mg/kg body weight. In this test sweating was only monitored at 0.5–1 min intervals in order to obtain continuous curves for the two sides of the forehead. Symptomatic/non-symptomatic side ratios were compared with right/left side ratios of forehead sweating in the control group.

The mean, unweighted symptomatic/non-symptomatic side ratio of heat-induced forehead sweating in cluster headache patients was significantly reduced (0.66 ± 0.39 (mean ± SD) g m^{-2} h^{-1}) above the inner canthus, as

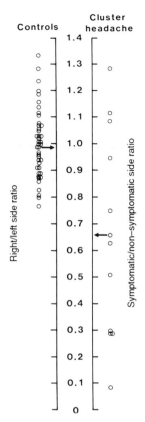

Figure 2.33 Heat-induced forehead sweating (weighted values; position I) in episodic cluster headache patients ($n = 12$) and controls ($n = 42$). Arrows indicate mean values. (From Saunte *et al.* (1983b). Courtesy of *Cephalalgia*.)

compared with controls (0.99 ± 0.11 g m^{-2} h^{-1}) (Figure 2.33). Only four of 12 ratios in the cluster headache group were above the lowest ratio in the control group. A typical example of such a heating test is demonstrated in Figure 2.34. The exercise test showed essentially the same trend. The mean, unweighted symptomatic/non-symptomatic side ratio of exercise-induced forehead sweating was 0.69 ± 0.32 compared with a mean control ratio of 1.06 ± 0.15 g m^{-2} h^{-1}; these values are significantly different. Vijayan and Watson (1982) later made findings similar to those obtained in our heating experiments. Using a non-quantitative method (the so-called Minor's method) they found that, when studied over time, cluster headache patients sweated less in the forehead on the symptomatic than on the non-symptomatic side. It should be mentioned that Drummond (1988) found no significant asymmetry in the 'lower' part of the forehead of cluster headache patients on body heating, but found an asymmetry (symptomatic<non-symptomatic side) in the 'upper' part of the forehead.

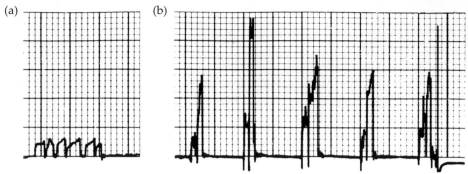

Figure 2.34 Heat-induced sweating in the middle part of the forehead in an episodic cluster headache patient in the interparoxysmal period, with slight residual pain. (a) Prior to heating. (b) Heating. Each heavy horizontal line represents $25\,g\,m^{-2}\,h^{-1}$ of sweating. Measurements were made on the right side first and then the left. Note partial lack of induced sweating on the symptomatic, i.e. right, side. (From Saunte *et al.* (1983b). Courtesy of *Cephalalgia*.)

One of our cases with left-sided headache attacks at the time had previously had right-sided attacks of cluster headache. He was later proven to have clear-cut signs of a right-sided, autonomic disturbance on the basis of pupillometric findings. At the time when the subjects for the heat-induced-sweating experiment were chosen, however, the pupillometric information was not available, so this patient was put into the wrong category, as far as the evaporimetric pattern is concerned. This patient was one of the exceptions indicated in Figure 2.33 (Sjaastad *et al.*, 1987b). The reason why there are exceptions to the rule of decreased, heat-induced, symptomatic-side sweating in cluster headache may partly be such occasional side shifts or bilaterality of the headache (Sjaastad *et al.*, 1985, 1988d). There may, therefore, be other similar cases in our material. The elucidation of the sweating pattern in connection with the shift of pain may deepen our understanding of the nature of cluster headache.

A further fact to be taken into consideration when evaluating these results is that the best way we felt we could evaluate forehead sweating in these cases was by comparing the two sides. We did not pay much attention to the absolute values because of the wide intraindividual variation in response. However, during attack the sweating does not seem to be within normal limits on the non-symptomatic side either (see above). This may indicate that there is also an abnormality on the non-symptomatic side, but to a lesser extent. Consequently, by employing the non-symptomatic side as a control, we may have introduced some error.

The autonomic fibres to the sweat glands are sympathetic in nature. Nevertheless, acetylcholine is the transmitter at the effector organ (muscarinic site). Hence pilocarpine, a parasympathicomimetic drug, was used to test the sweating in these patients. With pilocarpine, there was generally ultimately a clear increase in sweating on both sides of the forehead in all patients. However, there was a transitional stage starting a few minutes after the onset of

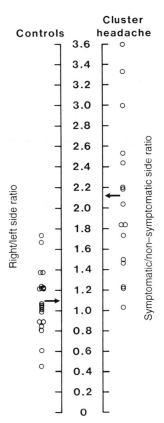

Figure 2.35 Pilocarpine induced sweating (weighted values; position I in episodic cluster headache patients (*n* = 16) and controls (*n* = 20). (From Saunte *et al.* (1983b). Courtesy of *Cephalalgia*.)

sweating and lasting for a few minutes, when there usually was clear asymmetry in forehead sweating, the sweating being more pronounced on the symptomatic side. If calculated at the time of the maximum difference, the pilocarpine test rendered a mean unweighted symptomatic/non-symptomatic side ratio of 2.07 ± 0.77 (right above the inner canthus), compared with a control right/left side ratio of 1.10 ± 0.32 g m^{-2} h^{-1}. These values are highly different statistically (Figure 2.35). Only one of the patient ratios (of a total of 16) was below the mean control ratio. The reason why the sweating was not calculated after a certain number of minutes, but at the time when the difference was maximimal, was that the asymmetry appeared after varying time intervals. The typical forehead sweating patterns in cluster headache on heating as well as pilocarpine stimulation are most marked in the beginning of the sweat test and fade to some extent during the later part of the test. Accordingly, the timing of the measurements is important (Salvesen *et al.*,

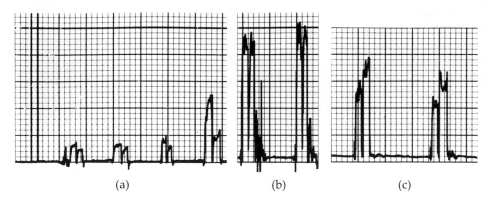

(a)	(b)	(c)

Figure 2.36   Pilocarpine test (0.1/kg body weight, s.c.) carried out in an episodic cluster headache patient in the interparoxysmal period (Horner-like picture). Measurements were made in the central part of the forehead. (a) At 6 min: sweating starts to increase on the symptomatic right side. (b) At 26 min: sweating is more or less symmetrical. (c) At 50 min: sweating is even higher on the non-symptomatic side. Each heavy horizontal line represents $25\,\mathrm{g\,m^{-2}\,h^{-1}}$. For control values see the legend to Figure 2.31. (From Saunte *et al.* (1983b). Courtesy of *Cephalalgia*.)

1988). We are presently searching for more adequate methods with which to express these differences. A typical example of a pilocarpine test in cluster headache is shown in Figure 2.36.

MECHANISMS UNDERLYING THE SWEATING ANOMALY IN CLUSTER HEADACHE

It has been postulated that in cluster headache there is a Horner's syndrome on the symptomatic side. Somewhat surprisingly, no attempt had been made to quantify one component of Horner's syndrome, i.e. the facial 'anhidrosis'. It was certainly a source of confusion in the past that, while 'anhidrosis' is an integral part of the Horner's syndrome, *increased* forehead sweating seemed to be a characteristic feature of the attacks in some cluster headache patients.

Heating and chemical stimulation (such as pilocarpine) reflect different mechanisms of sweat-gland activation (List and Peet, 1938; Antonaci and Sjaastad, 1988). The reduced, or in some cases, almost absent thermoinduced sweating in cluster headache may indicate a partial, functional or structural dysfunction of the sympathetic fibres to the sweat glands. List and Peet (1938) do not consider the pilocarpine test a valuable one for assessing the sweat function. In cluster headache, however, this test has proved useful. In most patients, there seems to be a transient hypersensitivity to pilocarpine on the part of the forehead sweat glands on the symptomatic side.

Such hypersensitivity may possibly be similar or identical to what Cannon (1939) has described as denervation supersensitivity. Sweating is also increased on the non-symptomatic side during attack, although to a lesser degree, which indicates that the underlying pathology is bilateral.

There may be various explanations for the bilaterality. If the primary disturbance in cluster headache is 'central', this may mean that the disorder in central 'autonomic' structures is also bilateral, but that the dysfunction on one side overshadows that on the other.

Theoretically, it is possible that the response on the other side is just part of a general response to a sweat-provoking factor. The fact that the sweating is sometimes generalized during attack (although not in any of our patients) adds weight to this option. Solomon and Guglielmo (1985) contend that facial sweating during an attack could be due to fear and emotion in connection with the attack. If this were the case, then a 'dry mouth' should be an accompaniment due to the same sympathetic stimulation. Sweating was, however, apparently present (assessed retrospectively) in a high proportion of their patients with seemingly normal salivation and even in patients with increased salivation. This discrepancy, if it can be verified by objective means, is clearly evidence against pure sympathetic stimulation being the underlying mechanism. Moreover, the asymmetry of attack-related sweating cannot be explained as being due to a *generalized* stimulus only. The regularity of the asymmetry as opposed to the infrequency of the generalized response makes the mentioned possibility an unlikely one as a general principle in cluster headache. Irrespective of the explanation for the increased attack-related sweating, *the asymmetry implies a local factor* (in addition to a general one?). In some patients, there may be stress/emotion-triggered sweating superimposed on the aysmmetric sweating caused by the attack mechanism *per se*.

The knowledge regarding the course that sympathetic fibres follow to the forehead is incomplete. Available evidence (Wilson, 1936; Vijayan and Watson, 1978) indicates that the sympathetic fibres to the sweat glands in the *forehead* (medial forehead?) follow the *internal* and not the external carotid artery, the terminal branches running along the supraorbital nerve. A lesion along the internal carotid artery (particularly in the carotid canal) causing a Horner's syndrome may, therefore, also affect the sympathetic fibres to the sweat glands in the forehead.

There is one serious objection to such an hypothesis: Cannon (1939) stated that 'When in a series of efferent neurons, a unit is destroyed, an increased irritability to chemical agents develops in the isolated structure or structures, the effect being maximal in the part directly denervated'. In the case of a lesion along the internal carotid artery or further out towards the periphery, the supersensitivity of the sweat glands should be maximal. However, although this line of reasoning seems to be relevant as far as the autonomic system in general is concerned, the sweat glands have been considered to be an exception to this rule. With lesions of the third sympathetic neuron, sweat glands have been considered to be more or less *unresponsive* to chemical stimuli such as pilocarpine. Schliack has over a prolonged period made contributions in this field (e.g. Schliack, 1962, 1974). It is, therefore, of more than passing interest that he is convinced that central lesions lead to hyper-responsiveness of the sweat glands to pilocarpine, whereas post-ganglionic lesions lead to lack of response of the sweat glands (*'die postganglionäre Läsion lässt jedwede Schweiss-sekretion versiegen'*). He compares the pre-ganglionic lesion with a motoric 'spastic' paresis, and the post-ganglionic one with a 'peripheral' motor paresis. There is evidence from human as well as animal experiments in favour of this supposition (Hyndman and Wolkin, 1941; Kahn and Rothman, 1942; Netsky, 1948; Janowitz and Grossman 1951; MacMillan and Spalding, 1969). The common belief was that the sweat glands were subject to atrophy in post-ganglionic lesions. Contrary to this belief, however, Janowitz and Grossman (1950) demonstrated that sweating did appear in the denervated skin when it was exposed to radiant heat. The consensus, nevertheless, seems to have been that sweat glands are an exception to Cannon's law.

Provided this information is correct, one may argue along the following lines. The fact that the sweat glands in the forehead of cluster headache patients do respond, not only during spontaneous attacks but also following pharmacological stimulation, show that they are functionally intact. According to the previous theories, there should consequently not be any major lesion of the third neuron in cluster headache. The lesion leading to the sweating anomaly in cluster headache would, still according to this line of reasoning, in all probability be located proximally to the third neuron.

In order to provide evidence for the localization of the process underlying the sweating anomaly in cluster headache, we have recently studied the same variables in patients with dysfunction of the first and second neuron. The first-neuron cases were mostly patients with Wallenberg's syndrome, the patients with a second-neuron dysfunction being cases of neck tumours, trauma, etc. (Salvesen *et al.*, 1986, 1987a). We have recently also had the opportunity to examine two patients with a probable third-neuron dysfunction (Salvesen *et al.*, 1989). In cases with a first-neuron dysfunction, we have found a pattern similar to that in cluster headache, i.e. with a clear hypersensitivity to pilocarpine (Figure 2.37). This does not, of course, *prove* that the lesion leading to the sweat anomaly in cluster headache is located along the first neuron (Salvesen and Sjaastad, 1987). It suggests, however, that the sweat anomaly in cluster headache is compatible with such a localization of the dysfunction. Our recent investigations seem to demonstrate that the same pattern is found in third-neuron dysfunction (Salvesen *et al.*, 1989), while second-neuron dysfunction seems to exhibit a less marked hypersensitivity pattern (Salvesen *et al.*, 1987a). It should be noted that the number of patients in these studies was small. Our data on the third-neuron dysfunction tend to show that the so-called exception to Cannon's law (i.e. that the sweat glands degenerate as a consequence of a third-neuron lesion) may not necessarily be a true observation. What has been studied in animal experiments and some human studies, is a complete third-neuron lesion, which has given rise to a complete loss of sweating. The situation in cluster headache may be a *partial*, and not complete sympathetic lesion. This may lead to a different picture. It, therefore, still seems theoretically possible that the sweat anomaly may be due to a lesion along—or rather a

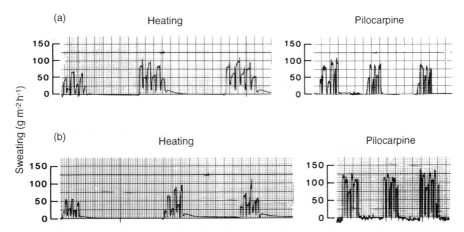

Figure 2.37 Sweating pattern in the forehead in Horner's syndrome, due to a *central neuron lesion*. (a) Forehead sweating patterns in a left-sided lesion. (b) Forehead sweating pattern in a right-sided lesion. The first, third and fifth peaks in each group of six peaks represent the right side, positions I–III (see Figure 2.30). The second, fourth, and sixth peaks in each group represent the corresponding positions on the left side. *Heat-induced pattern*: note the markedly smaller values on the symptomatic side in both patients. *Pilocarpine stimulation*: (a) there is a complete reversal of the pattern seen in the heating test, indicating supersensitivity of the symptomatic (left) side; (b) the right side has now more or less caught up with the left one, indicating supersensitivity (although there is no pattern reversal). (From Salvesen *et al.* (1987a). Courtesy of *Cephalalgia*.)

dysfunction of—the third neuron. Additional evidence for preserved forehead sweat glands in probable third-neuron lesions was recently obtained in the aforementioned study done by Salvesen *et al.* (1989), where pilocarpine gave rise to profuse sweating. It is worth noting that in dysfunctions of neurons I–III as well as in cluster headache, it is not a question of 'anhidrosis'; rather a 'hypohidrosis' is found (the sweating in these conditions is usually subclinical).

The reasoning in explaining the sweat anomaly in cluster headache has so far been based on the assumption that there is a typical Horner's syndrome in cluster headache. This may not be the case (see the following section). It should be emphasized that the central pathways from the hypothalamus distally are not entirely known in man (Appenzeller, 1970).

It should also be emphasized that what has been estimated in cluster headache is evaporation, i.e. total water loss. This consists of transepidermal water loss and sweating (perspiratio insensibilis). At high levels of water loss, sweating dominates. In our studies, we made the supposition that the 'excess' water loss is due to sweating. However, it is possible that a greater than expected fraction of the excess evaporation is not necessarily due to sweating *per se*.

In spite of the fact that the sweat anomaly demonstrated in cluster headache fits with a model of a supersensitivity reaction, the possibility also exists that it could represent other pathophysiological mechanisms. The release of the transmitter (transmitters?) from the third-neuron sweat fibre terminals may be much more complicated than is presently known. There may, hypothetically, also be several types of fibres to the glands.

A further point against the theory of third-neuron dysfunction is that the sweat changes seem to be bilateral. There are even indications that the sweating on the non-symptomatic side fluctuates *pari passu* with the severity of the headache. In addition, the locational dissociation of pain and sweating demonstrated in one case (see present section) is difficult to reconcile with a *pure* unilateral third-neuron lesion.

The evaluation of forehead sweating is a unique means of improving the understanding of cluster headache pathogenesis: it is, first of all, a *dynamic* test, reflecting the development and course of a single attack (unlike, for example, pupillometry which is carried out in the free interval only). Furthermore, there is an affected and a control side, although the latter is probably also moderately affected. This gives it some advantage above, for example, electrocardiographic recordings in this context. The latter also probably less frequently show gross abnormalities.

PUPILLOMETRY: 'HORNER'S SYNDROME'

A small pupil on the symptomatic side is found in a proportion of cluster headache cases (Kunkle and Anderson, 1960, 1961; Nieman and Hurwitz, 1961). If one were to apply the classical ideas concerning the automatic nervous system, this could result from either parasympathetic overstimulation or from sympathetic dysfunction. On the basis of supplementary tests, both Kunkle and Anderson and Nieman and Hurwitz felt that an oculosympathetic paresis was present.

The introduction of the electronic, infra-red pupillometer has added another dimension to the study of the pupil in cluster headache (e.g. Turner, 1969, 1975, 1980; Loewenfeld and Rosskothen, 1974; Bourne *et al.*, 1979; Smith *et al.*, 1979; Smith and Smith, 1983). Riley and Moyer (1971) found signs of a sympathetic deficiency when applying cocaine, adrenaline, and hydroxyamphetamine topically. Fanciullacci and co-workers (Fanciullacci, 1979; Fanciullacci *et al.*, 1982) have studied pupillary reactions in cluster headache in further detail. There was no definite mean side difference in pupil size in the basal state. Tyramine (2%), cocaine (4%), homatropine (0.1%) and phenylephrine (1%) eyedrops were used, one drop of each solution being instilled bilaterally. Application of indirectly acting sympaticomimetic agents, such as tyramine, a releaser, and cocaine, a re-uptake inhibitor ($n = 45$ and $n = 10$, respectively), invariably resulted in a definite anisocoria, with the smaller pupil on the symptomatic side. It was not defined what was exactly meant by anisocoria. Homatropine tests ($n = 7$) gave rise to a marked bilateral dilatation of the pupils, but with significantly smaller pupils on the symptomatic side. The persistent anisocoria with homatropine indicates that the cause of the pupillary abnormality is not solely to be found in the parasympathetic supply to the iris.

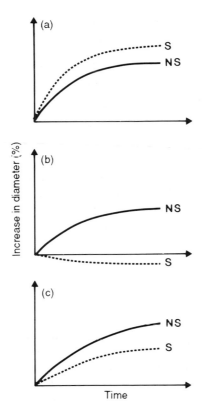

Figure 2.38 Horner's syndrome: pupillary response to indirectly acting sympathico-mimetics (like hydroxyamphetamine and tyramine) in patients with lesions in sympath-etic neutrons I–III, compared with the response in episodic cluster headache patients. Note that the pattern in cluster headache patients is not the same as any of the Horner's syndrome patterns. (a) First- or second-neuron lesion; (b) third-neuron lesion; (c) cluster headache. S, Symptomatic side; NS, non-symptomatic side. (From Sjaastad (1988a). Courtesy of *Cephalalgia*.)

A remarkable finding was that phenylephrine (a directly acting sympathicomi-metic agent) gave rise to an insignificant anisocoria with the smaller dilatation on the symptomatic side (a total of 15 tests).

Fanciullacci *et al*. (1982, 1988b) interpreted their tyramine studies as demon-strating a latent Horner's syndrome in cases where there was no manifest anisocoria in the basal state. Del Bene *et al*. (1985, 1987) found that even children of cluster headache patients showed anisocoria on tyramine stimulation. Such anisocoria was present in 78% of the children, a figure significantly higher than that found in controls (three of 12 children, i.e. 25%). A decreased response to indirectly acting sympathicomimetics is not consistent with a first- or second-neuron pattern, where the opposite trend is encountered (Thompson and Mensher, 1971; Thompson, 1987) (Figure 2.38). The reduced tyramine response on the symptomatic side should indicate a lack of noradrenaline in the peripheral sympathetic neuron. However, if the finding of no relative increase in dilatation of the symptomatic-side eye with the phenylephrine test is reproducible, there should not be a third-neuron dysfunction. If a regular third-neuron lesion were present, a considerable supersensitivity ought to be found on the phenylephrine test. The relative lack of response to phenylephrine administration is not compatible with a dysfunction of the first-neuron either. The best interpretation would then be that in cluster headache there is only a *functional* deficiency of the transmitter system; or, the miosis could be due to a co-involvement of other transmitters.

The results of the phenylephrine studies done by Fanciullacci *et al.* are, however, somewhat in opposition to the results obtained by other groups who found an exaggerated pupillary response to directly working sympathicomimetics on the symptomatic side in cluster headache (Thompson and Mensher, 1971).

In addition, Riley and Moyer (1971) have provided evidence for a supersensitivity to sympathicomimetics in five of their 19 cluster headache patients with an apparently complete oculosympathetic paresis: in these patients, the mean response to cocaine (4%) and hydroxyamphetamine (1%) was -0.10 and -0.32 mm, respectively. In the *very same patients* the response to adrenaline (0.1%) was $+1.78$ mm. The response to a directly acting sympathicomimetic drug was different by one order of magnitude from that following application of indirectly acting sympathicomimetic drugs.

Because of the existing inconsistencies, pupillometry in cluster headache patients has also been carried out by our group. The equipment used was the Whittaker binocular, infra-red pupillometer with television transmission and real-time recording. In our studies, the extent of the basal anisocoria was larger in cluster headache patients (many of whom were studied during a bout) than in control individuals ($p < 0.02$) (Figure 2.39). The anisocoria (with the smaller pupil on the symptomatic side) was significant in patients ($p < 0.01$) but not in controls. It is evident from Figure 2.39 that there was quite often a miosis on the symptomatic side in cluster headache patients. Eleven of 32 patients (34%) had an anisocoria exceeding the highest degree of anisocoria in the controls (Salvesen *et al.*, 1987b). Micieli *et al.* (1988) also found a moderate, relative miosis on the symptomatic side on both dark and light adaptation during the cluster period, but not during the remission. It should be emphasized that the degree of anisocoria in the basal state may influence the various pupillometric tests (Salvesen, 1989a).

Cluster headache patients on the whole had a lesser degree of anisocoria ($p < 0.001$) than patients with first-, second- or third-neuron lesions (Thompson and Mensher, 1971) (Figure 2.40). Contrary to the findings of Fanciullacci *et al.* (1982), we found a moderate, but clearly exaggerated, response to phenylephrine on the symptomatic side (Figure 2.41) (Salvesen and Sjaastad, 1987; Salvesen *et al.*, 1987b). The response to hydroxyamphetamine (an indirectly

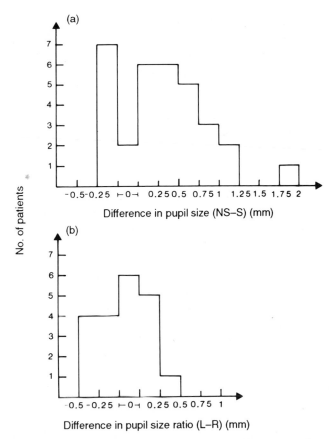

Figure 2.39 Nomograms showing the degree of pupillary inequality. (a) Episodic cluster headache patients outside attack and with no pharmacological manipulation (*n* = 32; mean anisocoria 0.32 mm); S, symptomatic side; NS, non-symptomatic side. (b) Male age-matched controls (*n* = 20; mean anisocoria 0.06 mm); L, left; R, right. (From Salvesen *et al.* (1987b). Courtesy of *Cephalalgia*.)

acting sympathicomimetic agent) was different, being most marked on the non-symptomatic side (Figure 2.42). The increased sensitivity, as also evidenced by our studies on sweating (Salvesen *et al.*, 1986, 1987b), does not imply that the response to the directly working sympathicomimetic agent is necessarily more marked on the symptomatic than on the other side in *absolute* terms. It suffices that the response to directly working sympathicomimetics on the symptomatic side is more marked in relative terms (i.e. when compared to the other side) than the response to indirectly working sympathicomimetic agents.

I feel that, until proven otherwise, there is an oculosympathetic supersensitivity reaction pattern in cluster headache. According to Riley and Moyer (1971), the response to light stimulation (using infra-red electronic pupillometry) was

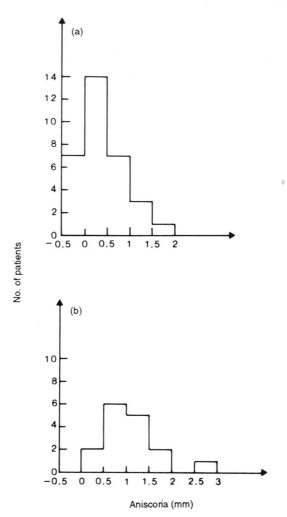

Figure 2.40   A pupillometric comparison of anisocoria (non-symptomatic side – symptomatic side, without any pharmacological manipulation) in: (a) episodic cluster headache patients (mean difference = 0.36 mm); (b) patients with Horner's syndrome, neurons I–III (mean difference = 1.03 mm) (Thompson and Mensher, 1971)—note the more marked anisocoria in Horner's syndrome. (From Salvesen *et al.* (1987b). Courtesy of *Cephalalgia*.)

one of 'delayed recovery toward its initial size' on the affected side. This is also indicative of—but does not prove—a sympathetic dysfunction on the symptomatic side (Loewenfeld and Rosskothen, 1974).

Even though a phenylephrine supersensitivity seems to be present, this does not *per se* unequivocally pin-point any location of the dysfunction. According to Thompson and Mensher (1971), dysfunction of the central (first), preganglionic

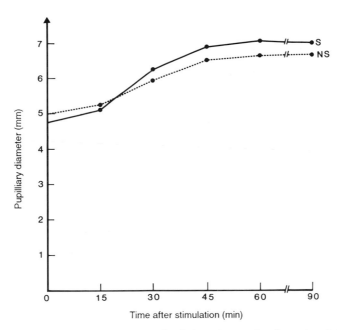

Figure 2.41 Pupillary diameter at standard time intervals after stimulation (phenyl-ephrine test) in episodic cluster headache patients ($n = 27$). Note the 'cross-over' phenomenon. S, symptomatic side; NS, non-symptomatic side. (From Salvesen *et al.* (1987b). Courtesy of *Cephalalgia*.)

(second) and the postganglionic (third) neuron are all associated with an exaggerated phenylephrine response on the symptomatic side. This means that it is impossible on the basis of the phenylephrine response alone to locate the lesion. Thompson and Mensher used a strong (10%) phenylephrine solution. Possibly, a better differentiation between the three neuron dysfunctions could be achieved with a weak solution (1%). In a recent study by our group, the response to a 1% phenylephrine solution (Figure 2.43) seemed to be more marked on the affected side in first- than in second-neuron affections (Salvesen and Sjaastad, 1987). In first- and second-neuron dysfunctions, the response to the tyramine test (and hydroxyamphetamine test which, quantitat-ively speaking, has a similar effect on the pupil) on the symptomatic side clearly outweighed that on the non-symptomatic side (Figure 2.44). This response thus contrasts markedly with the situation in cluster headache (Figure 2.38). The pattern in third-neuron lesions (adapted from Thompson and Mensher (1971)), also differs clearly from that in cluster headache (Figure 2.38). The pupillary response to hydroxyamphetamine in two cases of probable third-neuron lesions (Salvesen *et al.*, 1989) was similar to that described by Thompson and Mensher (1971) (Figure 2.38).

The hydroxyamphetamine pattern of cluster headache is, therefore, not identical to any of the patterns known in first- to third-neuron lesions. It bears

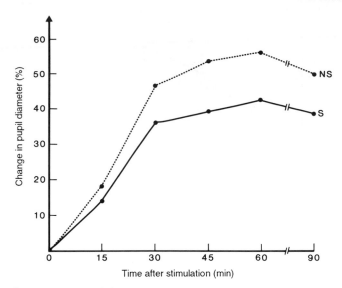

Figure 2.42   Increase in pupil diameter (as a percentage of the basal value) at standard time intervals after bilateral application of hydroxyamphetamine in episodic cluster headache patients (*n* = 23). S, Symptomatic side; NS, non-symptomatic side. (From Salvesen *et al.* (1987b). Courtesy of *Cephalalgia*.)

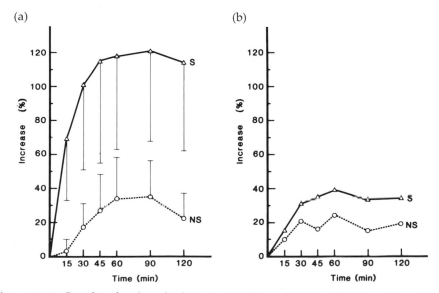

Figure 2.43   Results of a phenylephrine test (1%) in patients with Horner's syndrome due to: (a) central neuron lesion (*n* = 5); (b) preganglionic neuron lesion (*n* = 3). Values are mean ± 1 SD. S, Symptomatic side; NS, non-symptomatic side. (From Salvesen *et al.* (1987a). Courtesy of *Cephalalgia*.)

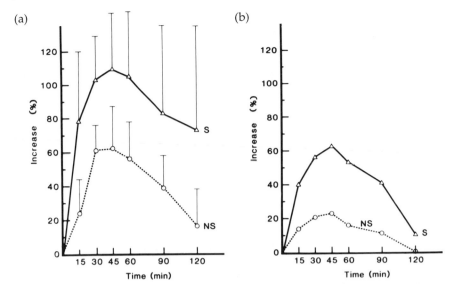

Figure 2.44 Response to a tyramine (2%, eyedrops bilaterally) test in patients with Horner's syndrome: (a) central neuron lesion ($n = 5$); (b) pre-ganglionic neuron lesion ($n = 3$). Pupillary dilatation was followed pupillometrically. Values are mean $\pm$ 1 SD. S, Symptomatic side; NS, non-symptomatic side. (From Salvesen *et al*. (1987a). Courtesy of *Cephalalgia*.)

some resemblance to the pattern of third-neuron lesions, but in these the response is absent. It should be stated that 'a third-neuron pattern' has been observed in some (approximately 15%) of our cluster headache patients (Figure 2.45). The reason for the incomplete response in cluster headache *might* be that the 'lesion' is only partial (cf. the lesser degree of anisocoria in cluster headache than in Horner's syndrome patients generally (Figure 2.40)). Another, and possibly more likely, explanation is that the pupil in cluster headache is not a regular 'Horner pupil'; it may resemble a Horner pupil but not be identical to it. Until more information is available, we prefer to term the pupil in cluster headache a 'Horner-like pupil'. It should again be stressed that the response to phenylephrine ('the crossover phenomenon', see Figure 2.41) is also much less marked in patients with cluster headache than in patients with first- or third-neuron lesions. This also attests to the label 'Horner-like pupil'. This could also be due to a lower degree of sympathetic dysfunction in cluster headache than in the ordinary Horner's syndrome. However, it may mean that the pupil in cluster headache is essentially different from that in Horner's syndrome. There seems to be good correspondence between the pupillary responses to hydroxyamphetamine and phenylephrine in cluster headache, both showing a low degree of sympathetic damage—if any.

It is remarkable that cluster headache patients with a marked degree of anisocoria (mean 0.9 mm) still show a considerable degree of dilatation (up to 37%) on hydroxyamphetamine stimulation (Salvesen *et al*., 1989a). In third-neuron lesion cases, studied by Thompson and Mensher (1971), with a lesser

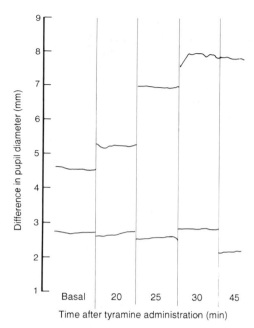

Figure 2.45 Results of a tyramine pupillometric test in an episodic cluster headache patient. Note the marked difference between the two sides, with a lack of dilation of the right, i.e. symptomatic, pupil. This pattern (a 'third neuron pattern') is exceptional in cluster headache, in that we have observed it in only approximately 15% of cases studied.

degree of anisocoria (mean 0.83 mm) there was no dilatation on hydroxyamphetamine stimulation. This observation also seems to indicate that the primary abnormality underlying the miosis of cluster headache may be at variance with that of a 'pure' third-neuron Horner's syndrome.

Patients showing the typical cluster headache pattern on pupillometry also tend to have the typical forehead-sweating patterns (see page 206). This combination of patterns was found in 16 of 29 cluster headache patients. In seven patients, there was a discrepancy between the two modes of examination, supersensitivity reactions being present in one system only, whereas in six cases no supersensitivity response whatsoever was found (Salvesen et al., 1988a).

One main problem in both our study and those done by others is that cases of verified third-neuron lesions are difficult to find. Progress in this line of approach to elucidating cluster headache pathogenesis is clearly in need of further, tenable information regarding the pupillographic pattern in definite third-neuron lesions. What has been used in previous studies as representatives for third-neuron lesions are cases of cluster headache (sic) and Ræder's syndrome (Thompson and Mensher, 1971; Maloney et al., 1980), and possibly post-carotid angiography cases. The circular argument type of reasoning is close when cases of cluster headache (where the location of the sympathetic 'lesion' is certainly not known beyond doubt) are used as substitutes for typical third-neuron lesions. Furthermore, the fact that a diagnosis of Ræder's syndrome has been employed in a total of 18 cases in one series attests to the suspicion that strict diagnostic criteria have not been used; Ræder's syndrome is a rare condition (see Ræder's Syndrome). The forehead- and facial-sweating pattern of Ræder's syndrome was not taken into consideration in that work (Riley and Moyer, 1971).

The results of the pupillometric studies on cluster headache patients are difficult to evaluate at the present time. First of all, the classic ideas of only two systems exerting an influence on autonomically innervated organs like the iris is probably too simplistic. Various other substances determine the pupil width, e.g. substance-P in the rabbit's eye gives rise to a small pupil (Bill *et al.*, 1979). It may, therefore, be that the tests carried out in cluster headache do not necessarily reflect changes in the sympathetic/parasympathetic system alone. Other transmitters may also be involved.

There is no consensus as to these interpretations. Fanciullacci *et al.* (1988b) found a more marked miosis on the symptomatic side than on the opposite side after intravenous administration of clonidine (an inhibitor of central sympathetic activity). They interpreted their findings as indicating a possibly reduced central sympathetic tone. Del Bene *et al.* (1985) and Del Bene and Poggioni (1987) claim that even children with cluster headache and cluster headache patients' children demonstrate a latent adrenergic neurone deficiency on pupillometric testing with indirectly acting sympathicomimetics.

It is likely that the pathological process that occurs in the various autonomically innervated organs studied in cluster headache is one and the same. One of the best studied organs in cluster headache is the forehead sweat glands. If a certain abnormality of the sweat glands in the forehead is uncovered, this will have a major impact on the reasoning also for the mechanism underlying the pupil abnormality.

NERVE STIMULATION AND PUPILLOMETRY: BLINK REFLEXES

The pupil dilates on painful stimuli. Sandrini *et al.* (1984, 1985) stimulated the sural nerve percutaneously and elicited the flexion reflex in cluster headache patients ($n = 11$, studied in a bout but between attacks) and controls ($n = 8$); they then assessed the influence thereof on the pupils. The threshold (T) for the flexion reflex was determined on both sides. Then stimuli of $\frac{1}{2}T$, T and $2T$ strength were applied. On the symptomatic side, there was an impaired dilatation as a consequence of painful stimuli. On the non-symptomatic side, dilatation was found, but of significantly lesser magnitude than in controls. There was a significant correlation between the magnitude of the stimulus and pupillary size. Later, this study was extended to include the remission phase

($n = 21$; cluster period $n = 28$). In principle, the same trend (but with less marked changes) was observed during remission (Micieli *et al.*, 1988).

This may be an important approach. First, it is possible that this test may be useful in uncovering a latent 'Horner's syndrome' in the headache-free phase of cluster headache. The test may thus conceivably be of diagnostic significance in questionable cases. Secondly, this test can help in clarifying the nature of the pupillary changes in cluster headache because it is a quantitative test.

Transcutaneous electrical nerve stimulation of the infratrochlear nerve causes an ipsilateral miosis. In healthy controls ($n = 16$), Fanciullacci *et al.* (1989) found a slow, long-lasting miosis. In migraine ($n = 15$) and cluster headache ($n = 26$) patients a similar response was observed in the pain-free stage. During the cluster phase, however, there was a difference in response, a normal response being obtained on the non-symptomatic side only. On the symptomatic side, the response was clearly reduced. These results may indicate that the trigeminal pathways are affected during cluster headache bouts.

Pavesi *et al.* (1987) studied the threshold of the blink reflex (the bilateral, late response) in 18 cluster headache patients and 15 matched controls. All values in the patient group were within the control range. However, during the bout (but not during remission) there was an asymmetry, with higher thresholds on the symptomatic side. The significance of these observations is uncertain; they may indicate a trigeminal dysfunction.

CORNEAL SENSITIVITY

Vijayan and Watson (1984) studied corneal sensitivity in cluster headache, employing the Cochet–Bonnet aesthesiometer. The length of the nylon mono-filament of this instrument can be adjusted: the shorter the filament, the stronger the pressure that is applied. The threshold for corneal sensitivity can accordingly be tested. Control individuals feel the sensation of a 6 cm long filament. Invariably, the patients ($n = 15$) also felt the stimulus at 6 cm filament length. There was no difference between symptomatic and non-symptomatic sides or between *symptomatic* and *remission* periods. Therefore, there do not seem to be any indications of discrete lesions of the trigeminal nerve.

CUTANEOUS SENSIBILITY

Russell (1978b) used a transcutaneous nerve stimulator and measured the pain threshold and 'pain-tolerance levels' (the level of pain that the individual was able to tolerate) in the symptomatic side of the forehead in 22 cluster headache patients, most of whom were inside a bout, and in control individuals. Pain thresholds did not differ between patients and controls. As regards pain tolerance, however, cluster headache patients showed significantly higher levels than did controls. There was accordingly no evidence to suggest that cluster headache patients show an excessive reaction to pain.

Tactile pain thresholds were tested in eight cluster headache patients (seven males and one female) (Nattero *et al.*, 1987b) in the upper and lower extremities and the forehead, at least 30 days after actual attacks. An electrical stimulator was used for stimulus generation. The procedure was carried out three times over the course of 3 weeks. No differences in sensory threshold were found between the two sides. As regards pain threshold, there was no asymmetry in the extremities. In the head, however, there was a significant reduction of pain threshold on the symptomatic side.

Procacci *et al.* (1989) studied the sensory function between attacks in a group of 27 drug-free cluster headache patients in a blind fashion. Sensory and pain thresholds, and thresholds to electrical stimulation were examined. With these stimuli, two types of sensation can easily be distinguished: a tactile and a painful sensation.

Cutaneous thresholds were found to be invariably within normal limits and without asymmetry in the temporal area and on the forearm. Cutaneous hyperalgesia was assessed with various methods and was found to be present on the painful side in 10 patients, sometimes only in the face. Deep hyperalgesia was present in 17 patients (only on the symptomatic side in 12). A forearm 'ischaemic' test seemed to result in *more* frequent and more long-lasting complaints (pain and paraesthesiae) on the symptomatic than on the non-symptomatic side. All in all, signs of lateralization were present in 20 of the 27 patients.

The authors speculate that ipsilateral facilitation in the central nervous system may explain the hemihyperalgesia in the entire hemisoma. Activation of reflex arcs may give rise to pain in peripheral structures.

A prevailing finding in these investigations seems to be that there is no asymmetry in sensory thresholds. There is thus no positive evidence for a 'sensitization' on the pain side. In this connection, it may be mentioned that Sinforiani *et al.* (1987) found no signs of interhemispheric imbalance and of cortical dysfunction when cluster headache patients underwent a set of neuropsychological tests. These patients were compared with carefully selected controls.

EVOKED POTENTIALS

Somatosensory evoked potentials

Firenze *et al.* (1988) have studied contralateral somatosensory evoked potentials (SEP) after median nerve stimulation in common migraine ($n = 34$), tension headache ($n = 30$) and cluster headache ($n = 10$) patients and in healthy controls (10 males, 10 females). The patients were studied prior to and in connection with unilateral headache attacks provoked by the intravenous administration of histamine. There were no significant differences in latencies or amplitudes between controls, tension headache or migraine patients in the basal state or after histamine administration.

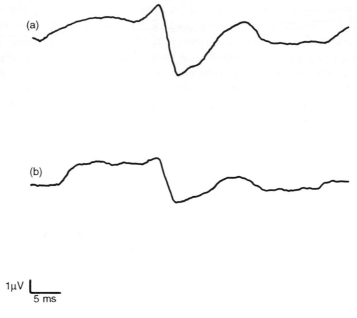

Figure 2.46 Somatosensory evoked potentials in a cluster headache patient (aged 39 years) during the attack-free interval (a) and during a histamine induced attack (b). (From Firenze *et al.* (1988). Courtesy of *Cephalalgia*.)

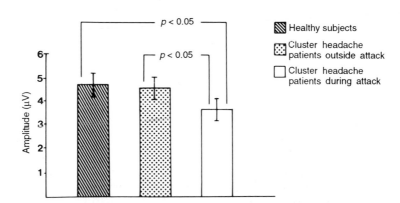

Figure 2.47 Mean somatosensory evoked potential amplitudes after median nerve stimulation in healthy controls and in 10 patients with cluster headache (stimulation on the side contralateral to the pain. (From Firenze *et al.* (1988). Courtesy of *Cephalalgia*.)

In the interparoxysmal period (Figures 2.46 and 2.47), normal SEP patterns were found in cluster headache. During attacks, the amplitudes of the N_1–P_2 complex obtained after stimulation on the side contralateral to the pain were significantly decreased (3.4 ± 0.7 μV), when compared to the amplitudes in healthy controls (4.5 ± 1.1 μV) as well as in cluster headache patients outside attack (Figure 2.47).

Such studies should be carried out during *spontaneously occurring* attacks as well. If the results are reproduced under such circumstances, they *may* furnish evidence for the validity of the 'central' theory of cluster headache.

Visually evoked potentials

If there are 'central' dysfunctions in cluster headache, they might be detected by visually evoked potential (VEP) examination. It, therefore, becomes important to study VEPs in cluster headache. Boiardi *et al.* (1986) (see also Boiardi *et al.*, 1988b) studied VEPs in 20 cluster headache patients with the episodic variety, 10 with left-sided and 10 with right-sided headache. All patients were in the remission period, and none of them were receiving medication at the time. Careful ocular evaluation including Goldman perimetry was carried out prior to study. Twenty age- and sex-matched controls were also studied. Each eye was tested separately, and the stimulus used was a black-and-white checkerboard pattern reversal.

No changes were observed as far as latencies are concerned between groups or between cluster headache patients with right- and left-sided pain. However, the P_{100} amplitudes were found to be significantly lower on the pain side than on the opposite side (9 out of 10 patients for both the right- and left-sided cases). The asymmetry which was significant and exceeded the normal variation appeared whether the right or left eye was stimulated.

In a similar study, Polich *et al.* (1987) could not reproduce Boiardi *et al.*'s findings. The VEPs were elicited with two different sizes of checker-board patterns. Their sample consisted of 10 male patients, headache- and drug-free at the time of testing, and a carefully selected matched control series. They found no differences between patients and controls.

The authors feel that the close matching of patients and controls in their material is the reason why they obtained a different (and more correct?) result from Boiardi *et al.* Without entering deeply into the discussion concerning which of these two research groups is right or wrong, I would like to add that the series studied by Polich *et al.* was small (seven had right-sided headache, two had left-sided headache, and one had headache on both sides). There seems to be a tendency that patients have smaller amplitudes than controls even in this series. Therefore, one wonders what would have been shown if a larger series had been studied in this setting.

It is futile to speculate further about the underlying mechanisms of the various findings, until it has been established beyond doubt whether or not VEPs are abnormal in cluster headache.

Brain-stem auditory evoked potentials

Brain-stem auditory evoked potentials in cluster headache were studied by Bussone *et al.* (1985). The sample consisted of 13 patients who were studied outside of attacks. All had normal hearing, and the clicks were presented monoaurally through an earphone. Twenty healthy individuals of the same mean age formed the control group. The interpeak latencies were similar in controls, migraine patients ($n = 26$) and tension headache patients ($n = 10$). A significant asymmetry was, however, noted in cluster headache: the I–V interpeak latency was prolonged on the pain side in 11 patients and on the contralateral side in two. The I–III and III–V latencies were proportionally increased, the I–III one being slightly larger. The latencies appeared to increase during attack ($n = 3$).

Later, Bussone *et al.* (1986) extended their studies to include 12 cases of episodic and three of chronic cluster headache (all male). Some patients were partly studied further, i.e. during untreated attacks ($n = 6$) and during lithium therapy, 900 mg day^{-1} ($n = 5$). Individual ipsi- and contra-lateral I–V interpeak latencies were measured to assess interaural differences. The interesting finding is that in all patients, regardless of the recording phase, the I–IV latencies were increased on the painful side. In control individuals ($n = 16$), some asymmetry was also found, but of a lesser magnitude. Criticisms of this study are that the number of patients studied was small and, above all, the huge interindividual differences in asymmetry in the patient group make it necessary to compare the *same patient* in the various phases. This, as far as one is able to understand, was only done to a limited extent.

If reproducible, these findings may, as indicated by the authors, suggest that a 'central' pathology is of importance in cluster headache pathogenesis.

PATHOGENESIS

GENERAL CONSIDERATIONS

The rather frequent, and sometimes regular, occurrence of attacks makes cluster headache apt for study. The fact that the headache is, in principle, unilateral, makes this headache favourable for study, because the symptomatic side can be compared with the non-symptomatic side. The similarity between the two headaches in the cluster headache syndrome, i.e. cluster headache and chronic paroxysmal hemicrania is so pronounced that many steps in the underlying derangement are probably identical in these two headaches. Chronic paroxysmal hemicrania lends itself even more readily to study than does cluster headache, because of the frequency of attacks, even during the daytime. In addition, the *onset* of attacks can be studied in chronic paroxysmal hemicrania and, perhaps more importantly, the period immediately prior to the onset of pain can also be studied. So, chronic paroxysmal hemicrania is easier to study than cluster headache, as far as the attack itself is concerned. It may, therefore, well be that various facts related to attacks in the cluster headache syndrome will first be established in chronic paroxysmal hemicrania. However, since there are differences between the two headaches, and even some marked ones, it is mandatory that even minor pieces of information concerning chronic paroxysmal hemicrania are proven to be applicable, or not, to cluster headache also.

As regards attack studies, there are methodological problems related to the investigation of cluster headache. The stage at which a particular attack has been studied (i.e. the beginning, the middle, or the end of the attack) may be of decisive importance for the outcome of a specific test. It will only occasionally be possible to study the initial phase of a spontaneously occurring attack. Waxing and waning of attack severity is usual, and this fluctuation probably also has an influence on many pathophysiological variables. An example of the great changes observed in the variables tested is provided by the recent pulse frequency studies of Russell *et al.* (1982, 1983) (see Electrocardiographic Rhythm Disturbances During Attack). Therefore, in future studies it may be necessary to state explicitly which part of the attack was studied. It may even, if refined details are to be clarified, be necessary to study in parallel the co-variation of two different variables, for example forehead sweating and pulse rate. It may also be opportune to relate the findings of other variables under exploration to one of the continuously fluctuating variables, e.g. sweating or pulse rate.

Next, due to the severity of the attacks it is difficult for patients to go through attacks without any medication. At least some tests should, nevertheless, be carried out in the drug-free state for every new parameter that is studied. The minimal necessary duration of the drug-free period prior to a study is another—partly unsolved—question. Furthermore, until proven that nitroglycerin, alcohol and histamine-induced attacks are identical to spontaneously occurring ones, it is mandatory that spontaneously occurring attacks are also studied for each new variable investigated.

The task of disentangling the pathogenesis of cluster headache may certainly be—and has been—approached in various ways. One feasible approach would be to try to delineate the *pain pathways* in cluster headache. This may be a fruitful route to follow. Demonstration of pathways for pain stimuli in general does not necessarily mean that these pathways, and these only, are the ones utilized by nociceptive impulses in this specific headache. To use this approach may, therefore, not be as simple as it may at first seem (Sjaastad *et al.*, 1987a). Another approach would be to try to define the 'shock organ', as Horton termed it. This is the most direct approach and is—as far as I am concerned— the ultimate aim of all approaches. Needless to say, this is the most difficult approach. There are naturally various routes that could be followed in trying to achieve this end.

A third line of investigation is the study of particular, abnormal variables, for example the autonomic or hormonal parameters. Autonomic phenomena are integral to the attack. Although the autonomic phenomena may be separated from the pain part of the attack (Sjaastad *et al.*, 1987b), these two parts are closely linked during attack, both temporally and usually also spatially. A complete attack, therefore, consists of pain and autonomic phenomena. The unravelling of autonomic signs may lead to an understanding of the origin and nature of the pain part (Sjaastad, 1985a; Sjaastad and Fredriksen, 1986). It is mainly *this* approach that I and my team have followed for the last 15 years or so.

MIGRAINE AND CLUSTER HEADACHE: A CONTINUUM OR SEPARATE NOSOLOGICAL ENTITIES?

Cluster headache was originally separated from the group of 'vascular' headache. At that time migraine was the prototype of 'vascular headache' ('vascular headache of the migraine type'). 'Vascular' in this connection was not only intended to imply that vascular phenomena *accompany* the attacks, but also that such phenomena could, in some vaguely understood way, be related to the mechanisms of the headache itself, and even might form the primary pathological steps in the chain of events leading to the attack.

Through Horton's seminal and fundamental work in this field, cluster headache gradually became accepted as a separate headache form. Over the years, the resistance towards such a distinction between migraine and cluster headache was apparently considerable. Kunkle *et al*. (1952, 1954) thus declared that, as long as the diagnostic boundaries of migraine and its variants were not clearly defined, there would be little justification for the segregation of cluster headache as a distinct and isolated entity from migraine.

Some clinical investigators still consider cluster headache to be merely a variant of migraine. Two relatively recent statements demonstrate the persistence of the 'unitarian' viewpoint even today: 'the three main types (of migraine) are: classical migraine, common migraine, and cluster headache or migrainous neuralgia' (Wilkinson, 1982). 'We look upon cluster headache as a form of vascular headache closely akin to migraine, but different from it chiefly in its clinical *pattern* of occurrence and in the *severity* . . .' (Graham 1975).

Cluster headache is thus still considered as only a variant of migraine in some circles. What can be the reason for this non-alignment among workers in the field? First of all, it may stem from observations that what could be termed 'transitional forms' (between migraine and cluster headache) seem to exist. Another factor may also be of importance. Some drugs e.g. ergotamine, methysergide and pizotifen, are effective in treating both types of headache. The most likely explanation for the latter phenomenon is that the therapeutic efficacy is due to a non-specific effect of the drug; the drug does not hit the nail on the head: rather it modifies some consequences of the attack, consequences that may be present in various types of headache, e.g. migraine and cluster headache. Another, somewhat less likely, explanation for the efficacy of a drug in two different types of headache is that different properties of the drug come into play in the two headache types.

Although the occurrence of intermediate, transitional, or mixed forms does not refute the possibility that two definitely separate clinical entities exist, their very existence seems to have obscured and confused the issue (Sjaastad, 1975b; Sjaastad *et al.*, 1984b). In the case of separate, independent entities, the following reasoning might seem appropriate: the same percentage of cluster headache sufferers as of individuals in the population at large should suffer from migraine. The only conceivable objection to this view would be that the very fact that a patient is already a cluster headache sufferer might prevent—or promote—the development of a migraine-like pattern when there is a disposition for this disorder also, or vice versa. Although it cannot be refuted that such possibilities exist, this would hardly seem to be the case. The prevalence of migraine in the population at large is not precisely known. A prevalence of 5% may not be too far off, if relatively moderate cases are included. Approximately 80–85% of ordinary cluster headache sufferers are male (Table 1.6), whilst only approximately one-third to one-quarter of migraine sufferers are male. One might, therefore, surmise that rather less than 5% of cluster headache sufferers would show a clinical picture with a mixture of migraine and cluster headache, if a chance co-existence is looked for.

If transitional forms were to exist, various attack patterns might, from a theoretical point of view, conceivably be apparent clinically: temporally dissociated, separate cluster headache and migraine attacks and/or attacks with ingredients of both types of headache. It may be that the clinical picture is so difficult to decipher that clinicians have partly refrained from attempting to do so. Some cases presenting features characteristic of both migraine and cluster headache have been described. Symonds (1956) and Friedman and Mikropoulos (1958) have described scintillation scotomas in patients with cluster headache. Horton (1944) described a case with 70% migraine and 30% cluster headache. In the series studied by Ekbom (1974b), only five of 163 patients seemed to have had migrainous features as well. Solomon and Cappa (1986) have looked into such cases in great detail; migraine usually preceded cluster headache.

From the foregoing, it might appear that it is probably impossible to establish, on the basis of the occurrence of intermediate or transitional forms, that cluster headache is merely a variant of migraine.

From a true clinical point of view, there are clear differences between the appearance of cluster headache and migraine, both with regard to sex distribution, temporal pattern, duration of attacks, unilaterality and severity of pain, as well as with regard to the accompanying phenomena such as nausea/vomiting, lacrimation, conjunctival injection, rhinorrhoea/nasal stuffiness, the occurrence of a Horner-like syndrome, etc. Clear differences also exist between the response to drugs of the two conditions: β-receptor blocking agents are of considerable avail in migraine, whereas they seem to be without any special potential in cluster headache. Lithium is one of the major drugs in cluster headache, but is without effect in migraine—the situation of the patient may even deteriorate on lithium (Peatfield and Rose, 1981).

There is another fundamental difference between the two headaches: in cluster-headache, all the accompanying phenomena (e.g. lacrimation and temporal vessel dilatation) generally appear on the same side as the pain. In migraine, accompanying phenomena, although of a different nature (such as cheiro-oral sensory disturbances), frequently seem to be present on the side opposite to that of the pain. If this assumption is correct, then there is *eo ipso* also a difference in pathogenesis between the two conditions.

In addition to the clinical, distinguishing features, the following supplementary tests indicate that there is a clear difference between migraine and cluster headache (the reader is referred to the various sections for details):

1. corneal temperature measurements;
2. intraocular pressure measurements;
3. corneal indentation pulse amplitude measurements; and
4. forehead sweating measurements.

Significant differences have also been demonstrated between migraine and cluster headache for other variables, i.e. cerebral blood flow (this concerns classic migraine; 'migraine with aura'), electrocardiograms and probably also electroencephalograms. Furthermore, differences in computed-tomography scans have also been found between the two headache forms. If the findings in the migraine group are true manifestations of the migraine process *per se*, there is reason to believe that there is a clear difference between the two headache forms in this respect also.

As a last example, the serotonin level in whole blood has been estimated by Anthony and Lance (1971a,b) and Anthony *et al.* (1969). They found that in migraine patients there was a marked fall in serotonin in platelet-rich plasma from an average of $0.72\,\mu g$ per 10^9 platelets prior to the attack to $0.45\,\mu g$ per 10^9 platelets during the attack. No significant changes were found in cluster headache (see elsewhere) (Anthony and Lance, 1971a,b).

It should be mentioned, however, that Waldenlind *et al.* (1985) found that platelet serotonin concentrations and the kinetics of serotonin uptake did not differ in cluster headache and migraine. Since the tests were carried out with platelet samples obtained during the remission, these findings suggest a constitutional property in cluster headache, characterized as low V_{max} and K_m of serotonin uptake into platelets.

In conclusion, it may be stated that appreciable differences have been found between migraine and cluster headache which suggest a dichotomy between the two headaches. Most likely, we are faced with two different nosological disorders and not only variants on a continuum or spectrum of two clinical pictures (cluster headache and migraine). The occurrence of symptoms of migraine and cluster headache in the same patient can probably usually be explained as the chance occurrence of both disorders in the same patient.

According to this view, pathogenetic aspects found to be generally applicable in migraine cannot be taken by analogy to be true for cluster headache also. The pathogenesis in its entirety will, accordingly, have to be worked out separately for cluster headache.

OCULAR ORIGIN OF THE PAIN?

In 1978, we proposed some hypotheses regarding the pathogenesis of cluster headache and, in particular, of the pain (Sjaastad, 1978). One of them was that the eye itself could be the origin of the pain. The background for this hypothesis was that:

1. the pain of cluster headache is centred in, around, or behind the eye;
2. there are multiple ocular signs that occur between and, in particular, during an individual attack, such as 'a partial' Horner's syndrome (e.g. Kunkle and Anderson, 1961) (or rather, as we see it now, a 'Horner-like syndrome'), and increased intraocular pressure and corneal indentation pulse amplitudes (Hørven and Sjaastad, 1977);
3. there are also more 'distant' signs, e.g. the attack-related bradycardia, which from a theoretical point of view might be secondary to changes taking place intraocularly ('oculocardiac reflex');
4. there are 'cold spots' in the vicinity of the eye on the symptomatic side in the pain-free phase (Wood and Friedman, 1974). Later, it was demonstrated that there are signs of disturbances in the autonomic nervous supply around the eye, with an abnormal sweating pattern in the forehead (Sjaastad *et al.*, 1981).

Logically, the *bradycardia* typical of a certain phase of the attack (Russell and Storstein, 1983) might be the expression of parasympathetic nerve stimulation or *sympathetic inhibition* or a combination of both, if the 'traditional' autonomic systems are involved. If the bradycardia were due to an oculocardiac reflex (e.g. Kirsch *et al.*, 1957), the parasympathetic system might be affected secondarily. However, the increase in intraocular pressure is only moderate, being clearly lower than that found in chronic paroxysmal hemicrania. The absolute levels of pressure are also clearly lower than those found in glaucomatous eyes. Whether the increase in *intraocular pressure* is sufficiently large to make this mechanism operative is doubtful. This problem may, however, be looked at from another angle: in glaucoma, the process of pressure increase is time-consuming; in cluster headache it may be hyperacute. This may indicate an important difference as far as symptom production is concerned. The possibility thus cannot be entirely ruled out that the bradycardia (e.g. Bruyn *et al.*, 1976; Hørven and Sjaastad, 1977; Russell and Storstein, 1983) observed during attack is caused by the increased intraocular pressure, i.e. as a result of the oculocardiac reflex. There may still be other factors pertaining to the eye that are responsbile for the bradycardia and not only the increment in intraocular pressure. I am, however, inclined to believe that the mechanism underlying the bradycardia is a different one.

The problem of the ocular origin of the *pain* was looked into by Rogado and Graham (1979) who searched for patients having a combination of enucleation and a cluster headache-like picture. In five such cases headache co-existed with ipsilateral enucleation, and this was also the case in later reported cases (McKinney *et al.*, 1983; Prusinski *et al.*, 1985).

It might be argued that in patients in whom the enucleation took place ahead of the development of headache attacks, the pain is not identical to the one in cluster headache and that the mechanism might be similar to that of 'phantom limb' pains (McKinney, 1983). The best proof for a lack of a causal relationship between eye and pain generation, as far as I am concerned, would, therefore, be in cases with enucleation *after* the onset of typical cluster headache. Rogado and Graham demonstrated that, even with this sequence of development, enucleation did not abort the headache.

The question of the identity of the above-mentioned cases with genuine cluster headache also arises. Thus, McKinney (1983), gave no information on the duration of single attacks and did not state how frequently nocturnal attacks occurred. The cluster phenomenon apparently was not present in the first phase of headache but seemed to be present later. The cluster phenomenon as such, however, seems to be a non-specific feature (Sjaastad *et al.*, 1988a). It would have been useful to have data on other typical cluster headache phenomena like attack-related forehead sweating and the effect of histamine/nitroglycerin in provoking attacks. The picture described by McKinney is at least cluster headache-like.

However, the data of Rogado and Graham (1979) enabled it to be concluded with reasonable certainty that the pain does not originate in the eye itself. The evidence available tends to show that the pain does not originate within the orbit either since cluster headache may co-exist with exenteration as well (McKinney, 1983).

WHERE DOES THE PAIN IN CLUSTER HEADACHE ORIGINATE?

This question cannot be properly answered at the present time. However, before outlining some possibilities, I would like to take the following roundabout approach: a comparison may be made with trigeminal neuralgia and sciatica. As far as such pain conditions are understood at the present time, the pain may be felt in an area quite distant from the area where the pathological process itself is located.

The importance of this point of view as regards cluster headache is illustrated by a case report by McKinney (1983). A patient had all the orbital contents exenterated on the left side due to a squamous cell carcinoma of the nearby skin. One year later, he started having bouts of left-sided headache, similar to ordinary cluster headache attacks. The fact that cluster headaches may 'co-exist with' a missing eye has been established previously (Rogado and Graham, 1979). The interesting fact in this connection is, however, the description of the pain in McKinney's case, which the patient located in the area 'where his eye would have been', despite the fact that the pain could not originate within the eye.

The pain of cluster headache may be felt over a wide area, but is usually *maximal in, around or—even more typically—behind the eye*. But this does not mean that it originates in these areas. The pain may be projected or referred to these areas, whilst its origin may be in a quite different site. To make a comparison with the other group in the cluster headache syndrome, i.e. chronic paroxysmal hemicrania, we have the following situation in a patient who can precipitate attacks mechanically. The most tender zone is in the neck, even outside attacks. From these tender areas, unilateral attacks (apparently 'regular attacks') can be precipitated. Such observations should be borne in mind when the origin of pain in cluster headache is discussed. Naturally, it is of great interest to elucidate or determine whether the pain of cluster headache is 'central' or 'peripheral' in nature.

The pain, may, in theory, have various causes and sources. It might be:

1. an autonomically mediated pain, for example through the implication of centripetally leading nerve fibres, like substance P fibres;
2. a pain due to involvement of vascular structures, the pain arising within the vessel wall or being due to secondary pressure on pain-sensitive structures (a 'vascular' pain in contradistinction to an 'ischaemic' pain?);
3. an 'ischaemic' pain';
4. a neurogenic pain; or
5. a 'central' pain.

There are no hard data to substantiate any of these suggestions. A 'central' theory has been discussed by e.g. Sjaastad (1978) and Medina and Diamond (1979). Sicuteria in his many publications has, over the years, also been a powerful supporter of the central theory (e.g. Sicuteri *et al.*, 1985). That pain may be created by intrinsic cerebral affections is known ('thalamic pain'). Raskin (1987) has also described head pain starting after electrode implantation in the periaqueductal grey area.

Some sources of pain can be excluded with reasonable certainty. The pain in cluster headache does not originate within the eye or the orbit (see previous section). Neither does the pain source seem to be intimately connected with extracranial vessels on the symptomatic side because, for example, the temporal artery has been removed in several cases without any tendency to abatement being seen. The fact that the temporal vessel on the symptomatic side is not infrequently involved during attack, but that its removal does not lead to any improvement of the headache, is in itself a remarkable phenomenon. Likewise, blockade of autonomic impulses (with atropine or β-receptor blocking agents) seems to have no influence on pain severity. On the other hand, impulses transmitted via the more recently discovered transmitters will not be blocked by these traditional blocking agents. Blockade of the superior cervical ganglion and stellate ganglion should, nevertheless, block transmitters other than noradrenaline. Blockade of the stellate ganglion does not provoke attacks (Lance, 1982). Other autonomic ganglia have also been mentioned as the source or mediator of pain. It has been claimed that cocainization of the sphenopalatine ganglion may be beneficial in cluster headache (Barré, 1982). If reproducible, this observation may be of importance when trying to outline cluster headache pathogenesis. There are, however, examples of removal of, for example, the sphenopalatine ganglion without any discontinuation of pain attacks (Meyer *et al.*, 1970).

What about the neck as a source of pain in cluster headache? A comparison with chronic paroxysmal hemicrania may again be in order: the relative regularity of attacks in some patients with chronic paroxysmal hemicrania may suggest that the initiation of attacks in this headache is 'centrally' governed. A certain regularity of attacks may also be present in cluster headache. The precipitation of attacks is a peculiar phenomenon; it is found in chronic paroxysmal hemicrania and cervicogenic headache but has so far not been demonstrated in cluster headache. Therefore, despite the special features that may point to a central origin, there remains a strong likelihood that the neck is involved in chronic paroxysmal hemicrania cases where there is a marked ability to precipitate attacks.

Although a dysfunction of a central 'metronomic' regulation might underlie the timing of attacks in chronic paroxysmal hemicrania, it seems as though this relative regularity of attacks is combined with a peripheral attack-generating mechanism. The attacks *may* even have a purely peripheral basis: time-consuming processes may occur repeatedly with the underlying mechanism being, for example, the accumulation and release of vasoactive substances; or the mechanical pressure upon peripheral nervous and pain-conducting structures may be exerted by, for example, venous pooling of blood. During attack, 'counter-measures' may take away the pathological pressure, only to lay the foundation for a new build-up. With these models, the attack *per se* may be viewed as a salutary process. These models may also be applicable in cluster headache, where the process seems to be slower (longer intervals between attacks).

If the headache is 'central' in nature, it may be that superior, regulating centres give the 'go-ahead signal'. For the manifestations of the pain, *peripheral* nervous structures may be played upon. The 'trigemino-vascular' system described by Moskowitz and co-workers (Moskowitz *et al.*, 1979; Moskowitz, 1984, 1986) is of considerable interest in this connection. The problem of antinociception also arises in this context.

One problem surfaces, however, if this is the solution: the good therapeutic response to glycerol around the Gasserian ganglion in chronic cluster headache cases (Waltz *et al.*, 1985; Ekbom *et al.*, 1987) and the apparently similarly good therapeutic response to injection of the major occipital nerve in the episodic form (Anthony, 1985). It is astonishing that two such different approaches, topographically speaking, can both lead to a striking improvement. If neck problems are present in cluster headache they seem, at least in the majority of cases, to be at a subclinical level. My guess is that one of these therapeutic trials is not going to stand the test of time. But, again to make a brief comparison with trigeminal neuralgia, the fact that an (admittedly transitory) effect is obtained in tic douloureux by injecting local anaesthetics around the peripheral branches does not mean that the site of pathology is just at this spot. Similarly, the beneficial effect of glycerol around the Gasserian ganglion does not mean that the ganglion is the site of pathology.

There is not sufficient basic knowledge to *exclude* the possibility that the primary pathology is 'central' in origin. The entire facial sensory and vascular systems may be so delicate and the 'central' processing of 'peripheral' impulses so intricate that multifaceted and multilocated stimuli can trigger the system. When certain impulses from the periphery are blocked, the threshold for setting off an attack may be heightened. The primary abnormality may, nevertheless, remain intact and unchanged. The pain may have its origin in the periphery only; it may also have combined 'peripheral' and 'central' origin (Sjaastad, 1988b) (see also Towards a Pathogenetic Synthesis).

THE MAJOR CHARACTERISTICS OF CLUSTER HEADACHE

The various clinical features of cluster headache have been dealt with in the foregoing. There are two typical traits of cluster headache that to some extent set this syndrome apart from others (i.e. these traits are also present in chronic paroxysmal hemicrania): the unilaterality of the attack and the various autonomic phenomena accompanying the attack. Other characteristics make it even possible partly to differentiate clinically between the ordinary form of cluster headache and chronic paroxysmal hemicrania: the cluster phenomenon itself (which is lacking in the non-remitting form of chronic paroxysmal hemicrania) and the male sex preponderance. These factors will be dealt with.

Cyclic nature of cluster headache: 'the volcano pattern'

The cyclic nature of cluster headache is not understood at present (e.g. Vijayan, 1989). In the early days it was believed that there was an absolute quietude between cluster periods. Scrutiny of the remission phase has shown that there are, at least in many cases, small reminiscences of attacks appearing to a greater or lesser frequency throughout the relatively silent phase, and occasionally there are more ferocious attacks, with a severity up to the level of the attacks that occur during regular bouts. There is thus no complete tranquillity in the remission phase.

The absolute timing set aside, the temporal pattern may seem to resemble that of a volcano: a 'volcano pattern' (Sjaastad, 1986c). Once in a while the molten lava is ejected (the cluster period). Then there are long periods of a relative outer inactivity (the remission phase). But the external, apparent calmness of a volcano does not entirely reflect the inner process. There is continuous interior activity, and this inner turmoil is occasionally reflected in small outbursts ('he is a little active again today'). The ferocity of the two headache disorders also seems to be comparable. I thus have a strong feeling that, at least frequently, the pathological *'process'* continues during remission, but at a significantly lower level than during a bout. Extrapolating this idea to chronic paroxysmal hemicrania, the difference between the temporal pattern of this headache and cluster headache may only be a relatively moderate difference between the level of the process in the two headaches during the ebb: the attacks break through in chronic paroxysmal hemicrania, although in a very weak form, but usually not in cluster headache (see also Figure 4.3).

However, the activity of the process in cluster headache is, qualitatively speaking, at such a level during the remission (as compared to the cluster phase) that the manifestations of the disorder cannot easily be provoked. Thus, attacks cannot be provoked by nitroglycerin in the remission. Furthermore, in some isolated cases, the remission may be of considerable length (up to 25–35 years); the disease process is apparently dormant (again like the volcano!), so that the patient has almost or completely forgotten the disease. The question also arises whether the headache may 'burn out' in some rare cases.

It remains a riddle why the process that continues at a low, discrete, subclinical level is activated at certain stages, whereas on other occasions there is only a small outburst, but no bout. Perhaps two factors have to be present to manifest this headache. It may be that long-term biological rhythms (circannual rhythms) are in some way connected with this process (Nappi *et al.*, 1983, 1985); it may be that hormonal, autonomic, environmental/seasonal or mental/emotional factors play a role in setting the scene (see under the various sections); or it may be that a combination of these factors may occasionally do the trick.

Male preponderance

The predominance of male cluster headache patients is bewildering, and there is no tenable explanation for this. Any theory aimed at explaining the pathogenesis of cluster headache must also explain this phenomenon. Theoretically, there may be several explanations for this phenomenon. Since there seem to be cases of true cluster headache in females, the male sex is not a necessary factor of the condition. The male preponderance could either be due to the sex hormones as such or it could be secondary to a specific behaviour of the male sex, in other words not directly related to male hormones (Sjaastad *et al.*, 1987a).

To deal with the last possibility first, the predominance of cluster headache in males might be due to a greater proneness of males to accidents (e.g. Manzoni *et al.*, 1983b). In particular, the liability to neck and head injuries may be of significance. The neck may be of crucial importance in the development of this headache. Lance (1982) found head injuries in eight of 60 patients, i.e. 13%. The nature and degree of the head injury were not specified. Friedman and Mikropoulos (1958) found a head injury frequency of 16% in their series (with or without loss of consciousness). The frequency of head injuries in the series studied by Manzoni *et al.* (1983b) may even be higher. Head injury with loss of consciousness had occurred in 11% of cluster headache patients and in 4% and 5% of age- and sex-matched migraine and tension headache patients, respectively. These figures are significantly different at the 2% (cluster headache versus migraine) and 5% levels (cluster headache versus tension headache) (χ^2 test). Head injury without loss of consciousness was found in 12% of cluster headache patients. The prevalence of headache without loss of consciousness did not differ in the three groups. The prevalence of severe head injury in cases of chronic cluster headache was even higher (21%).

Lance (1982) noted that in four of his cases there might be an association, both a temporal one and a locational one, between the head injury and the cluster headache picture. Manzoni *et al.* (1983b) found that in 12 (out of 20) patients in whom head injury with loss of consciousness had been unilateral, the side of the injury and the later headache corresponded. The mean latency period between head injury and onset of headache in these cases was 9.2 years. If this information is totally reliable, which is always a problem when patient memory is at stake, these figures mean that in eight out of 20 cases, i.e. in 40% of the cases, there was no correspondence between sides. It is also remarkable that among those patients who had undergone craniofacial surgery (such as mastoidectomy, correction of strabismus, removal of a maxillary cyst, and removal of infectious foci), the later occurring headache manifested itself on the side of the surgery in 11 of 15 cases. The average time interval between surgery and headache was about 5 years. The clinical picture in these cases seemed to be typical of cluster headache. It would have been desirable to have undertaken supplementary diagnostic tests for cluster headache in at least some of these cases.

The diagnosis of cluster headache has been considered to be easy, and it is straightforward in typical cases. In recent years, however, it has been observed that there are also cases which, from a diagnostic point of view, may seem like cluster headache patients, but in whom the pain attacks have frequently started after head and face trauma of different sorts, and also after operations. To the best of our understanding, pain is discernibly less marked in many of these cases than in ordinary cluster headache. Some autonomic phenomena, e.g. conjunctival injection and facial flushing, may also be more pronounced in such cases than in cluster headache patients. These patients do not exhibit to the same extent the autonomic function test patterns that are well established in cluster headache. Some such cases may bear some similarity to the pictures described by Bing (1913, 1930, 1945, 1952) and Brickner and Riley (1935).

It is not possible on the basis of the available evidence to rule out a possible role of head and neck trauma in the generation of clinically manifest cluster headache, or very similar clinical pictures. Abnormal sensory input from the injured area may thwart the usual central processing and integration of the total sensory input. Abnormal reflexes and axon reflexes may be established. However, that such trauma are the sole cause of cluster headache in general is highly unlikely. First of all, not all patients with cluster headache have undergone such trauma. In addition, such trauma occur fairly frequently in the general population and in other types of headache, without the development of cluster headache. We are, however, not on *terra firma* in this matter. Trauma to the neck and face and surgical procedures, including whiplash injuries, lead to clinical pictures, similar to cluster headache.

Anthony (1985) obtained pain relief by applying steroids locally in the area of the greater occipital nerve in patients with cluster headache. We have also tried to do greater occipital nerve/C_2 root injections in some hard-to-treat cluster headache cases in the course of the last 3–4 years, but without any appreciable success. Bigo *et al.* (1989) also applied methylprednisolone close to the greater occipital nerve on the symptomatic side in cluster headache patients (eight episodic cases, eight chronic cases). The results were less favourable than those obtained by Anthony. Altogether, there is a possibility of a connection between cluster headache and neck and head trauma, but there is no firm evidence to show this. It is interesting in this respect that many patients with cluster headache feel that holding the head in certain positions may ease the pain of attack to some extent.

There are, moreover, other possible differences between male and female behaviour which could be of importance in this connection. In Western countries, both the drinking and smoking habits may have had some detrimental effect on a particular age group. Kudrow (1980) has found some differences in drinking and smoking habits between cluster headache patients and the population as a whole. Whether or not these habits are of any *aetiological* importance in cluster headache is not known. Excessive drinking and smoking may be a direct reflection of the personality structure of prospective cluster headache patients. There may not be a causal relationship between these habits and the later development of cluster headache.

Another feature that may be significant is the negative influence of a heavy daily routine, and daily strain and stress factors (Selye, 1956). It would seem that these factors may be different between the sexes in certain age groups. Many cluster headache patients claim that there is obviously a relationship between the strenuousness of work and the start of another cluster period. This may also apply to initial onset of cluster headache. There is hardly a one-to-one relationship between stress and the initiation of cluster headache as such, or a particular bout. Emotional/psychological factors may help pave the way, making another cluster period 'permissible', if the other factors are tuned to initiate a cycle (a 'combination of provocative factors'; see 'The Cyclic Nature of Cluster Headache'). However, it is not as simple as a short-lasting, strenuous period or single emotional event precipitates an immediate outburst. However, over time, mental strain may produce the 'terrain' (by changing the central autonomic tone?) in which cluster headache may develop if the natural preconditions for developing the disorder are present (e.g. Sjaastad, 1987a).

Because of the expectations of them in modern society and/or because of their hormonal characteristics, males may be more vulnerable than females to certain external or internal influences (e.g. Sjaastad *et al.*, 1987a).

The male sex hormones *per se* may be important. Despite the hypermasculine appearance of cluster headache patients, if anything, low serum testosterone levels have been found in these patients (e.g. Facchinetti *et al.*, 1986), particularly during the cluster period. There thus seems to be a discrepancy between the hypermasculine appearance of these patients and the low testosterone levels. However, it would be of interest to know whether the patients studied really did have the 'leonine' appearance described by Graham (1975). Also, female patients may exhibit a virile physiognomy. It would be useful to know whether female patients exhibiting these masculine traits have changes in sexual hormones.

It is highly unlikely that the sex hormone levels *per se* are disease producing. The hormonal changes demonstrated in affected males are more likely to be the consequence than the cause of the headache. If the masculine physiognomy really is a reflection of testosterone activity, and the testosterone levels are decreased, abnormal reactions may be taking place at the receptor level (supersensitivity reactions) (Sjaastad *et al.*, 1987a).

'VASCULAR' MECHANISMS

Cluster headache was originally separated from migraine. Migraine was, and in many circles still is, considered to be a 'vascular' disease. The Ad Hoc Committee on Classification of Headache (1962) classified cluster headache as a subgroup of 'Vascular headache of the migraine type' (see above). This and the facts that the headache may be partly 'throbbing' (see Table 2.4) that the headache has been considered a 'red migraine' (i.e. with redness in the skin, as mentioned by the old clinicians (e.g. Heyck, 1981)), that conjunctival injection is an accompaniment of the attack, and that temporal vessels may be dilated, are probably some of the main reasons for the continued belief that cluster headache is a 'vascular' headache. Ekbom and Lindahl's (1971) observation of an improvement in angina pectoris during the cluster phase may also be consistent with such ideas. Hypertension during attack has also been described (Nattero and Savi, in press). It is probably worth mentioning that although 'large' vessels like the temporal vessels are occasionally affected in cluster headache, small vessels (like the conjunctival vessels) and not the major vessels are typically affected (Emblem, 1964).

The arterial territories involved have been pinpointed, but the locations reported by different workers are different. Furthermore, the vascular phenomenon of significance is supposed to be a dilatation, the dilatation being not only one of the processes that occur in a chain reaction during the disease process, but also being pain producing in itself. As a matter of fact, as shown below, the dilatation has been considered to be the main headache producing factor.

Medina and Diamond (1977) have claimed that '. . . during the headache phase, migraine involves mainly the external carotid circulation, and cluster headache the internal carotid distribution'. In addition, Anthony and Lance (1971b) reported that 'notwithstanding the difficulty regarding the classification of cluster headache, it is generally agreed that the headache is due mainly to dilatation of extracranial vessels, with some contribution from the internal carotid artery if some of the eye and nasal symptoms are to be accounted for'. Horton (1956a) has claimed that the pain of 'histaminic cephalgia' is chiefly extracranial in origin, owing to dilatation of the extracranial vessels. Ekbom (1975) found that approximately 50% of the patients experienced less pain on digital compression of the ipsilateral superficial temporal carotid arteries during the attack.

Apparently Ekbom's (1970) findings by angiography of an attack-related narrowing of the lumen of the internal carotid artery, presumably due to oedema of the wall, have stirred the imagination of many headache researchers in these respects. Therefore, questions regarding the interpretation of these findings arise. It should be noted that the mentioned changes were minor and were only found in a solitary case. The attack appeared after contrast injection, which may precipitate headache attacks, usually migraine-like in character (Hauge, 1954). A crucial question, therefore, is whether this was a spontaneously occurring attack. Would this finding be reproduced in spontaneously occurring attacks? Would it be reproduced in all cases? In other words, was it a characteristic of that very patient or is it a characteristic of the disease as such? I have a strong feeling that these aspects will have to be clarified before attaching too much importance to this finding.

For the sake of argument, let us assume that changes in the extracranial part of the internal carotid artery are characteristic features of cluster headache attack. How then do these changes come about? Are they primary vascular events? A 'spontaneous' vasomotion could be caused by intrinsic vascular wall circuits. Or is the signal brought to the vessel from somewhere else? If so, is the signal to the vessel of neurogenic nature or is it carried via the blood? In the latter case, abnormal levels of circulating vasoactive substances or abnormal sensitivity to vasoactive substances not occurring in excessive quantities could be the underlying mechanisms.

The systemic blood pressure is only very moderately changed during attacks (e.g. Russell and von der Lippe, 1982). The vascular reactions during attack may seem to be rather localized, i.e. in the facial area. Clear-cut, attack-induced changes (increased corneal indentation pulse amplitude and intraocular pressure) are also present during the attack, especially on the symptomatic side, and the temporal artery may be dilated. Is it then likely that vascular alterations (dilatation and other phenomena) start independently in these separate areas, or is it likely that there is a coordination of these events? One may have difficulty in understanding—and accepting—that arteries of this dimension, and situated 'rather far' apart topographically, should start 'operating' on their own. There are, so far, no indications to suggest that the one of these manifestations is caused by the other one, e.g. the internal carotid artery changes being primary to the ocular changes.

The following observations are relevant to the above-described sequence of events. Spontaneously occurring occlusive disease of the carotid artery as well as graded occlusion of the internal carotid artery give rise to a marked ipsilateral reduction in corneal indentation pulse amplitudes (Hørven *et al.*, 1971; Nornes *et al.*, 1971a,b). The opposite trend in corneal indentation pulse amplitudes (that is an increase) is found during attacks of cluster headache. It is, therefore, hardly likely that the demonstrated luminal changes in the internal carotid artery during attack have a causal relationship to the increase in corneal indentation pulse amplitude. The intraocular changes would rather seem to be occasioned directly by the disease process in some way. In other words, both attack manifestations (the ocular and carotid changes) may be due to the same pathogenic mechanism. This reasoning is still easier to accept if the 'internal carotid artery' is systematically substituted by the 'temporal artery'. The exact timing of the onset of ocular changes in cluster headache in relation to the onset of the attack itself is not known. The impulses to the eye may be mediated via either neurogenic or vasogenic stimuli.

In the closely related headache, chronic paroxysmal hemicrania, there is good reason to believe that a vasodilatation causes the intraocular pressure to increase during attack. It is, of course, not legitimate to conclude that, by analogy, the cause of the moderate intraocular pressure increase in cluster headache itself is also a vasodilatation (it may, to a lesser or greater extent, be due to oedema formation). The discrepancy between the two headache forms for this parameter may be just one of the features separating the two types of headache.

The most likely cause of a change in vascular diameter in a localized area is that it is mediated via neurogenic or haematogeneous (blood borne) routes. Since the theory of mediation via vasoactive substances was in vogue in the early stage of the cluster headache story, this possiblity is looked into more closely below.

VASOACTIVE SUBSTANCES

Since the pathogenesis of cluster headache has for decades been considered to involve vascular mechanisms, substances influencing the tone of vessels came to be of major interest as mediators. In principle, the tone of vessels may be influenced by circulating vasoactive substances, by locally active ones (formed *in loco* or liberated), or by neural (autonomic) impulses. There may of course also be some interplay between these factors. The autonomic impulses are dealt with elsewhere (see Pathogenesis).

The enormous problem we face at present (and, of course, even more so in the early years of the cluster headache story) is that we are only just beginning to acquire exact information on vasoactive substances. The solitary substance which may be of crucial importance as a mediator, and also as potential pain producer, may not yet have been detected. In the case of an interplay between substances, only one or two of these may have been detected. So, at present, it may be impossible to grasp the situation, however much energy is put into an attempt to do so.

Horton's original contention that histamine is the culprit in cluster headache must be seen in this light. Histamine had been detected long before Horton and co-workers' description of 'histaminic cephalgia'. The classical transmitter in the parasympathetic nervous system, acetylcholine, was identified as a neurotransmitter in 1936, whilst the one in the sympathetic nervous system, noradrenaline, was not identified as such until 1946. Adrenaline was isolated at the beginning of this century, but its role was not clear. Serotonin was not discovered until several decades later. The kinins were discovered in the 1940s.

Thus, at the time of the 'final discovery' of cluster headache (1939), not many vasoactive substances were known from which to choose one to explain the vascular phenomena of the disorder. Another feature that made histamine attractive in this respect is the flushing effect that histamine exerts when injected locally in the skin. Horton *et al.* (1939) had discovered that the temperature in the symptomatic side of the head increases during an attack. At that time it would have been quite natural in the search for a mediator which could convey the vascular response in cluster headache to choose histamine. No greater import than this should probably be attached to the choice of histamine alone.

Histamine is known to be an extremely potent substance, the amounts present in the human body being more than enough to kill its host, if liberated. Horton felt that cluster headache could be a manifestation of a 'localized anaphylactoid reaction' to histamine. In a vaguely understood and probably merely speculative way, histamine should give rise to both local and systemic symptomatology. Horton (1956b) thus claimed that 'it seems evident that histamine is released from the shocked tissues in the region of the pain and accounts for most local phenomena' of the spontaneous attacks. As evidence for the systemic effects exerted by histamine ('absorption of this agent in the blood stream') Horton mentioned the increased acidity of the gastric contents which, according to Horton, should be 'comparable to that which is induced by the subcutaneous injection of known amounts of histamine'. He claimed further proof for his hypothesis by being able to elicit genuine attacks with histamine and by obtaining a therapeutic effect through histamine desensitization (see elsewhere).

One of the points in Horton's reasoning that is very difficult to grasp is that he not only claimed that histamine liberated in the 'shocked tissues' may play a decisive role in the *spontaneous* attacks, but also stated (Horton, 1956a, 1961) that histamine liberation takes place in the 'shocked tissues' in the region of pain, also in attacks induced by histamine. Therefore, this theoretical model states that histamine should liberate histamine. To put it mildly, this contention would be difficult to prove.

One is bound to encounter enormous difficulties when attempting to establish a cause-and-effect relationship between the effects of a given vasoactive substance and the vascular changes of cluster headache. Even greater difficulties will be encountered in trying to explain the pain in this way. When two phenomena occur at the same time, the inference can of course not be made that one is the cause of the other. Needless to say, it may be the other way around, or it may be that the phenomena are not interdependent, i.e. that both are caused by a third factor. This is self-evident. Nevertheless, in headache literature, these elementary rules have quite often been violated.

As discussed elsewhere (see Histamine Metabolism), the moderate and sporadically occurring differences found concerning histamine or its metabolic products in and outside attacks do not allow the conclusion to be drawn that the histamine changes cause the attacks. The histamine changes are more likely to be consequences of rather than the cause of attacks.

Serotonin levels have been measured (in platelet-rich plasma) during and between attacks (see elsewhere) and, although the tendency was the same as for histamine (i.e. with a significant difference between the two phases), the changes did not quite reach statistical significance (Anthony and Lance, 1971a,b). In addition, no consistent changes related to attacks have been found for kinins (Sjaastad, 1970), prostaglandins (Bennett *et al.*, 1974), or other vasoactive substances.

One particular feature of cluster headache attacks speaks strongly, almost decisively, against blood-borne substances (in the general circulation) being the sole causative agents in cluster headache. Cluster headache is, in principle, a unilateral headache; a substance carried in the general circulation should cause as many symptoms and signs and as much of each one of them on both sides. A general factor of this nature cannot, therefore, account for the entire picture of cluster headache. If there is also a local factor involved this might explain the unilaterality. The liberation of a vaso-neuroactive agent into a local artery to the affected area might explain the unilaterality. However, this is a somewhat far-fetched idea. The constant involvement of autonomically inner-vated organs, and generally with a lesser degree of involvement on the non-symptomatic side, makes such an explanation of the pathology more or less unacceptable. In conclusion, therefore, blood-borne substances alone can with reasonable certainty be excluded as the sole pathogenetic agents.

The 'trigemino-vascular system' (Moskowitz *et al.*, 1979; Sicuteri *et al.*, 1983; Moskowitz, 1984; De Marinis *et al.*, 1984; Agnoli and De Marinis, 1987) with the substance-P containing neurons may be of importance in mediating the vascular responses that occur during a cluster headache attack. But then we have left the field of purely blood-borne substances as the source for signal mediation and have entered that of neurons as the substrate for signals between organs or structures.

THE SIGNIFICANCE OF AUTONOMIC INVOLVEMENT

The idea of a 'central' origin of cluster headache cannot flatly be rejected. For example, Raskin (1987) has proposed that the periaqueductal grey area and the somatosensory region of the thalamus may be pain producing zones. There is a considerable body of information that may be interpreted to fit with the idea of a central origin. Such evidence includes the circadian periodicity of attacks (Nappi *et al.*, 1983). Autonomic changes, such as in T-wave form and polarity and QTc prolongation (corrected QT-time) during hyperventilation have been interpreted as having a 'central' origin (Boccuni *et al.*, 1984). In recent years, however, the search for pathogenetic models in cluster headache seems largely to have concentrated on *peripheral* structures, vessels, nerves and ganglia. There are prominent and multifaceted autonomic features pertaining to the cluster headache syndrome. Any theory aimed at providing an acceptable explanation of the pathogenesis of cluster headache must, as a minimum, give an incontrovertible explanation of the accompanying autonomic symptoms and signs in their entirety. A complete understanding of these accompaniments of the cluster headache attack would lead directly to the core of cluster headache pathogenesis (Sjaastad *et al.*, 1987a, 1988a).

Since the first attempts to classify the autonomic symptoms and signs of cluster headache (Kunkle and Anderson, 1961; Nieman and Hurwitz, 1961), there have been two main theories for explaining the mechanisms underlying these disturbances: a sympathetic hypofunction theory and a parasympathetic hyperfunction one. At the present level of understanding, neither of these theories adequately explains the entire array of autonomic symptoms and signs that are present in cluster headache. A theory proposing a *combination* of these two concepts has also been advanced (Spierings, 1980). In the following discussion, I deal with the shortcomings of these hypotheses.

The carotid canal (Kunkle and Anderson, 1961; Nieman and Hurwitz, 1961; Ekbom, 1970; Vijayan and Watson, 1982; Drummond, 1988a), the intermedius and facial nerves (Sachs, 1968; Solomon and Guglielmo, 1985; Solomon, 1986), the greater superficial petrosal nerve and the sphenopalatine ganglion (Gardner *et al.*, 1947; Meyer *et al.*, 1970; Barré, 1982; Hardebo and Elner, 1987), to mention some of the structures, have been considered crucial in the causation of the autonomic phenomena of cluster headache. According to some authors, not only the conjunctival hyperaemia, the lacrimation, and the rhinorrhoea can be accounted for on the basis of an aberration in these structures, but even the pain (e.g. Gardner *et al.*, 1947).

Parasympathetic hyperactivity

Proponents of the 'parasympathetic barrage theory' hypothesize that the pain of cluster headache is brought about in one of two ways: parasympathetic, vasodilatory signals are conveyed to blood vessels, mainly the internal carotid artery (e.g. Drummond, 1988a), from which nociceptive impulses, in their turn, are conveyed via the trigeminal nerve; or pain impulses from tissues of the head/face are transmitted via parasympathetic afferent fibres.

Some of the autonomic features, e.g. lacrimation and nasal secretion, could theoretically be accounted for on the basis of the 'parasympathetic barrage theory'. This theory, however, has clear shortcomings. Forehead sweating

(Sjaastad, 1986c), although frequently *subclinical*, is one of the steadfast accompaniments of cluster headache attacks. The forehead sweating can hardly be explained as being caused by a direct parasympathetic stimulation. Alternative mechanisms have, therefore, been invoked: there is, supposedly, a change in internal carotid artery diameter during an attack, which subsequently (through, for example, oedema formation in the wall) could lead to a compression of the sympathetic network surrounding the artery. This should then give rise to a third-neuron sympathetic lesion (see later and Pupillometry). The reduced heat-induced forehead sweating on the symptomatic side could then be explained as signs of sympathetic deficiency in this overall picture of parasympathetic overactivity.

It would also be difficult to explain the heart-rhythm irregularities on the basis of a purely parasympathetic discharge theory. The bradycardia could possibly be explained as being due to attack-related intraocular pressure increase, via the oculo-cardiac reflex. However, there is a dilemma in this context in that the increase in intraocular pressure (and the corneal indentation pulse amplitude increment) is only moderate. As a matter of fact, notably higher values are observed in chronic paroxysmal hemicrania (Hørven *et al.*, 1989), in which there is less bradycardia (Russell and Storstein, 1984). The possibility exists that the increase in intraocular pressure may not be the decisive feature in eliciting the oculo-cardiac reflex; however, the pain in the ocular area *itself* may be. But, even the pain level seems to be as marked in chronic paroxysmal hemicrania as in cluster headache.

Moreover, the bradycardia is only poorly descriptive of the cardiac manifestations of cluster headache. There is, on the whole, a rather marked *tachycardia* in the initial phase of the attack, the tachycardia phase seemingly being as characteristic of the attack as the bradycardia phase (Russell and Storstein, 1983). The drastic *rhythm disturbances* during attack (atrial fibrillation, sinoatrial block and atrioventricular block (Russell and Storstein, 1983)), occurring in 19% of the cases, and the *rapid changes* between the various abnormalities probably represent the most conspicuous electrocardigraphic changes in cluster headache. These abnormalities are not easily explained as being caused by simple parasympathetic barrage, which should cause bradycardia alone and not the rhythm abnormalities. Such a variety of disturbances has, interestingly enough, also been observed in connection with cerebral vascular catastrophes (Vaisrub, 1975) and epilepsy (e.g. Blumhardt, 1986).

A further dilemma with regard to the parasympathetic barrage theory is the fact that, whereas lacrimation, nasal secretion and facial sweating may occur on the symptomatic side during an attack, salivation is generally not increased (Saunte, 1984a). With pilocarpine as stimulant, salivation is an even more sensitive indicator of incipient stimulation than is forehead sweating (Table 2.40). Although pilocarpine is considered to be a parasympathicomimetic (muscarinic) agent, it may, admittedly, not lead to 'pure' parasympathetic stimulation because it also seems to have some 'anticholinergic' properties

Table 2.40 Various autonomic functions in episodic cluster headache: response on the symptomatic side, during attacks and after pilocarpine provocation

	Attack	Pilocarpine
Lacrimation	++	++
Forehead sweating	++	++
Salivation[a]	−	++

[a]From sublingual and submandibular glands. Note the strikingly different response during the attack itself and after pilocarpine administration.

(Newsome and Loewenfeld, 1974). The major salivary glands (the sublingual and submandibular glands) receive their parasympathetic innervation from the facial nerve (intermedius nerve) via the chorda tympani (see Figure 2.48). If the stimulus to the lacrimal and nasal glands during attacks were parasympathetic in nature, the signals would be mediated via the intermedius nerve. Such a stimulus would not only reach the mentioned glands, but even the salivary glands via the chorda tympani. The lack of a salivation increase during attacks, therefore, strongly contradicts a theory implying parasympathetic traffic along these routes. The possibility that the attack-related, parasympathetic irritation causing lacrimation and/or rhinorrhoea arises even more *peripherally* is hardly valid, because then, for example, the cardiac-rhythm disturbances would be even more difficult to understand. However, the possibility remains that fibres other than purely parasympathetic ones pass along the parasympathetic structures, such as the intermedius nerve, and that these may be involved, either alone or in conjunction with a more composite involvement.

The operative procedures carried out on parasympathetic, autonomic structures in cluster headache have mostly been directed at the nervus intermedius (Sachs, 1968; Solomon and Apfelbaum, 1986), the major superficial petrosal nerve (Gardner *et al.*, 1947; Stowell, 1970), and the sphenopalatine ganglion (Meyer *et al.*, 1970). There seem to have been some encouraging results, although, in general, the results of these operations seem to have been discouraging. The lack of consistency between pre-operative findings and post-operative results in connection with procedures directed towards parasympathetic structures weakens the position of these structures as being of major pathogenetic significance in cluster headache.

Common to the parasympathetic (and sympathetic) structures in question is that they are located rather far away from the midline (where, it is suspected, structures of crucial pathogenetic importance are located). If the *primary* pathological condition were located in one of these areas, then one would also have to explain how autonomic phenomena (and pain?) can spread to the other side. Are there any cross-links? Would it not be necessary to conjecture a

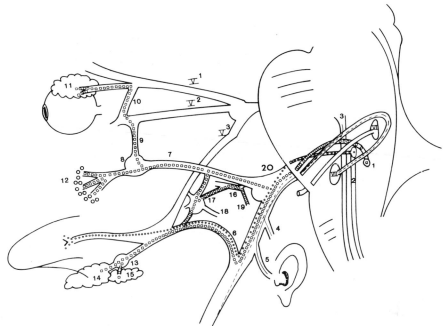

Figure 2.48 Parasympathetic innervation of lacrimal, nasal, sublingual and submandibular glands. (———) General somatic afferents (mechanoreceptors skin external auditory meatus and concha auriculae); (○) special visceral afferents (to nucleus gustatorius of solitary tract); (□) general visceral efferents (from nucleus saliv. superior to lacrimal, sublingual and submandibular glands and nasal mucosa secretory cells); (– – – –) special visceral efferents (mimetic facial muscles). The route of visceral efferents (and afferents) via the otic ganglion is an alternative possible mechanical variant. 1, Superior salivatory nucleus; 2, solitary tract; 3, descending spinal tract of the trigeminal nerve; 4, ramus postauricular VII; 5, ramus anastomoto cum ramus auricular X; 6, chorda tympani; 7, major superficial petrosal nerve; 8, pterygopalatine ganglion (sphenopalatine ganglion); 9, nervus pterygopalatinus; 10, nervus zygomaticus; 11, lacrimal gland; 12, glands, nasal and palatine mucosa; 13, Langley's ganglion; 14, sublingual gland; 15, submandibular gland; 16, minor superficial petrosal nerve; 17, otic ganglion; 18, anastomosis with tympanic nerve (IX); 19, anastomosis between 16 and IX; 20, geniculate ganglion. (From Bruyn (1984). Courtesy of *Cephalalgia*.)

'central' source (*'origo'*) with an extension to *both* sides? All these possibilities will have to be explored.

Sympathetic hypofunction

There are signs and symptoms that indicate a sympathetic autonomic dysfunction in cluster headache (Figures 2.49 to 2.51). Contrary to the case in migraine, no direct recording of sympathetic activity has been carried out in cluster headache. Muscle nerve sympathetic activity, as estimated by means of the microelectrode recording technique from the peroneal nerve, did not reveal any difference between spontaneously occurring attacks and the headache-free state in eight patients with common migraine (Fagius, 1985). It should be

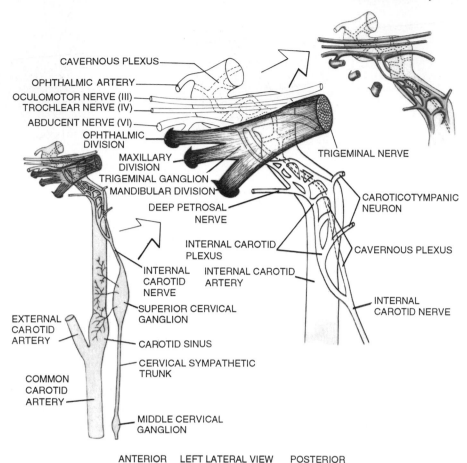

CAVERNOUS PLEXUS

OPHTHALMIC ARTERY

OCULOMOTOR NERVE (III)
TROCHLEAR NERVE (IV)

ABDUCENT NERVE (VI)

OPHTHALMIC
DIVISION

MAXILLARY
DIVISION

TRIGEMINAL GANGLION
MANDIBULAR DIVISION

DEEP PETROSAL
NERVE

INTERNAL CAROTID
PLEXUS

INTERNAL   INTERNAL CAROTID
CAROTID   ARTERY
NERVE

SUPERIOR CERVICAL
GANGLION

EXTERNAL
CAROTID
ARTERY

CAROTID SINUS

CERVICAL SYMPATHETIC
TRUNK

COMMON
CAROTID
ARTERY

MIDDLE CERVICAL
GANGLION

TRIGEMINAL NERVE

CAROTICOTYMPANIC
NEURON

CAVERNOUS PLEXUS

INTERNAL
CAROTID NERVE

ANTERIOR   LEFT LATERAL VIEW   POSTERIOR

Figure 2.49   Sympathetic innervation of the neck with special reference to the internal carotid artery. (From Vijayan and Watson (1982). Courtesy of *Headache*.)

emphasized that this type of study does not exclude the possibility of dysfunction in other parts of the sympathetic nervous system in migraine.

Signs of Horner's syndrome (or, rather, of a 'Horner-like syndrome') are an integral part of cluster headache (Table 2.41). It is widely believed that in cluster headache there are localized changes in the internal carotid artery in the carotid canal during an attack. The evidence of such a narrowing is meagre, to say the least. In one attack, which may have been precipitated by X-ray contrast medium, Ekbom (1970) found that the internal carotid artery was narrowed. This could be due either to oedema formation in the vessel wall or to a spastic condition, the latter alternative being favoured by Ekbom.

Strong statements have been made about the role of the carotid artery in the carotid canal in the production of autonomic phenomena in cluster headache on the basis of the rather meagre existing evidence; it has thus been claimed

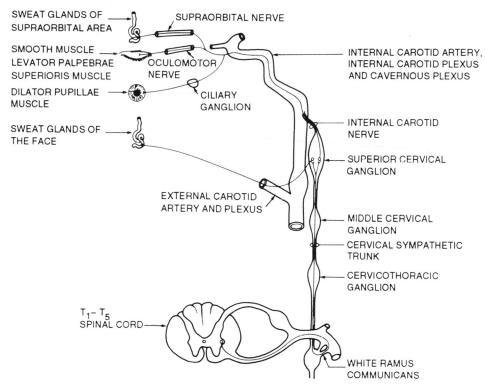

SWEAT GLANDS OF SUPRAORBITAL AREA

SUPRAORBITAL NERVE

SMOOTH MUSCLE LEVATOR PALPEBRAE SUPERIORIS MUSCLE

OCULOMOTOR NERVE

DILATOR PUPILLAE MUSCLE

CILIARY GANGLION

SWEAT GLANDS OF THE FACE

EXTERNAL CAROTID ARTERY AND PLEXUS

INTERNAL CAROTID ARTERY, INTERNAL CAROTID PLEXUS AND CAVERNOUS PLEXUS

INTERNAL CAROTID NERVE

SUPERIOR CERVICAL GANGLION

MIDDLE CERVICAL GANGLION

CERVICAL SYMPATHETIC TRUNK

CERVICOTHORACIC GANGLION

T_1– T_5 SPINAL CORD

WHITE RAMUS COMMUNICANS

Figure 2.50 Sympathetic pathways involved in the innervation of various organs in the forehead, eyes, and face. (From Vijayan and Watson (1982). Courtesy of *Headache*.)

Table 2.41 Possible involvement of the sympathetic nervous system in cluster headache

Increased sympathetic stimuli during attack?	Sympathetic dysfunction? (Horner's syndrome)
If so: the miosis between attacks should, during attack, be converted to a mydriasis *But:* there is no mydriasis *Ergo:* there is probably no increased sympathetic tone	In favour of this: miosis (frequent), ptosis (occasional), facial anhidrosis (±), phenylephrine pupillometric test shows 'cross-over' pattern (±) Counter-arguments: Hydroxyamphetamine pupillometric pattern (−)[a]

[a]This pattern does not quite fit with I, II, or III sympathetic neuron patterns (see also Figure 2.44). Salvesen *et al.* (1987b, 1988).

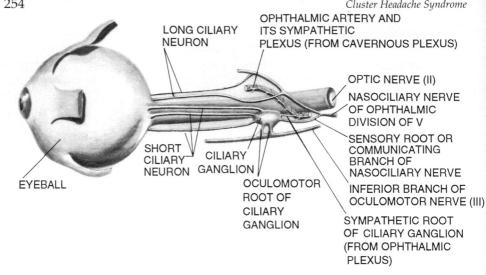

OPHTHALMIC ARTERY AND
ITS SYMPATHETIC
PLEXUS (FROM CAVERNOUS PLEXUS)

LONG CILIARY
NEURON

OPTIC NERVE (II)

NASOCILIARY NERVE
OF OPHTHALMIC
DIVISION OF V

SENSORY ROOT OR
COMMUNICATING
BRANCH OF
NASOCILIARY NERVE

SHORT
CILIARY
NEURON   CILIARY
          GANGLION

EYEBALL

OCULOMOTOR
ROOT OF
CILIARY
GANGLION

INFERIOR BRANCH OF
OCULOMOTOR NERVE (III)

SYMPATHETIC ROOT
OF CILIARY GANGLION
(FROM OPHTHALMIC
PLEXUS)

ANTERIOR   LEFT LATERAL VIEW   POSTERIOR

Figure 2.51 Sympathetic fibres in the orbit. (From Vijayan and Watson (1982). Courtesy of *Headache*.)

that the 'partial' Horner's syndrome seen in cluster headache *is* due to a dysfunction of the carotid periarterial, sympathetic nerve fibres. Our group has been opposed to accepting at face value the widely held belief that the pupillary signs in cluster headache are due to a *regular* sympathetic third-neuron dysfunction (post-ganglionic Horner's syndrome).

As we see it, the solitary case and the fact that the attack may not have been spontaneous indicate that conclusions based on this observation must be drawn with great caution. If there were oedema formation in the vessel wall, pressure could be exerted on the sympathetic plexus around the artery, which could result in a third-neuron sympathetic lesion (Figures 2.49 and 2.50). Other attack-related, local pathological events might also result in such a lesion. However, this chain of events represents different, unproven steps.

The occasional dilation of the temporal artery during attack may reflect the same pathological process as that observed in the internal carotid artery (Ekbom, 1970). From a theoretical point of view, these arteries themselves are hardly the source of pain. The surgical removal of the temporal artery at least does not lead to any improvement of cluster headache. According to Chorobski and Penfield (1932), the sensory input from the internal carotid artery is transmitted via the major superficial petrosal nerve and the geniculate ganglion (Figure 2.48). The finding that surgery directed towards parasympathetic structures has resulted in no clear, notable success in cluster headache might, to some extent, also disprove that the internal carotid artery is the source of the pain.

Some of the important facts when trying to implicate the sympathetic nervous system in cluster headache pathogenesis pertain to pupillometric findings. Fanciullacci *et al.* (1982) found no pupillometric signs of supersensitivity to a directly working sympathicomimetic agent (phenylephrine) on the symptomatic side during the remission stage or during a bout. This finding was made in the presence of a clearly pathological tyramine test result. The positive tyramine test indicates that there is a dysfunction of the ocular sympathetic system and of the third neuron at that. If so, this phenomenon ought to have been accompanied by a supersensitivity to directly acting sympathicomimetics; in other words, the phenylephrine test ought to have been positive. If reproducible, this combination of findings would definitely speak against a simple third-neuron sympathetic dysfunction. It should be emphasized, however, that, in accordance with our recent findings in patients who were mostly studied during a bout, there are, admittedly weak, signs of supersensitivity to phenylephrine (Salvesen *et al.*, 1987b). Our findings in *this* respect, therefore, are in conformity with the presence of a regular Horner syndrome.

The pupillary changes are, nevertheless, not easily explicable on the basis of a purely sympathetic involvement. With regular Horner's syndrome of the first- and second-neuron type, tyramine (or hydroxyamphetamine) eyedrops (Salvesen *et al.*, 1987a) cause *more* dilatation on the symptomatic than on the non-symptomatic side (Figure 2.38). In a third-neuron lesion, however, such eyedrops seem not to lead to dilatation. *Cluster headache does not follow any of these patterns* (Figure 2.38). This could be due to either of the following underlying mechanisms:

1. There is not a complete, but only a moderate, sympathetic dysfunction on the symptomatic side in cluster headache, for which reason the pupillometric pattern is not fully developed. In this case, the pattern in cluster headache would probably be very similar to a third-neuron pattern. Individual cluster headache patients with a tyramine pattern seemingly identical to the third-neuron pattern have, as a matter of fact, been identified (Thompson and Mensher, 1971; Sjaastad *et al.*, 1987b) but are unusual (approximately 15% of our cases; see Figure 2.45) (Sjaastad, 1988a).
2. The mechanism underlying the tyramine abnormality differs slightly or even fundamentally from that of the first-, second- or third-neuron dysfunctions. The finding that lithium may correct the anisocoria in cluster headache (Fanciullacci *et al.*, 1983) would, if reproducible, suggest an affection at variance with that of *ordinary* Horner's syndrome.

Not enough information is available at present to judge between these two possibilities. It should be emphasized that possibility (1) is not ruled out. The pupil in cluster headache can probably best be characterized as a 'Horner-like pupil'. In the case of a pure third-neuron sympathetic dysfunction, it would be difficult to explain the remaining autonomic phenomena which would then in all probability need to have another cause.

Another autonomic feature of cluster headache makes it difficult to accept a purely sympathetic theory. The pupil in cluster headache is reduced in width on the symptomatic side (mean anisocoria: cluster headache 0.32 mm; controls 0.06 mm (Salvesen *et al.*, 1987b)). Micieli *et al.* (1988) found a smaller average pupil width on the symptomatic side during the cluster period than in the remission (4.14 and 4.38 mm, respectively). We are not aware of any quantitative data concerning the pupil size during the attack, but from personal experience it may seem that the anisocoria becomes, if anything, more marked during the attack.

If the latter statements are true, it becomes difficult to reconcile them with, for example, the facial sweat findings, on the basis of a sympathetic 'barrage' theory. It is not unreasonable to assume that the autonomic stimulus to the ocular and forehead region during attack is one and the same. If the sweat glands are sympathetically innervated, the increased attack-related sweating in the forehead on the symptomatic side is consistent with a *hypersensitivity reaction* in deficiently functioning sweat glands (see the heating experiments described under Stimulation of Forehead Sweating).

One interpretation of the pupillary findings in cluster headache is that they, as already stated, reflect a third-neuron dysfunction. If, therefore, the above reasoning is correct, there ought to be a clear pupillary *dilatation* (and not a constriction) during attack (Table 2.41), due to a supersensitivity reaction, because this is particularly marked in third-neuron lesions (Salvesen *et al.*, 1989). If the previous reasoning is true, it can safely be excluded that what we are faced with in cluster headache is a sympathetic deficiency of a regular type (third neuron), combined with a sympathetic supersensitivity stimulation during attack. The possibility remains that the permanent dysfunction is sympathetic in nature whilst the attack-related stimulus is not, or possibly also vice versa (in which case the non-sympathetic disorder would probably dominate). Naturally, the premise may not hold true, i.e. the stimuli to sweat glands and pupils may be different. The fact that ptosis appears or increases during attacks is also difficult to fit in with this concept. The possibility exists that the ptosis may actually be a pseudoptosis (due to lid oedema, for example).

The forehead sweat glands and the pupil on the symptomatic side demonstrate supersensitivity reactions. The innervation of the dilator of the iris is supposed to be purely sympathetic, and supersensitivity reactions concerning the dilator function have been demonstrated. (This matter may, nevertheless, be more intricate. One interpretation of the lack of conformity of the hydroxyamphetamine test pattern in cluster headache with any of the patterns for neurons I–III (Salvesen *et al.*, 1987a, 1989) is that neurotransmitters other than the 'classic' ones are involved.) The post-ganglionic sympathetic nerves to the forehead sweat glands release acetylcholine as their transmitter acting on the muscarinic receptors. It is conceivable that the innervation of the sweat glands is also rather intricate. What we have demonstrated with regard to the forehead sweat glands in cluster headache is an increased sensitivity to pilocarpine (a parasympathicomimetic agent). The abnormality demonstrated in cluster headache may, therefore, seem to concern the sympathetic system, irrespective of the transmitter involved.

In conclusion, a 'pure' parasympathetic barrage theory can probably be discarded as an explanation of all the autonomic phenomena in cluster headache. Even *localized* lesions along the parasympathetic ganglia and fibres could hardly explain the entire array of autonomic symptoms and signs of a cluster headache attack.

Likewise, there are appreciable difficulties in explaining all the phenomena as being due to a sympathetic deficiency with supersensitivity manifestations. In conformity with these interpretations, Lance (1982) was unable to provoke attacks by anaesthetizing the stellate ganglion in two cluster headache patients during a bout. A supersensitivity reaction as far as the pupil is concerned would be the same as a reaction to sympathetic stimuli, i.e. a mydriasis (Table 2.41). If anything, there seems to be an even more marked miosis during attacks than otherwise. Accordingly, the pupillary changes during attacks do not point to a supersensitivity reaction or to a sympathetic hyperfunction. A 'combined' involvement of the parasympathetic and sympathetic systems might explain the phenomena somewhat better than would the involvement of one of these systems alone.

The most likely explanation of the autonomic phenomena at present would, however, seem to be an involvement of an autonomically functioning fibre system(s) at variance with the two traditional, classical systems. This system(s) could be involved alone or, which may seem more likely, there could be a co-involvement of the 'classical systems'.

THE CAROTID BODY AND CLUSTER HEADACHE PATHOGENESIS

Cluster headache attacks tend to occur during the night and also, according to Kudrow (1983), at high altitudes. Sleep apnoea also seems to occur frequently in cluster headache patients (Kudrow *et al.*, 1984). These observations could indicate that cluster headache attacks are induced by hypoxia. The usefulness of oxygen therapy in cluster headache adds *some* weight to this view. However, the fact that improvement takes place after addition of a given factor does not allow the inference that a lack of this factor is the cause of the ailment.

The above-mentioned viewpoints prompted Kudrow (1983) to propose an hypothesis concerning a possible role of the carotid body in cluster headache (Figure 2.52). The carotid body is a most sensitive chemoreceptor for hypoxaemia. Carotid body cells, glomus cells, afferent nerve endings or sheath cells seem to be stimulated by hypoxaemia, a lowering of the pH, and to some extent by hypercapnia. The superior cervical ganglion furnishes the carotid body with third-neuron sympathetic fibres.

The discharge rate from the carotid body increases with increasing hypoxaemia. Impulses from the carotid body (and the carotid sinus) are mediated through a special branch of the glossopharyngeal nerve (the carotid branch) and are conveyed to the nucleus solitarius. The incoming information is processed in the respiratory and cardiovascular centres. The respiratory centre

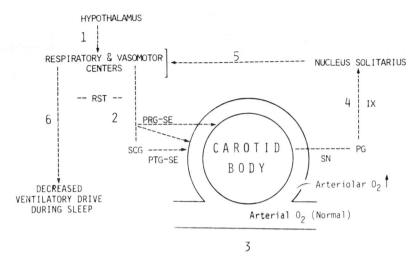

Figure 2.52 Schematic representation of the possible changes that occur in the carotid body reflex arc during the cluster period. The major physiological alteration of the cluster period is hypothesized to be due to inhibition of chemoreceptor activity, initiated in areas of the hypothalamus and resulting in diminished ventilatory responses, particularly during sleep. Affected respiratory reflex pathways are as follows. (1) Descending connections between the hypothalamus and vasomotor and respiratory centres. (2) Reticulospinal pathways (RST) to the carotid body via sympathetic efferent nerves. These include pre-ganglionic sympathetic efferents (PRG-SE) which innervate intrinsic carotid body structures and arterioles; and post-ganglionic sympathetic efferents (PTG-SE) having cell bodies in the superior cervical ganglion (SCG) and axon projections to carotid body arterioles. (3) Inhibition of sympathetic efferent stimulation may diminish chemoreceptive activity and increase total carotid body blood flow and oxygen delivery. (4) Carotid body afferent pathways (sinus nerve (SN) axons) to nucleus solitarius via petrosal ganglion (PG) of the ninth cranial nerve. (5) Afferent connections to the respiratory and vasomotor centres. (6) Descending efferent reticulospinal tract in the spinal cord transmitting impulses to peripheral motor nerves controlling respiration. Pre-ganglionic parasympathetic efferents to the carotid body and vagal parasympathetics contributing to respiration are not shown. (From Kudrow (1983). Courtesy of *Cephalalgia*.)

controls ventilation via phrenic and intercostal nerves, and the cardiovascular centre controls the heart activity via reticulospinal fibres.

Kudrow proposed that in cluster headache there is an inhibition of the sympathetic system and a disinhibition of the parasympathetic system influence on the carotid body. This is thought to diminish peripheral chemoreceptor activity. The cause of the solitary paroxysm is supposed to be oxygen desaturation, which leads to a hyperactivity in the chemoreceptor area and, thereby, a stimulation of the respiratory centre. Kudrow further claimed that this activity via the nucleus solitarius leads to stimulation of the nuclei of the seventh and tenth cranial nerves. A rise in P_aO_2 (or a change in blood pH) may determine the 'shut off' of the chemoreceptor activity, which terminates the attack.

There is evidence to show that there is a dysfunction in the sympathetic nervous fibres to the head in cluster headache. During the tranquil state, a hypofunction of various autonomically innervated organs in the head will prevail. When stimulated, however, the sympathetic fibres to many (all?) organs in this area should show supersensitivity phenomena, due to the dysfunction. Such supersensitivity could include *the chemoreceptor area (carotid body)*: a blunting of the carotid body chemoreceptor functioning could prevail during the non-agitated stage, the 'body' only reacting to marked blood gas changes, and *then* reacting with an overshooting (hyperventilation may be a part of the cluster headache attack *per se* (Sulg and Sjaastad, 1983)). During stimulation, the carotid body may conceivably start creating its own symptoms. In this model, the other autonomically innervated organs will be directly influenced by a common source, e.g. the hypothalamus or the 'periphery', and not only via the carotid body. In this model, the importance of the carotid body in pain production is reduced.

In my opinion, this hypothesis is too simplistic to explain the entire pathogenesis of cluster headache. It is, for example, difficult to grasp where the unilateral pain comes into the picture. There may still be a role for the carotid body (Kudrow, 1983) in the pathogenesis of cluster headache, a role which is more in line with the other autonomic dysregulations. In the peripheral organs, there may be several autonomic disturbances which appear in parallel and may depend upon supersensitivity phenomena, i.e. intraocular amplitudes, forehead sweating, heart rhythm, etc. The carotid body dysregulation also may be positioned at this level. The significance of the carotid body in the pathophysiology of this headache may, nevertheless, be somewhat more decisive than that of, for example, corneal temperature, because it is an important regulatory organ.

The possible nature of cluster headache

The pathogenesis of cluster headache is largely unknown (e.g. Sjaastad, 1986c). The attack consists of at least two components, i.e. the pain and the autonomic features. With regard to the main component of cluster headache, the pain itself, little information exists as to its origin or nature.

What is then the most likely nature of the basic autonomic abnormality? The most likely possibilities seem to be:

1. a primary disorder of the central regulation of autonomic functions;
2. a central dysregulation of the vegetative/endocrine/biorhythm interplay; and
3. a 'peripheral' affection with involvement of various autonomic ganglia and nerves.

The following features may speak in favour of a 'central' genesis of the attacks: the possible connection of cluster headache with emotional fluctuations and the possibly more than occasional linkage with rapid eye movement

(REM) sleep (Dexter and Weitzman, 1970; Dexter, 1974; Dexter and Riley, 1975); the possible spring–autumn type of undulation in symptoms in some patients (Friedman and Mikropoulos, 1958; Robinson 1958); and the effect of lithium therapy. It is possible that the increased exercise tolerance during the cluster phase in a patient with co-existing angina pectoris and cluster headache (Ekbom and Lindahl, 1971) also indicates a cerebral origin of the headache (altered autonomic 'tone'). Gruiloff and Fruns (1988) have recently proposed that the occurrence of limb pain during attack is due to a 'central' dysfunction. The applicability of each of these specifics may vary, and some of them may even possibly count in the opposite direction. Thus, for example, lithium may have a peripheral effect.

The various unilateral autonomic phenomena accompanying the attack are consistent with a 'peripheral' picture. As discussed elsewhere (see The Significance of Autonomic Involvement), the entire picture does not fit with a dysfunction of any of the two 'classic' autonomic systems.

Existing theories concerning cluster headache pathogenesis are rather unproductive. In the present context, pieces of evidence from seemingly totally unrelated fields which may possibly have a bearing on cluster headache pathogenesis are put into the melting pot in search of the crucial mechanism/ structure (Sjaastad, 1988b).

The tendency to bilaterality in cluster headache

Cluster headache is, in principle, a unilateral headache. Nevertheless, in approximately 15% of cluster headache cases the headache changes side at some point along the time axis (Manzoni *et al.*, 1983b). There thus seems to be a 'disposition' for the headache to develop on both sides in cluster headache.

The prevalence of cluster headache in a form that is severe enough to lead to medical consultations appears to be about 0.07% in Western countries (D'Alessandro *et al.*, 1986). The tendency for a patient to develop headache on the side opposite to the usual pain side is then around 200 times higher than the chance of an individual developing this type of headache *de novo* (Sjaastad *et al.*, 1987b). Side shift is thus a conspicuous feature of this disease. On rare occasions, the headache may even be bilateral.

The cluster headache *attack* consists of two components: the pain and the autonomic phenomena. The autonomic phenomena, such as nasal secretion, lacrimation, and forehead sweating (Sjaastad *et al.*, 1985) (see Tables 2.38 and 2.39) also show a tendency to bilaterality (Saunte, 1984a; Sjaastad *et al.*, 1985) and, in fact, much more regularly so than does the pain. In patients in whom the pain changes sides, there is sometimes a dichotomy between pain and autonomic phenomena (Sjaastad *et al.*, 1987b; Sjaastad *et al.*, 1988d), with the autonomic phenomena occurring on the side opposite the pain. Such a split between autonomic phenomena and pain creates some difficult problems with regard to determining the location of the abnormality. To explain this phenomenon by means of a pure *peripheral* aetiology of cluster headache, one may possibly be forced to accept two different foci, one for the pain and one for the autonomic phenomena, each being located on a different side.

It is conceivable that the process underlying the generation of pain is 'bilateral' but because the activity of this process is less pronounced on the contralateral side, it may be possible to perceive the pain on the most painful side only. It may be impossible to perceive a 'lesser pain' in the presence of a strong one; if the strong pain is removed, the lesser one will surface.

Some support for this idea may be derived from the results of surgical interventions. After operations on one side, pain attacks may recur on the opposite, previously pain-free side. This was thus the case in one of 12 cases treated with the so-called 'combined procedure', that is sectioning of the greater superficial petrosal nerve and neurolysis of the sensory root of the trigeminal nerve (Kunkel and Dohn, 1974). In our patient with a cluster headache-like picture and a Hageman factor deficiency (see Symptomatic Cluster Headache: Aneurysms), the headache shifted to the opposite side after removal of the giant aneurysm. Furthermore, in a patient with an arterio-venous malformation in the corpus callosum area, endovascular embolization led to the headache always appearing on the opposite side thereafter (Gawel *et al.*, 1989).

Most probably, the conspicuous unilaterality of the pain indicates a same-sided 'peripheral' abnormality. If there is, in addition, a 'central' disturbance, this central focus may 'play' on the peripheral anomalous structure.

However, in addition to explaining the unilaterality of the headache, a pathogenetic model of cluster headache must also explain the marked tendency to bilaterality of the pain and autonomic manifestations.

Symptomatic cluster headache

Cluster-headache investigators seem to belong to two categories, as far as their view of symptomatic cluster headache is concerned. One group claims that, since cluster headache does not have any recognizable macroscopic substrate, the 'symptomatic' cases, i.e. cases in which there is a macroscopic abnormality, are of no particular interest. The pain should either be ascribed to the substrate detected, with any resemblance to cluster headache being merely due to chance; or, the patient has both a regular cluster headache and a non-pain-giving pathological structure. Members of the other group contend that if a pain syndrome greatly resembles cluster headache, this may contribute important information concerning cluster headache itself (perhaps particularly as far as localization is concerned), irrespective of the fact that one is faced with two entirely different types of headache.

Symptomatic cluster headache as a group has been dealt with elsewhere. Suffice it to say in this context that not all the cases reported under this heading deserve to be categorized under it. The difference from cluster headache was often considerable. Some cases did not show a proper cluster phenomenon; some had other atypical features, alone or in combination. There are, however, clearly cases that deserve to be mentioned in this context (see Table 2.16).

In a case of pituitary tumour (Tfelt-Hansen *et al.* 1982), three typical features of cluster headache as such were present, i.e. a severe, unilateral pain accompanied by ipsilateral autonomic phenomena. Because of the similarity with cluster headache, the *substrate* of the pain becomes important: The carotid siphon on the symptomatic side was stretched and displaced anteriorly, a fact that *may* have been of importance in the symptom generation. Another case of pituitary tumour and a cluster headache-like picture has been reported (Hannerz, 1989).

A patient with Hageman factor deficiency and a cluster headache-like headache also had a giant aneurysm of the anterior communicating/A_1 arteries (Sjaastad *et al.*, 1988b; Sjaastad, 1988c). The only one of the five major characteristics of cluster headache (see Table 2.13) that was lacking was male sex. Male sex, however, is not a necessary condition for the diagnosis of cluster headache. The clinical constellation of symptoms and signs in this patient was similar to that of the regular cluster headache picture.

However, manifold atypical traits were also present. The role of the giant aneurysm in this picture is dubious. Principally, the significance of it may be either: (1) a chance co-existence with the cluster headache-like headache, in which case this headache is probably at variance with existing, well-defined headaches (since it does not seem to be identical to cluster headache); or (2) the aneurysm has played a fundamental role, for the generation of *pain* over the years. The aneurysm apparently did not touch the trigeminal nerve or the third cranial nerve, and pupillometry and evaporimetry demonstrated no third-neuron sympathetic lesion pattern. Conceivably, pain could have been produced through a stretching influence on the arterial wall itself.

In this case, we are faced with an abnormality clearly differing from that underlying cluster headache pathogenesis. It may, however, be located in or close to the area where cluster headache *per se* may be (or usually is) located. Such a case may, in other words, aid in defining the area of interest in cluster headache.

Orbital venous vasculitis and cluster headache

The Tolosa–Hunt syndrome is associated with pathological changes in the superior ophthalmic vein and cavernous sinus (Muhletaler and Gerlock, 1979; Hoes *et al.*, 1981), which can be visualized by venography. At autopsy, non-specific, granulomatous angiopathy (Tolosa, 1954) has been demonstrated. Hannerz *et al.* (1987a) have demonstrated that cluster headache and even chronic paroxysmal hemicrania (Hannerz *et al.*, 1987b) may be associated with similar venographic findings which are partly bilateral. From a nosographic point of view, the Tolosa–Hunt syndrome and cluster headache appear to be clearly different disorders. The finding that these clinically different headache forms nevertheless seem to have some common phlebographic changes, may be interpreted in various ways (see also Orbital Phlebography).

Conceivably, one could be approaching a similar situation to the one that arose with the Morgagni–Morel syndrome ('hyperostosis frontalis interna', Moore, 1955) some decades ago: when a pathological condition seems to be present in many different disorders, then it is probably of little or no significance in all of them. We are probably not quite at that stage yet, with regard to these phlebographic changes in the various headache types. Furthermore, if a pathological finding is of crucial importance in a given disorder, then it ought to be present in 100% of cases, and this does not seem to appear in cluster headache.

There is, nevertheless, a possibility that the phlebographically demonstrated abnormality may be of significance in all these headaches. The venographically demonstrated changes may not be an entirely true reflection of the angiopathy. What is demonstrable may only be the markedly abnormal changes. Pathological changes not giving rise to phlebographic changes that are sufficiently marked to be visualized may still be of pathogenetic significance. The observation that the phlebographic findings are not only bilateral but may also be as pronounced on the non-symptomatic as on the symptomatic side could be seen in this light. The figures for phlebographic changes on venography in these conditions may thus be minimum figures. Venography may only aid in demonstrating that there *is* an involvement of the major collecting system at the base of the brain; at the present stage of accuracy, this technique cannot be expected to differentiate between various disorders.

Although these headache forms seem to have a common denominator in the superior ophthalmic vein/cavernous sinus abnormalities, it may be the *nature* of these abnormalities that is different in cluster headache and the other headaches. The pathological process itself may differ; it may be inflammatory, autoimmune, etc. Structures outside the venous system may be affected and may contribute symptoms and signs, and the location of pathology may differ slightly as far as the venous system is concerned. If the demonstrated abnormalities are of any importance pathogenetically, the fact that indomethacin works to a full extent in chronic paroxysmal hemicrania but is not very potent in cluster headache or the Tolosa–Hunt syndrome, may be an indication of the diversity of the pathological processes involved.

Sinus cavernosus extends across the midline both anteriorly and posteriorly to the pituitary gland (sinus circularis). This *may* indicate yet another possibility for extending the pathological process across the midline in cluster headache. The cavernous sinus is a possible substrate for the pathogenetic process in cluster headache (see later). The fact that the first and second branches of the trigeminal nerve penetrate this structure does not detract attention from it in this context.

Relevant evidence from stimulation experiments

Many cluster headache patients are able to localize the maximum pain rather precisely: the point where the extrapolated lines from two fingers, one pointing directly into the eye from the front and the other pointing into the anterior/mid-temporal area, would meet is where the maximal pain resides. The pain is so severe that it feels as though the eye is being pushed forward, out of its socket. Which vascular segments or other structures will—when stimulated by pain-provoking stimuli—be able to reproduce the pain of cluster headache as accurately as possible?

A major portion of the knowledge concerning intracranial pain-producing structures stems from the experiments of Ray and Wolff (1940). According to them, pain in the *ocular area* might be produced by stimulation of different structures, such as the superior sagittal sinus and its tributary veins, the transverse sinus, sinus rectus, and the cavernous sinus. A *retroocular* pain was produced by stimulation of the proximal portions of major arteries, e.g. middle cerebral and internal carotid arteries, but also of the pontine arteries. Stimulation of the dura at the floor of the anterior fossa, of the diaphragma sellae, and of the tentorium cerebelli also gave rise to retro-ocular pain. Stimulation of the anterior cerebral artery also resulted in such pain; this artery was sensitive from its point of origin to a point 1 cm beyond the genu of the corpus callosum, a segment several centimetres long. Miller Fisher (1968) found no headache in cases of anterior cerebral artery occlusion ($n = 9$).

Ocular pulsatile flow studies

Corneal indentation pulse amplitudes (Hørven, 1970b) increase during attack, but asymmetrically, i.e. the increase is greater on the symptomatic side than on the non-symptomatic side (Hørven and Sjaastad, 1977). As has recently been shown, the corneal indentation pulse amplitudes are *lower* than the mean normal level on both sides in the interparoxysmal period (Hørven et al., 1989), and during attack they only just exceed the mean control level. In addition, the intraocular pressure is not particularly high during an attack either. The pulsatile part of ocular blood flow represents approximately 60–70% of the total ocular flow under normal circumstances. Ocular pulsatile flow, which can be quantified by dynamic tonometry, is significantly lower in the pain-free interval on both sides in patients than in controls ($p < 0.01$ for both variables). During an attack, the flow reaches average control levels on the symptomatic side.

The mechanism underlying these ocular flow changes may be found in feeding arteries, in the draining venous system, or in 'primary' intrinsic ocular circulatory changes. We have reason to believe that flow restrictions on both the arterial and the venous sides will lead to *reduced* corneal indentation pulse amplitudes, whereas such amplitudes are increased during the cluster head-ache attack. It is our considered opinion that the corneal indentation pulse amplitude increase during the attack is due to a primary vascular (arterial) intraocular vasodilatation. In the presence of an acute *venous* dilatation, the amplitudes would probably decrease. This latter point must, however, be viewed with some caution. The role of the cavernous sinus as for the ocular circulatory changes is thus probably not to hinder the drainage from the eye; the cavernous sinus is possibly the origin (or the mediator) of the signal to the intraocular vessels.

TOWARDS A PATHOGENETIC SYNTHESIS

Because of the change of pain and the bilaterality of the autonomic phenomena, the proximity to the midline may be a decisive factor in cluster headache pathogenesis. Side shifts may have one of two mutually exclusive explanations: (1) structures *in* or closely *adjacent to* the midline are the areas primarily involved, and spreading of the pathological substrate across the midline is thus highly facilitated; or (2) despite a 'considerable' anatomical distance between the structures on the two sides, they are so closely connected by nerve fibres that involvement of one side could implicate the other. Although the latter possibility cannot be rejected, the first model may seem more plausible. In this context, therefore, attention should be drawn to the 'midline concept' (Sjaastad, 1988b). How can this concept be reconciled with the theories concerning cluster headache pathogenesis that are presently in vogue.

In general there are at present two concepts concerning the pathogenesis: there is a 'central' origin of the essential steps of a single attack; or events take place on the 'periphery'. With regard to the central hypothesis, the hypothalamus has for a long time been the centre of attention; with regard to the peripheral hypothesis it is mainly various parasympathetic ganglia that have been of interest in recent years. A third possibility would be a combination of the above two hypotheses.

If the ideas that biological rhythms and the changes of seasons influence cluster headache stand the test of time, it will be hard to refute the concept of a central dysregulation in this headache. A cyclic dysregulation in the central mechanisms that regulate the endogenous biological rhythms, could explain the temporal pattern of cluster headache (Nappi *et al.*, 1981, 1987). This could again lead to a disruption of the temporal organization of hormonal secretions in cluster headache, such as with melatonin (Chazot *et al.*, 1984). Such a dysregulation would then probably be the *primary* abnormality (the 'permissive' anomaly) without which there would be no cluster headache.

A pain without peripheral autonomic accompaniments may be central in origin, and even in a headache like cluster headache, pain generation *may* theoretically be central. If, however, the headache has various autonomic accompaniments, such as lacrimation and a prominent temporal vessel, how is the interplay between central and peripheral factors then brought about? The signal to create these phenomena must under such circumstances be brought to the periphery. Both vascular (e.g. the dilatation of conjunctival vessels) and neurogenic (e.g. sweating and lacrimation) phenomena are integral parts of the attack. Although the occasionally occurring temporal vessel dilatation—and other attack-related phenomena—are clearly vascular in nature, the mediation of the signals to the vessel does not have to be, and hardly is, only vasogenic. A vasogenic background would be hard to explain, due to the unilaterality of the phenomenon. The signal is more likely to be neurogenic. There is a rather strong body of evidence to show that, during mechanically precipitated attacks of chronic paroxysmal hemicrania, the *signal* to the sweat and lacrimal glands is neurogenic in nature (Sjaastad *et al.*, 1986). Theoretically, the trigeminovascular system of Moskowitz (Moskowitz *et al.*, 1979, 1986) could mediate such impulses. Other similar, as yet unknown, systems may also be candidates for this role. In this model, there is thus a primary cerebral incentive and a secondary activation of autonomic functions (and possibly also of pain). It should be stressed that the likelihood that a neurogenic stimulus is primary to the vessel involvement does not indicate that *the pain* is neurogenic. The pain may well be 'vascular'. Or there may even be the following sequence of events: nerve impulses → vascular reaction → neurogenic pain due to vascular (compression?) phenomena.

Pain may also be triggered in the periphery, together with or independent of the autonomic phenomena. Admittedly, the fact that the pain and autonomic phenomena are usually on the same side is highly suggestive of a peripheral activation of both. In the case of a co-existence of a 'cerebral incentive' and a purely peripheral source of both autonomic phenomena and pain, the communication between the central structures and the 'periphery' must be accounted for. At present, it can only be guessed at. Also with this model, 'autonomically' mediated impulses may be primary to the pain: sensitization of autonomically innervated structures may take place through, for example, oedema formation (Sjaastad and Fredriksen, 1986).

Before trying to outline the area of interest, it should be emphasized that the various types of stimulation used by Ray and Wolff (1940) may not mimic the types of 'irritation' or 'stimulation' that the vessels and other structures are exposed to in human disease. For this reason alone, a one-to-one relationship between pain localization in the stimulation experiments and in cluster headache cannot be found. With this obvious reservation in mind, some reasoning as to the localization of the crucial substrate for the attack may be made.

The various structures located close to the midline that may give rise to ocular and even retro-ocular pain include structures located at the base and the top of the brain and structures in the anterior and posterior fossa. The anteriorly located main vessels (anterior cerebral and internal carotid arteries, and perhaps also the middle cerebral artery), the cavernous sinus and the adjacent dura seem to be structures capable of producing pain in the ocular area as a consequence of stimulation. In laboratory animals, these arteries are richly endowed with nervous structures (e.g. Edvinsson, 1985). These autonomically functioning nerves may have diverse functions, which at present can only be speculated upon. The possibility exists that the autonomic dysfunctions of cluster headache are partly or wholly linked to the dysfunction of these structures.

I have some reservations about including posterior fossa structures (and, for that matter, the venous drainage system on the superior surface of the brain) among the candidates for pain generation in cluster headache. Midline structures such as the 'posterior portions of the circle of Willis' (Stowell, 1970) can, however, not be completely rejected as candidates.

Since the dura at the base of the brain and the cavernous sinus may generate ocular pain on stimulation, the findings of Hannerz *et al.* (1987a) of cavernous sinus (and the ocular tributary vein system) involvement in cluster headache may be important. The cavernous sinus may theoretically contribute to the pain in various ways:

1. through venous wall or perivascular infiltrations;
2. through distention of the venous channel system;
3. through spasms;
4. through involvement of the two upper trigeminal branches, penetrating the sinus; and
5. through involvement of other structures passing through the sinus.

Could there be any connection between the cavernous sinus abnormalities observed by Hannerz *et al.* (1987a) and the ocular findings in cluster headache? Increased corneal indentation pulse amplitudes on the symptomatic side constitute an integral part of the attack. An excess of blood is pumped into the eye during each pulse beat during attack as compared with the pain-free interval. If distention really were to take place in the cavernous sinus, which anatomically speaking is a duplication of the dura, then the dura could be stretched and cause pain. The increased amplitudes could possibly represent an effort to overcome an increased resistance. However, if venous obstruction were the cause of the ocular circulatory disturbances in cluster headache, various attack-related phenomena would be difficult to explain. Why then, would, for example, normal intraocular pressure (or even levels in the low normal range) and not papilloedema be part of the picture? However, as demonstrated in one case by Hannerz *et al.* (1987a), the venous obstructions may be periodic in cluster headache. This might explain why papilloedema does not develop. I do not know whether constrictions of the superior ophthalmic vein/cavernous sinus *per se* can cause pain. Granulomatous infiltrations in this area apparently can (cf. Tolosa–Hunt Syndrome).

The Tolosa–Hunt syndrome, in which the symptoms may be long-lasting and not only periodic as in cluster headache, is not accompanied by papilloedema. To clarify whether the pressure in the cavernous sinus is increased in cluster headache, ocular venous pressure should be assessed. This should be possible. The fact that cluster headache may persist after enucleation on the symptomatic side (Rogado and Graham, 1979) more or less excludes a causal relationship between ocular circulatory changes and *pain generation*. Cavernous sinus changes may, through neurogenic impulses, give rise to the ocular, vascular changes which are clearcut enough, but neither result from nor cause the pain.

Although various arteries and veins close to the midline may give rise to ocular pain during disease or stimulation experiments, cluster headache as such is likely to have one single cause; it is not likely to be due to involvement of diverse structures with various locations, since its symptomatology is so stereotypical. Areas at the base of the brain near the midline and mainly in the middle cerebral fossa are of particular interest in cluster headache.

In cluster headache as such, there sometimes seems to be an involvement of both arteries and veins—the bulging temporal artery and the narrowed superior ophthalmic vein. Could *one type* of neurogenic stimulus influence both kinds of vessel and over such a widespread area? Or is it more likely that involvement of one vessel is secondary to that of another? In addition to a neurogenic factor, there are definite vascular factors inherent in cluster headache symptomatology. As stated previously, however, we feel that the *signal* from the primary 'origo' to the vessels is neurogenic, the vascular factors being of secondary importance under these circumstances. Nerve fibres connected to the vessels, either extrinsically or intrinsically, may be involved. This may or may not be the reason for the dual involvement, i.e. of both vessels and nerves.

The animal experiments done by Bill using substance-P fibres in the eye (Bill *et al*. 1979, 1987) are pertinent in connection with cluster headache pathogenesis. Stimulation of such fibres and the subsequent release of substance-P leads to miosis, extravasation and increased intraocular pressure. Miosis and relatively increased intraocular pressure are inherent features of the ocular pathology of the cluster headache attack. Involvement of substance-P fibres and/or of transmitters having a similar action, intraocularly or in the orbit, could accordingly explain many of the ocular phenomena of the attack (Sjaastad, 1986). Hardebo (1984), Sicuteri *et al*. (1983, 1985), Sicuteri (1985) and Fanciullacci *et al*. (1988) have also hypothesized that there may be involvement of substance-P in cluster headache itself. Sicuteri *et al*. (1983) attributed the beneficial effect of morphine during attack to an influence on substance-P neurons.

However incomplete and vague much of the evidence is in this field, and however few inferences really can be made on the basis of the available information, some evidence seems to point towards middle fossa structures close to the midline as being of possible significance in symptom production in cluster headache (Sjaastad, 1988b). The cavernous sinus accordingly seems to assume a prominent position in cluster headache pathogenesis. It should be mentioned that Moskowitz (1988) has recently proposed similar ideas.

3

Chronic Cluster Headache

Horton *et al.* (1939) unfortunately did not recognize or acknowledge one of the main characteristics of cluster headache—the cluster phenomenon itself. The term 'cluster headache' stems from 1952 (Kunkle *et al.*, 1952). However, the phenomenon itself was probably alluded to as early as 1936 by Harris, and the tendency to clustering was clearly described by Ekbom Sr in 1947.

Later, Symonds (1956) described a patient in whom the cluster phenomenon was absent, in other words, a chronic variety of this syndrome. Lovshin (1961) observed this special temporal pattern in several patients. Rooke *et al.* (1962) also observed chronic cases as did Balla and Walton (1964), Earl and McArdle (1968) and McArdle (1969), who described six cases of this variety. Somewhat later de Fine Olivarius (1970) described cases having the chronic variety of cluster headache, using the term 'hemicrania neuralgiformis chronica' for this condition. More strict diagnostic criteria for this headache were set out by Ekbom and de Fine Olivarius in 1971, a prerequisite in their estimation being that in 'chronic' cases attacks were to appear more or less continuously for 1 year or more.

The chronic variety has been divided into *primary* and *secondary* forms. 'Secondary' chronic cluster headache is understood to mean that a 'cluster' pattern antedated the chronic disorder, i.e. the headache was non-*chronic* in the beginning. 'Primary' chronic cluster headache is understood to mean that separate, well-defined bouts did not precede the chronic stage.

TERMINOLOGY

The term 'cluster headache' as introduced by Kunkle *et al.* (1952), is not merely a catchy term; it possesses the essential characteristics of a good name. It describes one essential manifestation of this disorder, i.e. the temporal accumulation of attacks. It also possesses another important feature: it is 'neutral', as far as the nature of the headache is concerned. It is essential that terms used for disorders, including headaches, where the aetiology and pathogenesis are largely and entirely unknown should be non-biased and non-trend-setting, otherwise they may hamper progress in elucidating mechanisms, etc. The adjective 'vascular' should, for example, not be used for headaches, unless the vascular component *is* (not only seems to be) essential, preferably causal, in the pathogenesis. The term 'sphenopalatine' neuralgia (as elaborated upon elsewhere) should *not* be used for headaches in which there is no proof of an involvement of this ganglion. Until the aetiology and pathogenesis of a disorder have been established — and may be even after that — only neutral terms should be used.

Whereas 'cluster headache' thus in many ways seems to be an ideal term for this headache, 'chronic cluster headache' may seem to be a *contradictio in adjecto*; the term implies a *non-clustering cluster headache*. If it is a cluster headache, i.e. an intermittent or cyclic headache, how can it then be chronic? There are, nevertheless, strong reasons why this term should be retained. The term cluster headache is in common usage even outside the domain of migrainologists. Furthermore, if chronic cluster headache and the remitting, non-chronic form are two varieties of the same disorder, it is all the more important that this relationship be indicated in the nomenclature. The term 'chronic cluster headache' should, therefore, indicate the chronic variety of cluster headache, irrespective of the meaning of the words. This should be the preferred term.

One reservation to this view stems from the (slight) suspicion that the *primary chronic* variety of the chronic form may show some dissimilarities to cluster headache as such. With this variant, we may thus be facing more than semantic problems (see below).

The term 'chronic migrainous neuralgia' has been used by some clinicians (e.g. Pearce, 1980). de Fine Olivarius (1970) used a similar term (hemicrania chronica neuralgiformis) when first describing his series of cases. This term was heavily criticized by the experienced Danish migrainologist Dalsgaard-Nielsen when it was first introduced (at the annual meeting of the Scandinavian Migraine Society, 1970). The term 'chronic migrainous neuralgia' is certainly far from being an ideal one and may even be an example of ill-conceived nomenclature. It should not be used for this headache for the following reasons. First, it has not been proven that a 'neuralgia' is a factor of essential significance in this headache. If words pointing to aetiology/pathogenesis are to be used, then it must be ascertained that they represent facts. For this reason alone, this term is clearly incorrect for chronic cluster headache at the present time. This reasoning must not be taken to indicate that the pain of cluster headache is not neuralgiform; it may still well be.

The term 'migrainous' may, if possible, be even more misleading. It purports to the idea that one is faced with a sort of migraine or a migraine-like condition. As discussed earlier (see Cluster Headache), there is every reason to believe that the pathological process that occurs in cluster headache differs clearly from that in migraine; the same goes for the chronic variety. To align this headache with migraine in such a sensitive matter as that of terminology, would accordingly be wrong. Moreover, and this is probably the most important single point, if the chronic and the episodic varieties are closely linked aetiologically and pathogenetically, it would be wrong to use totally different designations for the chronic and episodic varieties. A marked discrepancy in terminology would set them apart, even aetiologically and pathogenetically, and alienate them from one another in the minds of the users. If we really believe that the chronic disorder is connected with episodic cluster headache clinically, aetiologically, and pathogenetically, then this should be obvious from the terms applied. The two terms 'cluster headache' and 'chronic migrainous neuralgia' have no words in common; there is thus nothing to suggest a relationship between the disorders. Therefore, for the non-expert, the link between these two headache forms will not be obvious.

An interesting observation is that some of the most sincere advocates of the non-unitarian view on the interrelationship of migraine and cluster headache, nevertheless advocate the use of the term 'chronic migrainous neuralgia'. According to the principles already mentioned, the usage of the term 'chronic migrainous neuralgia' should be discontinued, the clearly preferred term being 'chronic cluster headache'.

DEFINITIONS

Ekbom and de Fine Olivarius (1971) have given a definition of 'Chronic cluster headache'. The patient should suffer from 'typical headaches', i.e. attacks of typical character, duration and pain level and the associated phenomena, the difference from the ordinary 'cluster' form mainly being the chronicity. A series of attacks should have lasted at least 1 year, and attacks should appear at least twice a week.

Some features of this headache should probably be more accurately defined. The upper limit of the frequency of attacks should tentatively be defined, because of the differential diagnostic difficulties versus chronic paroxysmal hemicrania, with which it may be confounded. If possible, objective evaluation criteria should be used in order to characterize these headaches more clearly. The reason why this is of the utmost importance is that one may not be faced with a homogeneous disorder, but with several disorders. These various problems of definitions will be dealt with in greater detail later. The mentioned inadequacies pertain in particular to the primary chronic variety, which ultimately may prove to be a real nosological problem.

According to the *Taxonomy Committee of the International Association for the Study of Pain (IASP)* (Merskey et al., 1986), *Chronic cluster headache* should be described as follows (with the permission of the committee chairman, Prof. H. Merskey): the features of chronic cluster headache are the same as those for cluster headache with the following differences.

Definition: bouts of unilateral pain usually in males, principally in the ocular, frontal and temporal areas occurring at least twice a week for more than 1 year.

Main features: chronic cluster headache is much more rare than cluster headache; the diagnosis requires at least two or more attacks per week over a period of more than 1 year. The pattern may arise from the beginning as regular attacks of more than two per week or a chronic pattern may supersede an ordinary intermittent cluster headache pattern.

Relief: the same measures as for cluster headache are effective, but lithium carbonate tends to work relatively better for chronic cluster headache.

Differential diagnosis: sinusitis, chronic paroxysmal hemicrania, cluster headache, cluster tic syndrome and migraine.

Code: 004.X8b Note: see note on cluster headache.

The classification of chronic cluster headache of the *International Headache Society (IHS) Headache Classification Committee* is as follows.

Description: Attacks occur for more than 1 year without remission or with remissions lasting less than 14 days.

Chronic cluster headache unremitting from onset. Previously used term: Primary chronic.

Chronic cluster headache evolved from episodic. Previously used term: Secondary chronic.

Comment: during a cluster period and in patients with the chronic form attacks occur regularly and may be provoked by alcohol, histamine or nitroglycerin. Pain is maximal orbitally, supraorbitally and/or temporally, but may spread to other regions. Pain usually recurs on the same side of the head during an individual cluster period. During the worst attacks, the intensity of pain is excruciating. Patients are unable to lie down and typically pace the floor. Age at onset is typically 20–40 years. For unknown reasons men are afflicted 5–6 times more often than women. The mechanisms of the pain are incompletely known despite abnormalities demonstrated by studies of corneal indentation pulse, corneal temperature, forehead sweating, lacrimation and nasal secretion or by pupillometry, thermovision, extracranial and transcranial Doppler.

CLINICAL SERIES

Series of chronic cases are small. The only exception to this is Kudrow's (1980) series (Table 3.1). In the various series, from 4–20% of the total cluster headache group have been made up by chronic cases (Table 3.1). In addition, Andersson (1985) in his series of 127 cluster headache patients found 114 patients with the episodic form, versus 13 patients with the chronic form (10%). The fact that the ratio between chronic and episodic cases seems to vary by a factor of 5 between

Table 3.1 Clinical characteristics of chronic cluster headache[a]

Authors	Size of series, n Chronic cluster headache	Size of series, n Total cluster headache	Relative frequency of chronic form (%)	Primary/ secondary chronic form	No. females/ males	Age at onset of headache (years)	No. of attacks per 24 h	Duration of attacks (min)	Duration of chronic symptoms (years)
Ekbom and de Fine Olivarius (1971)	17	167	10	9/8	0/17	Range 17–56 (mean 30)	<1–3	30–180	2–13 (mean 4.4)
Kunkel and Dohn[b] (1974)	31	185	17	19/12					
Heyck (1976)	5	48	10						
Pearce (1980)	4[c]	101	4	2/2	1/3	Range 47–61 (mean 57)	Usually 1–2		2/3–4.5
Kudrow (1980)	87	425	20	45/30[d]	12/75	F 36; M 33 (means)			
Manzoni et al. (1983b)	19	180	11	12/7	1/18	Almost 50% > 40 (mean 39)	1–5	30–120	3–9
Solomon and Guglielmo (1985)	17	146	12						

[a] Quality of pain is as with episodic variety (Ekbom and Olivarius, 1971; Manzoni et al., 1983b).
[b] Some of these patients, i.e. 6 of 31, had an attack frequency of <1 per week.
[c] Series of six patients, but two with attack periods of <1 year in duration.
[d] Obviously from another series (Kudrow, 1980: p. 15).

the various series is apt to make one wonder. This *may* indicate, but does not prove, that the criteria used for inclusion in the chronic group may not have been strictly the same in the various series. I have, as a matter of fact, seen only 3–5 cases where this diagnosis was suspected, if the diagnostic requirements regarding the temporal aspects were to be strictly followed. One may suspect that this diagnosis might have been favoured in some cases which might belong to categories such as cervicogenic headache and/or chronic paroxysmal hemicrania. Some might belong to still unclassified groups of unilateral headache.

The original criterion for chronicity (i.e. >12 months duration), set forth by Ekbom and de Fine Olivarius (1971) has not been adhered to invariably in all series. For example in Bussone *et al.*'s (1977) series comprising 20 patients (one female and 19 males), cases with a symptomatic period duration of down to 3 months have apparently been included. Cases exhibiting less than 1 year duration (down to 8 months) were also included by Pearce (1980) (Table 3.1).

The relative frequency of the primary and secondary forms is generally quite uniform in the various series, with slightly more cases in the primary than in the secondary subgroup (Table 3.1).

SOME CLINICAL CHARACTERISTICS

It is obvious from the following that the amount of exact information available on the chronic and the episodic varieties is quite different.

AGE OF ONSET (OF HEADACHE AS SUCH AND OF THE CHRONIC PHASE)

The age of onset *tends* to be higher in chronic than in episodic cases. Only in the series studied by Ekbom and de Fine Olivarius' (1971) was the age of onset in the chronic variety approximately the same as in the episodic one (Table 3.1). In Pearce's (1980) series, there was a relatively high age of onset, not only of the chronic phase, but also of headache as such, the mean age of onset of the latter being 57 years (Table 3.1). The youngest patient was female, and she did not satisfy the usual criterion for chronicity (i.e. duration ≥1 year; in her case 8 months). If she is excluded, all other cases were aged ≥47 years at onset of headache.

A comparison of age of onset in the chronic and episodic forms of cluster headache is shown in Figure 1.2, the mean in the episodic form being 28.9 and in the chronic form 39.0 years. The age of onset of headache as such, therefore, seems to be somewhat higher in chronic than in episodic cluster headache. It would be interesting to see whether this higher age is particularly connected with one of the subgroups or one of the sexes. Two of the cases in Pearce's (1980) series were primary chronic cases. In the four secondary chronic cases, the time from the appearance of the episodic to the appearance of the chronic form varied between 1.5 and 8.5 years, with a mean of 5.5 years.

SEX PREPONDERANCE

The prevalence of males seems to be as marked (or even more marked) in the chronic form as in the episodic form (Table 3.1). Again, however, the difference between the various series is appreciable, i.e. a ratio of 3:1 in one series (Pearce, 1980) and a ratio of 18:1 in another (Manzoni *et al.*, 1983b). The male preponderance in chronic cluster headache as such seems definite enough. Due to the variation between series of this parameter it would, nevertheless, be desirable to have more and bigger series to be able to define the ratio more accurately. In the series studied by Manzoni *et al.*, the one female patient had the primary chronic variety. Due to the paucity of data, no firm conclusion can be made as to the precise sex ratio in the subgroups.

ATTACK FREQUENCY

In the series of Ekbom and de Fine Olivarius (1971) and Manzoni *et al.* (1983b), representing a total of 35 patients, a frequency of attacks of <1–5 per 24 h was given (Figure 2.6; Table 3.1). The *upper limit* of the attack frequency can at the present time not be given accurately. Manzoni *et al.* (1983b) stated explicitly that the attack frequency is higher in the chronic than in the non-chronic variety.

In chronic paroxysmal hemicrania, the *lower* limit of the frequency of attacks is now fairly well known (Antonaci and Sjaastad, 1989): 3% of the cases have a maximum 24 h attack frequency of <5, and 18% have <9 attacks per 24 h. This is of considerable importance, since the treatment of these two chronic pain disorders differs fundamentally, chronic paroxysmal hemicrania being clearly adversely affected by lithium, and chronic cluster headache generally not being positively influenced by indomethacin. It is noteworthy that Bussone *et al.* (1977) included a case with an attack frequency of 15 attacks per day among their cases of chronic cluster headache. In a recent report by Bogucki and Niewodniczy (1984), a male patient of 29 years of age suffered from what may appear to be a secondary chronic form of cluster headache. He had an attack frequency of up to 30 attacks per 24 h, each attack lasting for up to 20 min. The location of the pain may have been slightly atypical in this case. The response to indomethacin was totally negative and the response to lithium positive. The diagnosis of chronic paroxysmal hemicrania, therefore, seems rather remote in this case. This case probably shows that an attack frequency, above—maybe even far above—8–10 per day in the exceptional case may appear in cluster headache, perhaps mostly in the chronic variety (or at least in a headache that has many similarities to cluster headache). An investigation of forehead sweating and pupillary parameters, etc., would have been useful to categorize this patient properly. These observations demonstrate that there is a certain overlap between chronic cluster headache and chronic paroxysmal hemicrania as far as attack frequency is concerned.

The *lower* limit of the attack frequency in the chronic variety of cluster headache was given as at least 2 attacks per week (Ekbom and de Fine Olivarius, 1971). Kunkel and Dohn (1974) are of the opinion that there may be up to 1 week or more between attacks in the chronic form. They divided their series of 31 cases into two groups, i.e. 25 with <1 week intervals between attacks and 6 with >1 week interval.

Nocturnal attacks have been described by Pearce (1980) and were also mentioned by Ekbom and de Fine Olivarius (1971). Whether nocturnal attacks are as typical as in the ordinary episodic form is not known.

PAIN QUALITY AND LOCALIZATION

On the whole the symptoms of the chronic variety seem to be rather similar to those of the episodic variety. The quality of the pain seems to be similar to that of the episodic variety (Manzoni *et al.*, 1983b). In Pearce's (1980) series, the pain occurred partly in the areas typical of episodic cluster headache. In other patients, however, the pain occurred in slightly atypical areas, such as the upper jaw, maxilla and malar region.

ASSOCIATED FEATURES

Ekbom and de Fine Olivarius (1971) noted that the typical associated phenomena of the attack of episodic cluster headache are also present during an attack of chronic cluster headache. Typical traits of regular cluster headache, such as watering of the eye and nasal stuffiness/rhinorrhoea, were noted in only half of the cases studied by Pearce (1980).

VARIOUS OTHER TRAITS

Manzoni *et al.* (1983b) found that *peptic ulcer* occurred significantly more frequently in the chronic than in the episodic form (37 versus 12%, respectively; $P < 0.01$). In addition, antecedent *head injuries* both with and without loss of consciousness were more frequent in the chronic than in the episodic form of cluster headache. The series studied were, however, small. There was also a tendency for *facial surgical procedures* to have been carried out more frequently in patients with the chronic form than in those with the episodic variety.

Tension and stress seemed to be trigger factors in the chronic variety (Manzoni *et al.*, 1983b). *Alcohol* seemed to be a triggering factor even more frequently in the chronic than in the episodic variety. It should, however, be noted that de Fine Olivarius (1971) observed that some chronic cases became addicted to alcohol. It is conceivable that moderate amounts of alcohol may have a precipitating role as far as attacks are concerned, whereas considerable amounts of alcohol and steady abuse may have a dampening effect on the tendency to attacks. This may be so even in the episodic form of cluster headache.

VARIOUS STUDIES CARRIED OUT IN CHRONIC CLUSTER HEADACHE

SLEEP APNOEA

Dexter (1984) studied four patients with chronic cluster headache during symptomatic and symptom-free nights over two nights for each pattern. There was no definite difference in sleep characteristics between the two periods. There were no nights that could be labelled as having the characteristics of sleep apnoea, i.e. >70 apnoea episodes per night. Kudrow *et al.* (1984) studied chronic cluster headache patients and found that only one out of five patients showed signs of sleep apnoea. This contrasts with what they (Kudrow *et al.*, 1984) found in episodic cluster headache in which disorder all the patients ($n = 5$, with a total of 11 attacks) displayed sleep apnoea phenomena. This could point to a difference between the chronic and episodic cluster syndromes.

HLA HISTOCOMPATIBILITY SYSTEM

The histocompatibility complex may seem to be different in the chronic and episodic types (Cuypers and Altenkirch, 1979), in that HLA-A$_1$ invariably was found in the chronic type ($n = 5$), but not in the episodic type. If this proves to be the case in a good-sized clinical series, it may indicate that these two forms of cluster headache are fundamentally different.

TREATMENT

The same treatment modalities have largely been tried in chronic cluster headache as in the episodic form of cluster headache. Generally speaking, the results of drug treatment are clearly inferior in the 'chronic' form as compared to the 'episodic' form.

DRUG THERAPY

Ergotamine, prednisone, and methysergide

Ergotamine in daily dosages of 1.5–4 mg, divided in 2–3 oral or rectal portions, seems to be a useful drug in many cases (Ekbom and de Fine Olivarius, 1971). A good or satisfactory result (i.e. an improvement of ≥50%) was found in around

70% of cases when an individualized treatment regime was adopted, partly with ergotamine administration centred on attacks of regular timing. In Pearce's (1980) series, the efficacy of ergotamine, although definite, was rather moderate.

Prednisone has also been tried in some cases ($n = 15$) by Kudrow (1980). The initial dosage was 40 mg, and this was then tapered off over the course of 3 weeks. Prednisone was found to be clearly superior to methysergide ($p < 0.001$). Pearce (1980) found that methysergide given in circumscribed courses seemed to be a reliable drug.

Methysergide treatment must follow the strict rules of dosage (preferably not more than 3–6 mg day^{-1}) and duration (intercalated drug-free periods of 2 months after 4–6 months of therapy).

Neither ergotamine nor prednisone therapy is unproblematic in the chronic variety of cluster headache: due to the limited effect of ergotamine, high dosages are often used. With relatively high dosage and prolonged periods of treatment (due to the fact that the chronic variety is not circumscribed in time like the episodic one) toxic side-effects may appear. Toxic effects of both drugs are of such a nature that the usefulness of these drugs in the chronic form is reduced. There has, therefore, been a search for other treatments to be used for the non-clustering variety of cluster headache.

Lithium

Lithium therapy is one result of a search for new drugs. It was originally tried, independently, by Graham (1973) and McGregor (1973) (for information: Graham, 1974) at the same time. Ekbom (1974c) also tried lithium therapy. Lithium has been shown to have a beneficial effect in other cyclical disorders, i.e. manic-depressive psychosis.

Lithium has been tried in both the episodic and chronic forms of cluster headache. It was originally thought to have a better effect in the latter form. The effect of lithium in the chronic form has been confirmed by Bussone *et al.* (1979) and by Kudrow (1977). The improvement sets in quite rapidly: according to Bussone *et al.* (1979), improvement is evident within 1 week, and Manzoni *et al.* (1983a) found a clear improvement within 2 weeks. Kudrow administered lithium over a period of 32 weeks and found >60% improvement in 96% of 26 cases. No difference was found between the primary ($n = 17$) and secondary ($n = 11$) forms of chronic cluster headache in this respect. The results of Mathew (1978) were as follows: in a total of 31 patients (14 episodic and 17 chronic cluster headache patients) 55% of the patients demonstrated a >90% effect, but 20% of patients demonstrated no definite improvement.

A carefully conducted study has been carried out ($n = 22$) by Manzoni *et al.* (1983a). The initial improvement (i.e. within 2 weeks) was more than 90% in 80% of the patients. Only two patients improved less than 60%. The mean weekly headache index dropped from 32.8 to 6.0 (Table 3.2). The long-term

Table 3.2 Results of lithium treatment in chronic cluster headache patients ($n = 22$)[a]

Initial results			Long-term results
Improvement (%)	>90	18 → 11	Improvement constantly maintained
		→ 7	Improvement maintained with transient worsenings
	60–90	2	
		→ 4	No benefit
	<60	2	

Mean improvement 82.9%

Adverse effects	*n*	Adverse effects	*n*
Severe, requiring discontinuation	0	Severe, requiring discontinuation	2
Mild, requiring continuation	7	(goitre 2)	
(tremor 4, diarrhoea 2, abdominal pain 1, olfactory hallucination 1, insomnia 1, vertigo 1, increased thirst 1)		Mild, allowing continuation (tremor 2, nausea 1, diffuse headache 1, lethargy 1)	4

[a]From Manzoni *et al.* (1983a). Courtesy of *Cephalalgia*.

effects were somewhat poorer. In 50% of patients the initial beneficial effect remained. In patients with a moderate initial effect this response vanished. In the remainder there were exacerbations of a periodic or more permanent nature. Although the series was small, there seemed to be a tendency for the primary chronic cases to fare worse than the secondary ones.

The influence of drug discontinuation was studied in nine of Manzoni *et al.*'s cases with chronic symptoms (Table 3.3). In six cases there was an exacerbation of the headache, whereas in three there seemed to be a reversal to the episodic form with long-lasting periods of remission. Lithium seems to give a greater degree of improvement than does prednisone (Kudrow 1977, 1980).

Calcium blocking agents

Nimodipine. A double-blind, cross-over study ($n = 8$) with nimodipine was carried out by Meyer and Hardenberg (1983). The dosage was 60 and 120 mg day^{-1} for 2 months each. After 4 weeks of therapy, the attack frequency had invariably declined, and this tendency continued for the rest of the trial period. The mean monthly attack frequency was reduced to approximately one fifth of the original frequency ($p < 0.002$). Breakthrough attacks had the usual severity and duration. Adverse effects (gastrointestinal complaints, muscle

Table 3.3 Course of chronic cluster headache after interruption of lithium treatment[a]

Patient No.	Age (years)	Diagnosis	Duration of disease (years)	Treatment duration before interruptions (months)	Course of headache after interruption
1	60	Primary	2	5	Rebound headache
2	54	Primary	10	21	Periodic course
3	53	Primary	6	8–16	Rebound headache
4	38	Primary	8	14	Rebound headache
5	29	Secondary	10	42	Periodic course
6	26	Secondary	4	7–21	Rebound headache
7	31	Secondary	5	5–14–31–42	Rebound headache
8	61	Secondary	3	6	Periodic course
9	39	Secondary	9	12–18	Rebound headache

[a]From Manzoni *et al.* (1983a). Courtesy of *Cephalalgia*.

aches, menstrual discomfort, skin changes, etc.) occurred in 40% of the patients. None of them were severe, and all subsided upon discontinuation of the drug.

These findings seem interesting; however, the number of cases studied was small. The question of a place for nimodipine—and other calcium antagonists—in the therapy of cluster headache should, therefore, be considered to be *sub judice*. It may be added that our own, admittedly limited, experience has not been encouraging so far.

Verapamil. Gabai and Spierings (1989) treated 15 chronic cluster headache patients with verapamil (isoptin) in an open study, the average dosage being 572 mg (range 120–1200 mg). A total of 60% of the cases improved (>75% after an average of 5 weeks, range 1–20 weeks); these results were of the same order of magnitude as those obtained in the episodic group.

In another study, attacks were induced by nitroglycerin in 15 chronic cluster headache patients. Acute intravenous verapamil administration at the time of maximum pain led to a reduction of the pain (Boiardi *et al.*, 1986b).

Ketotifen

Split *et al.* (1983) have tried ketotifen prophylactically, a mast cell stabilizer. Fifteen patients were treated over 8 weeks after 1 week of placebo treatment. The dosage was 1 mg three times daily, and the study design was single-blind. The number of attacks in these two periods was compared. The drug seemed to have a good (moderate to excellent) effect in all but two patients. When compared with the placebo period the number of attacks decreased by 68%. In 53% of the patients, the attacks disappeared or almost disappeared. The improvement achieved during the ketotifen period continued for the 8 weeks following withdrawal of the drug. Although these results seem promising, they need to be corroborated by other studies. The results obtained do not prove that histamine *per se* plays a pathogenetic role in cluster headache.

Other drugs: drug therapy—concluding remarks

Other drugs such as *pizotifen, flumedroxone* (Ekbom and de Fine Olivarius, 1971), and *cyproheptadine* have also been tried on small groups with limited success. It has been reported that the headache was 'abolished by cimetidine' in one single case (Pearce, 1980). In all probability this was a fortuitous event, since the case presented seems to be a fairly typical one, and cimetidine has been shown not to be effective in episodic cluster headache (Veger *et al.*, 1976).

The treatment of chronic cases is one of the tough challenges of the migrainologist. There are patients in whom, after many years, none of these conservative measures seem to be of any avail any more. There is a clear need for a safe drug of persistent efficacy. Kudrow (1985) defined 'treatment resistance' as a lack of responsiveness to all conventionally accepted, prophylactic cluster headache medications. In a group of 113 cluster headache patients Kudrow found 24 patients in this category.

SURGICAL TREATMENT

The various surgical approaches to cluster headache, both those of historical interest and those in current use, are reviewed in the following sections. Surgical therapy in cluster headache should be reserved for patients that are refractory to all kinds of cluster headache drugs and combinations of such drugs. Suffering is usually much more marked and protracted in the chronic than in the episodic form. Many of the surgical therapeutic alternatives, therefore, have relevance only to the chronic cases. In some chronic cases, the suffering may be so high that one may even have to resort to somewhat untraditional methods in an endeavour to alleviate the pain.

Resection of the temporal artery

According to Kunkel and Dohn (1974) this approach may give rise to 'surprisingly long periods of remission' in isolated cases. Watson *et al.* (1983) resected the artery in five patients and carried out cryosurgical destructive lesions in a sixth patient, all without any benefit. White and Sweet (Watson *et al.*, 1983) only obtained three successful results out of 24 patients. Temporal artery resection *per se* is generally considered to be rather ineffective. Even ligation of the common carotid artery has been tried, and apparently pain relief was obtained (Safer, 1962).

Supra- and infra-orbital nerve blockades and avulsions

Harris (1936) treated some patients with alcohol injections of the supra- or infra-orbital nerves or both. There were some instances of success, but there were also some relapses. Sachs (1968) carried out a supraorbital neurectomy on one patient without much benefit. Stowell (1970) reported on 21 patients treated with alcohol blockade or avulsion of the supraorbital nerve; only five cases showed no response. Watson *et al.* (1983) injected alcohol into the infra- ($n = 1$) and supra-orbital ($n = 1$) nerves and obtained good anaesthesia but no pain relief. It was emphasized that the pain in each case extended beyond the sensory areas of these nerves. *Avulsion* of the infraorbital nerve was carried out in five cases; in three cases with pain predominantly confined to the infraorbital nerve territory, benefit lasting 5 months to 7 years was obtained. In two cases, both with an area of pain by far exceeding the infraorbital nerve innervation area, no relief was obtained.

Auriculotemporal nerve resection

The auricolotemporal nerve was resected in conjunction with the superficial temporal artery in two cases with ensuing relief lasting for several months (Watson *et al.*, 1983). Since temporal artery excision *per se* is mostly considered to be ineffective, one might speculate that the improvement observed may have been due to the resection of the auriculotemporal nerve. The improvement following auriculotemporal nerve resection is not necessarily specific.

Nervus intermedius resection

Sachs (1968) sectioned the intermedius nerve on the symptomatic side (partly also the seventh and eighth nerves) and obtained freedom from pain in all four cases, lasting from 10 months to 15 years (and still persisting at the time of publication). In his critical report, he considers various possibilities of why such sectioning is effective in relieving pain (e.g. by inhibiting the tendency to ipsilateral parasympathetically mediated vasodilation upon stimulation of the seventh and tenth cranial nerves, after sectioning of nervus intermedius, as demonstrated by Chorobski and Penfield (1932)). The only summary description hampers the clinical classification of Sachs' cases; probably one of them (and possibly three of them) suffered from cluster headache. Despite the favourable results obtained, Sachs warns against using this procedure in routine cases. An interesting observation made was that lacrimation, which was generally greatly reduced post-operatively, remained normal in one case. In addition, Furlow (1942) found that the lacrimation remained intact after nervus intermedius sectioning, whilst taste was abolished on the anterior two-thirds of the tongue and salivation was reduced to one fifth. In Furlow's case, the diagnosis was nervus intermedius neuralgia (Hunt), and there were trigger zones; the neuralgia was cured by the sectioning.

Kunkel and Dohn (1974) resected the intermedius nerve in one case. They warn against complications such as deafness, facial palsy and loss of taste. Kunkel and Dohn do not recommend this operation. Some theoretical considerations regarding putative nervus intermedius involvement in cluster headache have been presented by Solomon (1986).

Decompression of the seventh cranial nerve

Solomon and Apfelbaum (1986) carried out surgical decompression of the seventh cranial nerve in five patients; in two cases they also decompressed the trigeminal nerve and in one case the glossopharyngeal nerve. In two cases, a compression due to an artery was observed, whereas in the other cases there was compression due to vein and artery, vein, and bony spur. In two cases there was an improvement, lasting >1.5 and 2.5 years, respectively. The authors felt that the observed effect exceeded that of a placebo procedure. They advocate a return to sectioning of the intermedius nerve if decompression does not give optimal results.

Sphenopalatine ganglionectomy

Meyer *et al.* (1970) treated 13 cluster headache patients with sphenopalatine ganglionectomy (Figure 2.48). The patients were invariably unresponsive to medical treatment and were severely afflicted by their headache. Pre-operatively, attacks were induced by alcohol, and an anaesthetic blockade of the ganglion was then carried out, with immediate pain relief. The ganglion was exposed through the maxillary sinus. The post-operative period ranged from 3–4 to 11 months. The follow-up results were as follows: 'Seven patients no better, four improved, and two having no pain at all, although the time intervals in the last two cases are too short to be certain of the outcome'. The authors themselves recommend that this procedure should be used in only carefully selected patients.

Greater superficial petrosal nerve resection

Gardner *et al.* (1947) resected the greater superficial petrosal nerve on the symptomatic side (Figure 2.48). A total of 17 operations were performed in 13 patients. Three patients had bilateral headache. Apparently, 'excellent' results were obtained in 25% of the cases, fair results in 50%, and failures in 25%. At a later stage Gardner apparently became disappointed with his own results and stopped doing the procedure. Stowell (1970) operated on 37 patients over the course of 20 years; 32 of them experienced a complete relief for a period of time, whereas in four cases no relief at all was obtained. Fifteen patients experienced subsequent recurrence of attacks. Of these, four were reoperated on and three had complete, permanent relief.

One of Sachs' (1968) cases underwent this operation (chronic cluster headache) and remained pain free for 3 years. A repeat neurectomy produced a 2 year disappearance of pain. Sweet (1988) divided the major superficial petrosal nerve together with the lesser one in 13 patients. Full relief was obtained in five patients with a duration of 6–27 months (average 18 months), after which there was a complete recurrence.

This procedure may seem to have *some* assets. However, it involves major surgery, and the likelihood of recurrence is considerable.

Tractotomy: 'small lesion' in the lower end of the medulla oblongata

Malmros (1973) treated three chronic cluster headache patients with medullary trigeminal tractotomy a.m. Sjøquist, i.e. a transection of the spinal trigeminal tract at the level of the obex (e.g. Brodal, 1969). The long-term results did not seem to be encouraging.

In patients in whom cutting of the greater superficial petrosal nerve and the intermedius nerve in addition to a trigeminal rhizotomy did not lead to any relief, Sweet (1988) made a 'small lesion' in the lower end of the medulla oblongata. In this area, trigeminal pain pathway fibres are joined by pain conducting fibres from the intermedius and glossopharyngeal/vagal nerves. A lesioning in this area would, therefore, lead to an analgesia without anaesthesia in the distribution of the trigeminal nerve, as well as in the deep cephalic structures. In three patients treated in this way the results were, on the whole, equivocal.

Various therapeutic procedures directed towards the trigeminal ganglion, nerve and roots

'Combined procedure' (sectioning of the greater superficial petrosal nerve and neurolysis of the trigeminal sensory root). Kunkel and Dohn (1974) have carried out this combined procedure in 12 cases, all males, nine of whom experienced immediate relief upon operation. In three patients, headaches continued as before. Three of the patients who originally improved later experienced a recurrence of attacks. Six of the original 12 patients were relieved of their symptoms for a considerable period; the time of follow-up is not stated but may have been up to 3–4 years. Later, Kunkel (1981) stated that this procedure had been carried out in 20 patients, two-thirds of whom experienced a remission 'for varying periods'. Some patients, previously unresponsive to medical therapy, again responded to medical therapy when they experienced a partial post-operative recurrence of symptoms. White and Sweet's (Watson *et al.*, 1983) observation that the greater superficial petrosal nerve may carry sensory fibres may provide a rationale for treating chronic cluster headache with a 'combined' procedure directed towards this nerve and the trigeminal ganglion. In summing up their surgical experiences with this syndrome, Watson *et al.* (1983) also arrived at this conclusion.

Injections of the trigeminal ganglion. Harris (1936) treated some cases with alcohol injections of the ganglion, with only partial success. Horton (personal communication) also used this treatment in some cases, but with only moderate or no success. McArdle (1969) carried out alcohol injections of the trigeminal ganglion in six cases with 'complete success' over an observation period of up to 5–6 years. Alcohol injections of the Gasserian ganglion have also been tried by others: Maxwell (1982) described such injections in eight patients in whom he obtained a transitory abatement. Alcohol injections in cluster headache patients should no longer be carried out.

Trigeminal nerve neurectomy. Stowell (1970) cut the first division of the trigeminal nerve in five cases, with complete, permanent relief of pain. The time of observation was not given.

Radiofrequency trigeminal gangliorhizolysis. Radiofrequency waves cause a selective destruction of pain fibres, which are poorly myelinated, sparing the myelinated touch fibres.

Maxwell (1982) treated eight chronic cluster headache patients with percutaneous radiofrequency trigeminal gangliorhizolysis. These cases were carefully selected on the basis of case histories, characterized by unilaterality of pain and long-lasting and severe complaints. A trigeminal anaesthetic blockade was tried initially to familiarize the patient with the post-operative status. There was a 'subjective and objective evidence of complete anaesthesia in the distribution of the ipsilateral trigeminal nerve following lidocaine blockade', and the corneal reflex was absent in each case during the blockade. This group was compared with another group of 15 patients having severe, intractable craniofacial pain, with a female predominance, bilaterality of pain, vomiting, as well as a positive family history of headache. In this group, response to the local anaesthetic trigeminal ganglion blockade was considered negative.

In the eight chronic cluster headache patients, complete, initial pain relief was obtained. In five of the eight patients, pain relief persisted for a mean of 32 months (range 7–59 months). Two patients, working full-time 25 and 12 months post-operatively, had occasional, mild headache attacks, not requiring any continuous medication. In one patient, the chronic headache reverted to a cluster pattern. Propranolol, which was of no avail pre-operatively, abated the post-operative attacks. There seemed to be a close association between the sensory loss in the trigeminal area and the diminished corneal reflex on the one hand and the beneficial result of the gangliorhizolysis on the other. A most interesting observation was that in one of the completely pain-free patients, a '*forme fruste*' type of attack seemed to exist, with hemifacial flush, lacrimation, and nasal stuffiness. This strengthens the view of the duality of the autonomic phenomena and pain in the cluster headache syndrome, as advocated by our group (Sjaastad *et al.*, 1987b, 1988d; Sjaastad, 1988b). None of the patients developed anaesthesia dolorosa or painful facial dysaesthesia. If carried out in larger series, this operation would probably give rise to complications of this type in a small number of cases.

Onofrio and Campbell (1986) treated 26 patients with percutaneous radiofrequency thermocoagulation trigeminal gangliorhizolysis or by retrogasserian sensory rhizotomy. The patients were aged 19–65 years, and the follow-up period ranged from 10 months to 5 years. Fourteen of these patients exhibited an excellent result of surgery, 13 of them showing corneal anaesthesia and one showing marked corneal numbness. Two patients showed 'good' and two 'fair' results, whereas the last eight patients showed 'poor' results. Strikingly, three patients had corneal anaesthesia post-operatively, but did not benefit from the operation.

Mathew and Hurt (1988) treated 27 intractable chronic cluster headache patients with percutaneous radiofrequency trigeminal gangliorhizolysis. The average follow-up time was 28 months, with a range of 6–63 months. The results were as follows: excellent 15; very good 2; good 3; fair 1; and poor 6. Complications included anaesthesia dolorosa, stabbing pains, and corneal infection. The complications were generally mild, and the benefit derived from the surgery by far outweighed the discomfort. The patients with excellent results exhibited analgesia within the V_I and V_{II} zones, and the corneal reflex was also reduced.

Sweet (1988) treated 20 patients with thermal trigeminal rhizotomy. Eleven of these patients who were followed post-operatively for an average of 5.3 years (range 10 months to 20 years) obtained continuous relief.

These results seem encouraging. This procedure may seem to be one to be resorted to in intractable cases, but not for the ordinary case. For the achievement of optimal results, Mathew and Hurt (1988) recommend that the headache should be strictly unilateral, that the patient is stable mentally, and has a low, what they termed: 'addiction proneness'.

Glycerol injection in the trigeminal cistern. With Håkanson's (1981) method, glycerol 0.40 ml (range 0.35–0.5 ml) is injected transovally into the trigeminal cistern (cavum Meckeli). In order to make sure that glycerol is deposited in the cistern, the trigeminal cistern is visualized by means of metrizamide. Pure glycerol is hypotonic; the partial, neurotoxic effect on trigeminal sensory fibres may possibly be explained on this basis. Sweet *et al.* (1981) have used a similar technique. This technique was originally intended for the treatment of trigeminal neuralgia. Later, it was also tried in chronic cluster headache.

Dalessio *et al.* (1983; Waltz *et al.*, 1985) reported on glycerol treatment in five chronic cluster headache patients. None showed complete relief of symptoms, four showed partial relief, and one patient no relief. Ekbom *et al.* had by 1987 treated seven patients who had failed to respond to ordinary drug treatment, oxygen inhalation or various nerve blockades and resections. Three cases were partly or wholly improved for periods up to 12 months, whereas two cases failed to improve. Two of the patients were virtually symptom free after 5.5 and 3 years, respectively. The chronic course seemed to be substituted by a mild, cyclic one in these cases, similar to what may occur after radiofrequency gangliolysis (Maxwell, 1982). The occasional breakthrough attacks in these cases could be abated with drug therapy. The glycerol treatment was repeated one or two times. A notable observation is that there seemed to be a good correlation between the degree of sensory loss in the innervation area of the first branch of the trigeminal nerve and the degree of improvement. The headaches seemed to recur *pari passu* with the gradual return of facial sensibility.

Transitory aseptic meningitis may occur with this therapy, and the corneal sensibility as well as the corneal reflex may be lost (Ekbom *et al.*, 1987). In no instances were neuroparalytic keratitis or anaesthesia dolorosa observed. A further disadvantage with this method is the development of arachnoiditis in the trigeminal cistern, which is due to the procedure itself; this hampers further injection therapy after the first 2–3 injections. Because of the recurrence of pain, which may take place when this method is applied, it will probably not be an adequate method for use on chronic cluster headache patients in future.

SURGERY: CONCLUSIONS

Many of the methods mentioned are only of historic interest. Many of them have proven to be ineffective, and some of them carry great risks. A surgical approach may, nevertheless, be indicated in the treatment of resistant chronic cluster headache patients. Section and avulsion of nerves should generally not be carried out, and the same goes for alcohol injections of the Gasserian ganglion.

To me, it seems that the procedures directed towards the Gasserian ganglion or the fifth cranial nerve seem to give the best long-term results. Possibly, 'the combined procedure' (Kunkel and Dohn, 1974) will stand the test of time.

In general, it is important that surgical intervention of this type leads to a clear reduction of sensation, and it seems to be of major importance that the sensory deficit corresponds to the area of pain. Since the pain is mainly located around the eye, anaesthesia in this area is crucial. When pain is present in the second branch of the trigeminus, clear reduction of sensation of the corresponding area becomes important. However, pain may not be abolished despite apparent complete anaesthesia (e.g. Onofrio and Campbell, 1986).

In recent years, two different approaches have come to the fore: (1) Cavum Meckeli injection of glycerol; and (2) radiofrequency trigeminal gangliorhizolysis. Seemingly, the radiofrequency method is marginally better than the glycerol one as far as long-term results are concerned. Recurrences may seem to occur sooner with glycerol injections. In addition, radiofrequency thermocoagulation seems to have advantages over the glycerol injections in Meckel's cave, since it may be easier to control the extent of destruction with radiofrequency thermocoagulation. After a few glycerol injections, arachnoiditis will appear in the cave, and this prevents further treatment of this sort.

It is of the utmost importance that patients for radiofrequency therapy are carefully selected and that the ground is prepared before the intervention through information/question rounds with the prospective candidate. The possible complications, including sensory and motor deficits, anaesthesia dolorosa, and even death, must be made clear to the candidate for operation. As already outlined, it is important that the headache is unilateral, that the patient is stable mentally, and that the patient's inclination to drug addiction is of the lowest possible level. The patient should be completely unresponsive to medical treatment.

In this context it may be worth mentioning that one of Onofrio and Campbell's (1986) patients who got anaesthesia dolorosa post-operatively, with recurrent keratitis and 'off-bite', has 'instituted litigation'.

THE STATUS OF CHRONIC CLUSTER HEADACHE

In the definition of chronic cluster headache (Ekbom and de Fine Olivarius, 1971), the lower limit of the duration of an attack series was arbitrarily set at 1 year. Pearce (1980) for example, has included cases of only 8 months' duration. If a continuous succession of attacks has taken place over a 6–9 month period, this pattern seems to have a tendency to continue. There are exceptions to this rule, as there are when applying the rule of 12 months. The limit for chronicity could probably safely be moved downwards, probably not to 6 months at this time, but probably to 9 months. It has been advocated (Kudrow, 1987) that a subgroup of 'subchronic' cases be interposed between the episodic and chronic groups. In my opinion, the difference in symptomatology between this new and the two existing groups is not sufficiently marked to justify this extra group. Instead of clarifying the situation this extra group will probably lead to confusion.

The classification of primary and secondary forms of chronic cluster headache may be a useful one. The secondary form is readily linked to regular cluster headache and may be viewed as a further development of the ordinary disorder. The differences between the two forms, i.e. the secondary chronic and the episodic forms, may be only minor and the transition between them fleeting. With this type of evolution, the elements are the same as in the development of many cases of chronic paroxysmal hemicrania, i.e. with a remitting ('pre-chronic') and a chronic stage; the relative importance of the two stages at the present time may seem to be an inverse one in cluster headache and chronic paroxysmal hemicrania (Antonaci and Sjaastad, 1989).

Some differences between the episodic and chronic forms have been observed. The HLA histocompatibility system possibly differs in the chronic and episodic forms (Cuypers and Altenkirch, 1979). The combined results from various sleep studies (Kudrow *et al.*, 1984; Dexter, 1984; Mathew and Frost, 1984) may indicate that sleep apnoea occurs in the episodic form but not to the same extent in the chronic variety. The more marked resistance to therapy among the chronic cases may also point to a real difference between these two varieties. However, this may only reflect a difference in severity between the two clinical manifestations.

These are only pieces of information and even together are nowhere near enough to come even close to proving that chronic cluster headache differs essentially from the ordinary episodic form.

Whereas there should be no major obstacles to accepting secondary chronic cluster headache as a variant of the ordinary episodic form, the situation is rather different with regards to the primary chronic variety. In this variety, one highly characteristic, crucial feature of cluster headache has never been found to be present: i.e. the periodicity of the attacks—the cluster phenomenon. If one diagnostic hallmark has never been present, the diagnosis becomes much more difficult than usual, and the chances of diagnostic error in the solitary case are then considerably increased. As a matter of fact, experienced workers in this field agree that the cluster phenomenon is so important diagnostically that during the first bout the information at hand is generally insufficient to make the diagnosis acceptable clinically. Only when a second bout appears and only when the typical temporal pattern emerges can a reliable diagnosis be made.

The question consequently arises of whether the primary chronic variety really is a cluster headache. There are, as far as we are concerned, five main diagnostic pillars of the cluster headache syndrome, i.e. the cluster phenomenon, the male sex, the unilaterality, the excruciating severity, and the accompanying autonomic phenomena. The entire constellation of symptoms and signs is not present in every case of cluster headache. Thus, there probably are genuine female cases of cluster headache, although in our experience there seem to be few of them. Furthermore, most female patients in our series seem to exhibit atypical traits, such as long-lasting attacks, less typically outlined bouts, more nausea and vomiting than usual, and occasionally rhinorrhoea and lacrimation are scanty or absent.

There are other, distinct features characterizing cluster headache: the duration and frequency of attacks, the presence of nocturnal attacks, the age of onset, etc. How do the clinical pictures compare in the two varieties of cluster headache? As for the purely clinical variables, many features in Pearce's (1980) case histories of chronic cluster headache cases seem to be the same as in the 'episodic' cases. Such features were: nightly attacks and attacks during naps; and regular timing of attacks, also during the night. However, there were atypical cases: partly, the pain seemed to be (located) primarily in areas slightly different from those of cluster headache. The associated features may seem to have been present less regularly than in the episodic variety. There are no data to suggest that the *unilaterality* is a less prevalent feature in the chronic than in the episodic form.

What factors are *sine qua non* as far as the diagnosis of this headache is concerned? In my opinion one of the criteria—and this probably concerns each one of them—may be absent, without discrediting the diagnosis: there may be bilateral cases of cluster headache (although such cases are rare); there are probably 'mild' cases of cluster headache (Sjaastad *et al.*, 1988c); and occasionally the number of autonomic phenomena present has been few.

However, if *two* of the main criteria are absent, one may be on thin ice diagnostically, but such cases may still exist. For example, a male patient may have 'mild' attacks and the ipsilateral autonomic phenomena may be absent. What then is the situation with the diagnostic status of a female patient seemingly belonging to the rarely occurring group of primary chronic cluster headache? Manzoni *et al.* (1988) have mentioned several cases (*n* = 7) showing this combination of factors. A tenable answer as to the *sine qua non* factors cannot be given until the substrate of cluster headache, including that for the chronic form, is identified.

It is to be suspected that the group of primary chronic cases as such, as diagnosed and presented in various series, may be heterogenous. A substantial fraction of the patients may suffer from disorders slightly or wholly at variance with cluster headache. In particular, 'cervicogenic headache' (Sjaastad *et al.*, 1983c) may probably be confused with the primary, chronic variety of cluster headache. The chances for error may seem to increase if the patient is female. The possibility exists that there are subgroups within this panorama that will eventually be isolated and identified.

A subgroup such as the primary chronic cluster headache group is, needless to say, going to be very small in any series, and the subgroup of female primary chronic cluster headache cases will be even smaller. It would, therefore, be difficult for a single investigator to acquire experience in this field. Data on the rare cases in these subgroups should be collected in a multicentre manner, if further progress is to be made in this special field. Details of each of the case histories, including data on the various supplementary parameters, should be collected. The only investigator who has so far given case histories of his cases, seems to be Pearce (1980). Another feature that is *not* known is the long-term fate of chronic cases. How is the condition influenced by age? Does the pattern revert to the ordinary episodic one in the sporadic case (except in, for example, lithium treated and surgically treated ones)? If so, how frequently does this happen?

Studies of more patients and, maybe above all, more *detailed case histories* are needed to fill the gaps in the information. It is highly desirable that in chronic cases intraocular pressure, corneal indentation pulse amplitudes, forehead sweating, pupillometry, and other variables such as the response to nitroglycerin, are monitored in order to establish the correspondence to ordinary cluster headache, or in order to separate the solitary case from ordinary cluster headache. This would be important work. And it should be done soon!

4

Chronic Paroxysmal Hemicrania

NOMENCLATURE AND TERMINOLOGY

Chronic paroxysmal hemicrania was first described in a preliminary report in 1974 (Sjaastad and Dale, 1974), with the following comment: 'a new (?) treatable headache entity'. At the time of the full report (Sjaastad and Dale, 1976), the term 'Chronic paroxysmal hemicrania' was coined. This term was chosen for the following reasons: once the typical headache pattern had developed, it seemed to be a lasting one (at least over a number of years), unless modified by drugs. There was headache every day (or maybe almost every day). Hence the term 'chronic' was used. There was also a constant succession of solitary, rather clearly delineated attacks (hence 'paroxysmal'). The headache was strictly unilateral and did not shift side (hence 'hemicrania'). In this chapter the term 'chronic paroxysmal hemicrania' is abbreviated to CPH, for convenience.

In other languages, other terms have been constructed to convey the same meaning. Thus:

Italian: *Emicrania cronica parossistica* (Nappi and Savoldi, 1983);
French: *Hemicranie paroxystique chronique* (Thevenet et al., 1983);
German: *Chronisch paroxysmale Hemicranie* (Pfaffenrath et al., 1984b);
Spanish: *Hemicránea paroxistica crónica* (Guerra, 1981; Espadaler, 1986); and
Portuguese: *Hemicrânia paroxística crônica* (Raffaelli, 1984).

Since only two and three cases, respectively, were reported in our first two communications (Sjaastad and Dale 1974, 1976), it was hardly to be expected that the *complete* clinical picture would be known from the very beginning. In all likelihood, new facets would be discovered at a later date. In the very beginning, it was thus not known that a stage with another attack pattern (i.e. a remitting course) frequently antedated the typical, chronic stage, in that the first cases seemed to have started abruptly, following a non-remitting course. This 'atypical' stage was later termed the 'pre-chronic stage' (Sjaastad *et al.*, 1977) (see also later). This 'non-continuous' ('remitting') stage may in the long run prove to be as frequent and typical a manifestation of this disorder as the first discovered, chronic stage. A number of patients, in other words, will not make the transition to the chronic form. The term 'pre-chronic' should, accordingly, in these cases probably be substituted by the term 'remitting' (see later).

THE HISTORY OF THE EMERGENCE OF A 'NEW' HEADACHE

The first case of chronic paroxysmal hemicrania (CPH), a female aged 44 years with a 9-year history of headache, was brought to our cognizance in 1961, with a diagnosis of 'typical cluster headache' (Sjaastad and Dale, 1974, 1976). However, the patient was a female (which, of course, may be consistent with a diagnosis of ordinary cluster headache, although females are admittedly rarely affected). There was another trait that, upon scrutiny, did not seem to be quite typical: there was a *multitude* of attacks per 24 h, i.e. up to 24 or more per day. Another remarkable feature was the intractability of the headache prior to the admission to our hospital (Rikshospitalet, Oslo University Hospital). Over the course of the following years, every feasible drug was tried on her. Prior to each admission, she had discontinued her usual drug (mainly acetylsalicylic acid) which kept the attacks at a reasonable level. Each drug trial ended either with an absolutely negative response, or—more usually—with an adverse reaction. The latter response pattern was so typical that for almost every new drug that was tried she was brought from a stage of moderate or weak attacks to a stage of incapacitating and excruciatingly severe attacks. This happened usually within from less than 24 h to 2–3 days. She then felt ill not only in the head, but in the entire body. For these reasons, every new drug that was tried usually had to be discontinued within a few days. After such an experience, she was usually at this lower level of functioning for weeks. For this reason, it took a long time to test the various remedies at hand. But she would not give up the hope that there was a solution to her problem. And she was the one who motivated us to try new approaches, not the other way around. Without the persistence of this lady and her intent resoluteness never to take no for an answer, we in all probability would not have reached any goals.

The extra suffering that she endured due to these trials was considerable. To make matters even worse, she was diagnosed as being an hysterical person—and even accused of it—and she was told time and again that she 'invented' the symptoms, despite the unilaterality of the pain, lacrimation, rhinorrhoea, etc. She was told that she should go home and pull herself together.

In the course of these years, we simultaneously, during her numerous and partly long-lasting stays in our department, investigated many other aspects that we hoped could contribute to our understanding of the headache and, eventually, to formulating therapeutic approaches. Since the patient steadily complained that the pain was at its maximum in the ocular area and because of the multitude of ocular signs associated with the attack, a major aim of the investigations was the disentanglement of ocular symptomatology using such methods as intraocular pressure measurements, corneal indentation pulse amplitude measurements, and corneal temperature measurements (Broch *et al.*, 1970; Hørven *et al.*, 1971, 1972, 1977). In addition, the following parameters were studied: urinary histamine excretion and histamine catabolic pattern (Sjaastad and Sjaastad, 1970, 1977a), cutaneous forehead blood flow (Sjaastad *et al.*, 1974) etc. Due to the seriousness of her situation it was even considered necessary to carry out cerebral angiography, pneumoencephalography (Sjaastad and Dale, 1976), CBF studies, a study of flow velocity through vessels to the eyes, etc. (Broch *et al.*, 1970).

The patient was so set on therapeutic approaches that she underwent various surgical procedures elsewhere. The reason for this was partly that, during the worst periods, she felt 'sick in the entire body' and also had abdominal complaints. Due to these complaints she underwent a Billroth II operation in 1968. Bilateral ovariectomy was carried out in 1964. Several molars were also extracted on the symptomatic side. None of these procedures led to any substantial improvement of the headache. She claimed, however, that after the abdominal operation, she had less abdominal complaints when she was 'sick in the entire body' (during the worst attacks).

Despite these extensive complaints, the patient felt that everything centred on the eye, and we found some clear-cut abnormalities concerning the eye. We did, however, at no time feel convinced that the intraocular pressure increase could in itself readily explain the pain and, in retrospect, we are even more convinced that the pressure increase did not cause the pain.

At the time, however, we had arrived at a point where we were running out of arguments when trying to reject the patient's contention that an enucleation of the right (symptomatic side) eye would perhaps solve her pain problem.

Fortunately, the following developments took place simultaneously. The patient had from the start claimed that salicylates seemed to give her some relief, not to the extent that the pain disappeared, but at times when they were not maximal the paroxysms could be modified by salicylates. Perhaps the paroxysms became even more rare during such medication. We thought that a lot of drugs would be more promising than salicylates as potential therapeutic agents. The anti-inflammatory agents were therefore put rather far down on our list of potentially effective drugs worthy of trial. In sorting out the relative efficacy of the various anti-inflammatory agents, my previous co-worker, Dr Inge Dale, was most helpful. When in late 1972 we finally arrived at indomethacin on our list, the response was no less than miraculous. The work with this patient had then taken us close to 12 years, with numerous annual in- and out-patient consultations.

We contended at the time—and continue to contend—that a blind study of a drug with placebo in a case like this is not mandatory in order to ascertain the drug effect. First, a multitude of drugs had been tried already and had not only given a totally negative response but, on most occasions, a clear adverse response was found. Next, as far as indomethacin is concerned, the response was shown to be absolute and it was *permanent*, unlike a placebo effect. As far as headaches of maximal severity are concerned, placebo trials are probably not indicated to the same extent as in headaches of moderate to mild degree, like migraine and the more moderate cases of tension headache. Finally, the effect of a drug is much easier to evaluate in a chronic disorder like this with a constant flow of attacks than in a cyclic disorder with an unpredictable sequence of attacks. In CPH cases at an early stage with only moderate complaints and an intermittent pattern, the situation may differ. Nevertheless, a single-blind, cross-over trial with indomethacin and identical looking indomethacin capsules was carried out using our two first patients and a convincingly positive result was obtained.

At the time of the therapeutic breakthrough, another patient with a similar headache was referred to us. This patient proved to have a similar response to indomethacin. We then started to understand that we could be faced with a new variety of cluster headache—or even a new headache altogether. The first mention of this headache in international fora was at the meeting of the American Association for the Study of Headache in New York in 1973. The first published communication concerning the first two cases appeared in 1974 (Sjaastad and Dale, 1974).

In 1976, we ventured to call this headache 'chronic paroxysmal hemicrania' (Sjaastad and Dale, 1976). By this time the first non-Norwegian patient had been discovered, i.e. a female patient from the USA (W. Caskey, Boston). Patients have been discovered in the following countries (in chronological order as given): Norway (Sjaastad and Dale, 1974); USA (1976); Czechoslovakia (Nebudova, 1978, not published until 1987); Denmark (Christoffersen, 1979); Italy (Manzoni and Terzano, 1979; see also Manzoni *et al.*, 1981); France (Leblanc *et al.*, 1980); Mexico (Guerra, 1981); Canada (Pelz and Merskey, 1982); Sweden (1982, unpublished); Australia (Kilpatrick and King, 1982); UK (Petty and Rose, 1983); Germany (Pfaffenrath *et al.*, 1984b); Poland (Bogucki *et al.*, 1984a,b); India (Dutta, 1984); Spain (1985, unpublished); Brazil (1985, unpublished); South Africa (Joubert *et al.*, 1987); and New Zealand (MacMillan and Nukada, 1989).

By 1979, a total of eight cases had been diagnosed (Sjaastad *et al.*, 1980). By 1982, a total of 20 cases had been published (Table 4.1). Even at that time, a female preponderance appeared rather obvious. Forty four cases had been published or related to us in detail by 1985. We now have information on 84 cases throughout the world (Antonaci and Sjaastad, 1989). For many of the reported cases, however, only fragmentary evidence is at hand, the reports on CPH cases partly being hidden, for example, within communications on surgical aspects of headache (Watson *et al.*, 1983). We are, therefore, not in a position to give a verdict on whether or not all these cases are genuine (see later). The real number of recognized and treated cases of CPH by now probably exceeds this number by a factor of 2–5, since new cases are usually not

Table 4.1   The first published case reports of CPH

Authors	*n*	No. of females	No. of males
Sjaastad and Dale (1974)	2 ⎫ = 3	2	0
Sjaastad and Dale (1976)	1 ⎭	1	0
Price and Posner (1978)	1	0	1
Christoffersen (1979)	1	1	0
Manzoni and Terzano (1979)	1	1	0
Sjaastad *et al.* (1979)	1	1	0
Stein and Rogado (1980)	2	2	0
Leblanc *et al.* (1980)	1	1	0
Sjaastad *et al.* (1980)	2	2	0
Hochman (1981)	1	0	1
Rapoport *et al.* (1981)	1	0	1
Guerra (1981)	2	0	2
Pelz and Merskey (1982)	1	1	0
Jensen *et al.* (1982)	1	0	1
Kilpatrick and King (1982)	2	2	0
Total No.	20	14	6

Table 4.2   Relatively large clinical series of CPH patients

Authors	*n*
J. Graham *et al.* (personal communication)	4
Manzoni *et al.* (1983b)	4
J. M. Espadaler (personal communication, 1987)	6
Kudrow (personal communication, 1987)	9
Own series	9

reported in the literature or related to us. Even some 'large' series have been collected (Table 4.2).

CPH is, as discussed further in the following, in many respects similar to cluster headache. Despite this similarity the two headache forms clearly differ from each other in some rather important respects. Most workers in the field, therefore, feel that CPH is a separate entity, but there is still no consensus on this matter.

CPH has been mentioned as a separate headache disorder in various textbooks since 1976 (e.g. Prusinski, 1976; Bousser and Baron, 1979; Kudrow, 1980; Lance, 1982; Nappi and Savoldi, 1983; Selby, 1983; Adams and Victor, 1985; Dalessio, 1987; Blau, 1987).

CLASSIFICATION

Chronic paroxysmal hemicrania (CPH), although similar to cluster headache (or Horton's headache) is probably a distinct headache entity. There are, nevertheless, many similarities between ordinary cluster headache and CPH. CPH and cluster headache should, therefore, probably, at least for the time being, be classified under the common heading of 'the cluster headache syndrome' (Sjaastad, 1986a). This grouping together may need to be changed when the pathogenesis of the two headaches is disentangled. The relative frequency of the two headaches, as well as the order in which they were discovered, are of little or no significance in this context. This should be indicated by placing them on an even footing (see Table 4.3). Right at the beginning we linked this headache to an *absolute* indomethacin effect (Sjaastad and Dale, 1974). As far as we know today, a complete and lasting indomethacin response is one of the crucial criteria of CPH. It seems difficult, at the present stage, to imagine what would justify the diagnosis in a case where there is no indomethacin effect. This feature sets CPH apart from cluster headache. The increase in the intraocular pressure and intraocular pulse amplitudes on the symptomatic side during attacks are also crucial features of CPH. It has, however, not been ascertained whether the last two criteria are necessary for the diagnosis. It may be that in the mild case (or mild attack) the increment in corneal indentation pulse amplitudes is only moderate or even absent.

We have given many descriptions of the clinical picture (Sjaastad and Dale, 1976; Sjaastad *et al.*, 1980; Sjaastad *et al.*, 1983b; Sjaastad, 1986b, 1987b). The first complete description of the criteria was given by Merskey (1983). A complete description of criteria in a total setting of headache descriptions is the one given by the Taxonomy Committee of the International Association for the Study of

---

Table 4.3   Classification of the various forms of chronic paroxysmal hemicrania[a]

   I. *Chronic paroxysmal hemicrania (CPH)* (Sjaastad, 1986a)
      (A) Pre-chronic form
      (B) Chronic form

  II. *Chronic paroxysmal hemicrania (CPH)* (Sjaastad, 1989)
      (A) Unremitting form
           (a) Unremitting from onset
           (b) Evolved from the remitting form
      (B) Remitting form

 III. *Cluster headache and chronic paroxysmal hemicrania* (Headache Classification
      Committee of the International Headache Society, 1988)
      (A) Cluster headache (with its subgroups)
      (B) Chronic paroxysmal hemicrania[b]
      (C) Cluster headache-like disorder not fulfilling the above criteria

---

[a]Courtesy of *Cephalalgia*. See also Table 1.1.
[b]This is the only form accepted by the Headache Classification Committee of the International Headache Society (1988).

Pain (IASP), headed by Professor Harold Merskey, London, Ontario (1986) (printed with the permission of H. Merskey):

Chronic paroxysmal hemicrania (chronic stage): multiple daily attacks of pain usually in females and principally in ocular, frontal and temporal areas by day and night, usually with lacrimation and nasal stuffiness and/or rhinorrhoea, with absolute relief from indomethacin.

Site: ocular, frontal and temporal areas. Occasionally the occipital, infraorbital, aural, mastoid and nuchal areas. Pain may also be felt in the neck, arm and upper part of the chest. Invariably unilateral and the side does not change.

System: uncertain. Possibly vascular or autonomic nervous system. Central nervous system changes may be fundamental.

Main features: rare, 80–90% females, age of onset probably above 20, but pre-CPH stage may appear about time of puberty. Daily attacks at maximum of 12 or more per 24 h, usually 15–30 in 24 h. Range 1–30 attacks per 24 h. Patients have attacks every day. Characteristically there is marked fluctuation in the severity of attacks and their frequency. 1–2 attacks per day which are barely noticeable may alternate with frequent severe attacks every day, thus providing a modified cluster pattern. Attacks last 5–45 min, maximum 60 min, the most usual duration being 10–30 min. At maximum they are excruciating. Some patients walk around during attacks, others sit quietly, still others curl up in bed. The pain is pressing, knife-like, boring, occasionally throbbing. Attacks occur at regular intervals all through day and night. The patients are awakened by the nocturnal attacks.

Associated symptoms: nausea is rare and vomiting very rare. Slight ipsilateral ptosis/miosis may occur during attacks, sometimes also oedema of the upper lid. Ipsilateral conjunctival injection and lacrimation probably occur in most patients and so do ipsilateral nasal stuffiness and/or rhinorrhoea. Bradycardia and extrasystoles occur in some patients during severe attacks. Attacks may be precipitated in some cases by bending or rotating the head, particularly when at the peak of the attack curve. Attacks disappear partly or even completely during the greater part of pregnancy, to reappear immediately post-partum.

Signs: ptosis/miosis, tearing, rhinorrhoea and blocked nose.

Relief: immediate absolute and permanent effect of continuous indomethacin treatment.

Pathology: unknown.

Diagnostic criteria: absolute response to indomethacin.

Differential diagnosis: sinusitis, chronic cluster headache, cluster headache, cluster-tic syndrome, migraine and psychiatric illness.

Code: 006.X8c (see Cluster Headache).

The description of the Headache Classification Committee of the International Headache Society (IHS) (1988) is as follows.

Chronic paroxysmal hemicrania: previously used terms: Sjaastad's syndrome.

Description: attacks with largely the same characteristics of pain and associated symptoms and signs as cluster headache, but they are shorter lasting, more frequent, occur mostly in females, and there is absolute effectiveness of indomethacin.

Diagnostic criteria:

A. At least 50 attacks fulfilling B–E (see below).
B. Attacks of severe unilateral orbital, supraorbital and/or temporal pain always on the same side lasting 2–45 min.
C. Attack frequency above 5 a day for more than half of the time (periods with lower frequency may occur).
D. Pain is associated with at least one of the following signs/symptoms on the pain side:
    1. conjunctival injection,
    2. lacrimation,
    3. nasal congestion,
    4. rhinorrhoea,
    5. ptosis,
    6. eyelid oedema.
E. Absolute effectiveness of indomethacin ($150 \, \text{mg day}^{-1}$ or less).
F. At least one of the following:
    1. history, physical- and neurological examinations do not suggest one of the disorders listed in groups 5–11; [Groups 5–11 denote headaches with organic background and associated with drug withdrawal, metabolic disorders, etc. (see Headache Classification Committee of the IHS, 1988).]
    2. history and/or physical- and/or neurological examinations do suggest such disorder, but it is ruled out by appropriate investigations;
    3. such disorder is present, but chronic paroxysmal hemicrania does not occur for the first time in close temporal relation to the disorder.

IHS comment: most attacks last 5–20 min and the frequency may be as high as 30 per 24 h. Although longer lasting remissions are not seen in chronic paroxysmal hemicrania, frequency, duration and severity of the attacks may vary. Nausea and vomiting rarely accompany the attacks. There is great female predominance. Onset is usually in adulthood. The chronic stage may probably be preceded by an episodic stage similar to the pattern seen in cluster headache, but this has not yet been sufficiently validated.

THE VARIOUS FORMS OF CHRONIC PAROXYSMAL HEMICRANIA

THE PRIMARY CHRONIC FORM: UNREMITTING FORM, THAT IS, UNREMITTING FROM ONSET

Our two first patients belong to the primary chronic group (Sjaastad and Dale, 1974). The patients had headache every day from the onset (see Table 4.3).

However, there was a marked fluctuation in attack frequency and severity. During the worst periods, the attack frequency was 16–24 per 24 h. During the lenient periods, there might be 1–2 very moderate pain episodes during 24 h, or maybe just a discomfort only barely different from zero. The important feature in our estimation is that the discomfort never faded away completely. A soreness in the most painful areas persisted interparoxysmally.

This developmental pattern seems to be the predominant one in chronic paroxysmal hemicrania (CPH) (Antonaci and Sjaastad, 1989). In a few series, the remitting group seems to dominate, quantitatively speaking. A situation with an apparent dominance of the remitting form may arise if inadequate emphasis is placed on the lenient, but still existing, discomfort in the troughs. It is clearly not a requirement that a pre-CPH stage is present in an individual patient (Sjaastad and Dale, 1976; Bogucki *et al.*, 1984a,b; Antonaci and Sjaastad, 1989).

THE SECONDARY CHRONIC FORM: UNREMITTING FORM, THAT IS, EVOLVED FROM THE REMITTING FORM

By 1979 (Sjaastad, 1979; Sjaastad *et al.*, 1980), retrospective evidence had been obtained that many of the patients who at the time of diagnosis had been in the chronic stage, had previously passed through a non-chronic (remitting) stage. No patient has been *observed* to make such a transition. The disease process in this early stage is presumably the same as in the full-fledged syndrome, in the absence of the typical temporal attack pattern. Accordingly, the response to indomethacin must be assumed to have been complete even at this stage. However, none of the later chronic cases have been given indomethacin at this stage. We thus have no definite information at hand to indicate that indomethacin could stop the disease process at the pre-chronic stage.

Attacks during the early, non-chronic phase often seem to be more short-lasting and somewhat less severe than those that occur during the later stage. In other cases the solitary attack appears to be undiscernible from that at the later, chronic stage. In cases that have become chronic, the intervals between 'cluster' phases appear to shorten, the headache attacks eventually becoming chronic. There are some interesting reports that demonstrate the increase in attack frequency over time before the chronic stage is reached (e.g. Davalos, personal communication). The recent development in one of our own cases in this stage with steadily shorter remissions may indicate that the chronic stage is approaching.

A few of our cases have had migrainous symptoms in the pre-stage, that is scintillating scotoma and obscurations. In retrospect, we tend to believe that in these cases there has been a chance co-existence of migraine and CPH. In other words, migrainous symptoms like these are probably not an integral part of the CPH picture.

'REMITTING FORM': 'PRE-CHRONIC STAGE'

In many instances, there seems to have been a stage of varying duration (1–19 years) with a less characteristic attack pattern ante-dating the stage of a daily, continuous attack pattern. We originally termed this stage the 'pre-CPH stage' (Sjaastad *et al.*, 1980). In recent years, cases have been diagnosed while in the pre-CPH stage (Stein and Rogado, 1980; Sjaastad and Russell, unpublished observation, 1979; Pelz and Merskey, 1982; Jensen *et al.*, 1982). Later, Kudrow *et al.* (1987) added some more, non-chronic cases to the list.

The term 'pre-CPH stage' should probably be substituted by the term: 'remitting form' of CPH, since it may well be that some (many?) of these cases will never reach the chronic stage (Table 4.3). The relative importance of the remitting stage has increased in recent years. This stage may be as important as, or even more important than, the chronic stage (Sjaastad, 1987b,e). At present (Antonaci and Sjaastad, 1989), only 17 out of 84 known cases (i.e. 20%) are in the remitting stage (see Relative Frequency of the Chronic and Remitting ('Pre-chronic') Forms).

SYMPTOMATOLOGY AND CHARACTERISTICS OF CHRONIC PAROXYSMAL HEMICRANIA

AGE OF ONSET

In a previous series ($n = 8$), the mean age at onset of the chronic stage was 29 years and the range 23–39 years (Sjaastad *et al.*, 1980). In 41 patients seen at a later stage, the mean age of onset was 33.7 years (Table 4.4). Later, a range of 11–81 years was found (Antonaci and Sjaastad, 1989). Recently, Kudrow and Kudrow (1989) have described the onset of chronic paroxysmal hemicrania (CPH) at 6 years of age in a male. The 'unremitting from onset' group has a somewhat higher mean age of onset (36.8 years) than those with a remitting stage, i.e. 26.9 years. The mean age of onset in the entire CPH group thus seems

Table 4.4   Age at onset of chronic paroxysmal hemicrania[a]

	Age group (years)						
	10–19	20–29	30–39	40–49	50–59	60–69	>70
No. of patients	11	10	6	3	8	2	1
Mean age at onset 33.7 years (range 11–71 years)							

[a]Based on published and unpublished reports, where this information is available.

to correspond largely to the mean age of onset in cluster headache as such. The age of onset in the chronic form of cluster headache seems to be somewhat higher than that of the episodic form (Manzoni *et al.*, 1983b; Ekbom, 1986). The age of onset of a clear, fully fledged CPH pattern in those who have been through a pre-stage is sometimes difficult to assess accurately, retrospectively. The remitting stage seems, on an average, to have lasted around 17 years in those who have made the transition (Antonaci and Sjaastad, 1989).

Since CPH is mainly a female disease, it may also be of interest to compare the age of onset in CPH with that in female cluster headache patients: the mean age of onset in Ekbom and Waldenlind's (1981) series was: 30.9 years and in Manzoni *et al.*'s (1988) series it was 27.7 years. There is thus apparently no considerable difference between cluster headache and CPH in this respect. The distribution of the age of onset of cluster headache in females seems to be diphasic, possibly indicating a heterogeneity (Ekbom and Waldenlind, 1981).

SEX DISTRIBUTION

CPH has been considered to be a female disease. It was, however, evident at a rather early stage that there are *definite* male cases (Price and Posner, 1978; Rapoport *et al.*, 1981). By 1979, eight definite cases had been reported world-wide: seven females and one male (Sjaastad *et al.*, 1980). The accumulative Norwegian series consists of nine cases (seven females and two males). In 62 cases, on whom we have ample information, there were 31% males (Table 4.5).

The sex distribution in this series is, therefore, significantly different from that in the population as a whole ($p < 0.0002$, binominal test). In Ekbom and Waldenlind's (1981) cluster headache series, there were 215 males (86%) and 34 females (14%). Evidently, the sex distribution in CPH is even more significantly different from that in cluster headache than from that in the population as a whole (χ^2 test; addition law of probability). With time, however, more and more male cases have been described. It is, therefore, entirely possible that, over time, the sex ratio in CPH will approach that in the general population, although a difference will probably remain. The sex ratio in conditions like cluster headache is so different from that in CPH that this discrepancy will, in

Table 4.5 Sex distribution in chronic paroxysmal hemicrania[a]

Total no. of cases	Females		Males	
	n	%	*n*	%
62	43	69	19	31

[a]Cases published, or presented to the author in person or cases on which fairly detailed accounts have been given to the author.

all likelihood, remain. There thus seems to be a real discrepancy between the two disorders of the cluster headache syndrome in this respect.

LOCALIZATION OF PAIN

The pain is, generally speaking, strictly unilateral, and the attacks always recur on the same side. Only a couple of exceptions to the latter rule appear to have been published (e.g. the Canadian case (Pelz and Merskey, 1982)) where the pain at an early age may have been on the side opposite to where it later appeared. The question of memory deficits in such cases always comes up. A couple of patients have noted that, when the pain has been exceedingly severe, the pain may have been felt slightly beyond the midline. The frequency of side-shift in cluster headache (i.e. approximately 15% of 161 cases (Manzoni *et al.*, 1983b)) and CPH, i.e. three cases out of 84, differs significantly (standardized normal deviate, $P < 0.007$). One possible bilateral case has been reported (Pöllmann and Pfaffenrath, 1986).

The painful areas as described by the first eight patients are detailed in Table 4.6. The patients generally complained of pain in several areas, for which reason the number of areas involved exceeds the number of patients. All patients, except one, indicated the temporal/ocular areas, the maxillar, or the supra- and retro-aural areas as the site of maximum pain. Occasionally the patient reported maximum pain in the back of the head. In a recent survey, 75% of patients had pain in the ocular area and 44% complained of forehead pain (Antonaci and Sjaastad, 1989). The pain in mechanically precipitated attacks was located in the same areas as that in spontaneous attacks (Sjaastad *et al.*

Table 4.6 Areas of the sites of maximal pain indicated by the first eight chronic paroxysmal hemicrania patients[a]

Area	No. of patients
Temporal	5
Ocular	4
Above or behind ear	3
Maxillar	3
Forehead	2
Neck[b]	2
Jaw	1
Occipital	1

[a]From Sjaastad *et al.* (1980). Courtesy of the *Upsala Journal of Medical Sciences* (*Stockholm*).
[b]During the most severe attacks, three more patients complained of pain in the neck and two of them in the shoulder and arm also.

1979). The pain may occasionally, or more regularly, spread to the neck and ipsilateral shoulder and arm in some patients.

CHARACTER OF PAIN

The pain at the peak of the curve is generally *excruciatingly severe*. We have in the past considered the at least occasional occurrence of excruciatingly severe attacks to be a diagnostic criterion. It is as clear that many (all?) patients at times experience attacks of more moderate severity. Many patients thus experience a distinct 'modified cluster pattern' (see later), and it is in the valleys of this pattern that the moderate attacks appear. As shown by Russell (1984), however, more moderate attacks may also appear between severe attacks. We have reason to believe that there are also cases having a more moderate attack pattern throughout, with regard to both the severity and the frequency of attacks. This is similar to what is found in cluster headache (Sjaastad *et al.*, 1988c).

In the initial phase of an attack, the pain may have a pulsating quality. The pain is usually piercing, boring, or claw-like. Some patients pace the floor during attack, but usually their behaviour during attack is different from that of cluster headache patients: they sit quietly, hold the head in their hands or even curl up in bed (Stein and Rogado, 1980). Some of our patients have experienced short-lasting, lightning-like pain attacks in the head (Sjaastad, 1979; Sjaastad *et al.*, 1979), which we have termed 'jabs and jolts' (see elsewhere).

DURATION OF ATTACKS

The attacks are generally more short-lasting than in ordinary Horton's headache, i.e. usually between 10 and 30 min (mean 20.9 min) (Antonaci and Sjaastad, 1989), with a range of 5–45 (occasionally 60) min (Sjaastad *et al.*, 1980). Some patients have relatively short-lasting attacks (i.e. 5–10 min), and others have more long-lasting attacks (i.e. 20–40 min). Nine out of 84 patients experienced attacks of more than 30 min duration, and one of them experienced attacks lasting up to 2 h (Antonaci and Sjaastad, 1989). In individual patients there is often a tendency towards relatively short-lasting attacks during periods of mild attacks, whereas more long-lasting attacks occur during the worst periods. In other patients, the attack duration seems rather constant despite the variation in severity and frequency. Russell (1984) has corroborated our previous, purely clinical impression of an intraindividual relationship between the frequency and duration of attacks on the one hand and the severity on the other.

In estimations based on accurate timing, Russell (1984) found a mean duration of attacks of 13.3 ± 7.6 (mean ± SD) min and a range of 3–46 min, based on 105 attacks in five CPH patients, in contrast to a mean duration of

49.0 ± 35.5 min based on 77 attacks in 22 cluster headache patients (Russell, 1981).

ACCOMPANYING PHENOMENA

Lacrimation on the symptomatic side seems to be the most frequently occurring autonomic accompaniment of attack (52/84), and *nasal stuffiness* (35/84) and *conjunctival injection* (30/84) also occur frequently (Antonaci and Sjaastad, 1989). *Rhinorrhoea* on the symptomatic side also accompanies the attack in many cases (34/84). There is occasionally a clinical impression of slight *swelling of the eyelids* on the symptomatic side during attacks, and sometimes there is a manifest swelling (usually in bad periods). This may be the reason why one gets an impression of ptosis in some of these cases. Photophobia occurs in some cases (18/84).

A particularly puzzling phenomenon observed in two of our first four patients was telangiectasia of the most distal parts of the eyelids. The telangiectasia was present on both sides, but seemed to be most marked on the symptomatic side. The inherent difficulties of assessing such phenomena quantitatively bars any definite statement as to the influence of attacks on these structures. The telangiectasia seemed, however, to fluctuate, being most pronounced during periods with severe attacks. A remarkable observation has recently been made in one of these patients, i.e. the one who can readily precipitate attacks (see later). A long-lasting remission took place after many years of suffering (Sjaastad and Antonaci, 1987), and some months after the onset of the remission the telangiectasia had disappeared completely. A similar, but even more marked telangiectasia is an integral part of the 'short-lasting, unilateral neuralgiform headache attacks with conjunctival injection . . .', recently described by us, the so-called 'Sunct' syndrome (Sjaastad *et al.*, 1989b). The latter article also gives an illustration of this.

In some cases, the pupil on the symptomatic side appears slightly contracted (Sjaastad *et al.*, 1979). Whether the pupil width changes as a consequence of attacks remains uncertain. A *'closed-box' feeling*, reduced hearing, as well as a hypersensitivity to sounds are occasionally experienced on the symptomatic side during attack (Sjaastad *et al.*, 1977, 1980). Dizziness and vertigo have not been overt complaints of our patients.

Nausea may be present on rare occasions (12/84) when the attacks are particularly severe, frequent and/or long-lasting. It never seems to be pronounced and does not really bother the patient. *Vomiting* is almost non-existent (2/84). Rarely occurring symptoms and signs are generalized sweating, V_1 hypersensitivity, and temporal artery dilatation.

It should be emphasized that the figures given for the associated phenomena are probably minimum figures, since such information was not always given in all the articles used (Antonaci and Sjaastad, 1989). A further circumstance contributing to an incorrectness of these data is the fact that attacks frequently have not been observed by the investigators themselves.

THE TEMPORAL PATTERN

Rhythmicity of attacks

Attacks may, in some patients and on some occasions, occur with a rather regular rhythm. During the worst periods, attacks may, on average, appear as frequently as every hour, during both the day and the night. This does not mean that attacks appear exactly on the hour; for example, when there are, say, around 24 attacks per 24 h, attacks *may* appear on the hour (±5 or more minutes). At other times, the attacks appear more randomly.

In patients with a marked ability to precipitate attacks, attacks may appear in rapid succession. It would, for example, not be difficult to precipitate five attacks in an hour. There does not seem to be any refractory period after an attack in such patients.

Nocturnal attacks

There does not seem to be any *preponderance* of nocturnal attacks in CPH. Nocturnal occurrence of attacks is, nevertheless, a typical trait of CPH, so typical that the lack of or only rare occurrence of nightly attacks has, until recently, been considered as a lack of conformity with a diagnosis of CPH. However, it can presently be stated with reasonable certainty that nocturnal attacks are not obligatory for a diagnosis of CPH to be made. There are patients who only rarely (or even never) are awakened at night due to attacks. This may or may not be due to a relative mildness of attacks.

In Russell's (1984) study, the patient triggered a timer at the onset of all attacks so that presumably exact information on attack frequency was obtained. The 24-h distribution of day and night attacks, i.e. 105 attacks in five patients, was as follows: 32 attacks occurred between midnight and 8 a.m., whereas 33 attacks began between 8 a.m. and 4 p.m. and 40 attacks between 4 p.m. and midnight (Figure 4.1). On the premise that the 'hours of sleep' were from approximately 23.00 to 07.00 h (i.e. 8 h or one-third of the 24 h period), less than one-third of the attacks occurred during sleep, i.e. 33 of 105 attacks (31%) (see Figure 4.1). There was thus no period with a definite increase in attack frequency, although there seemed to be a slight increase in frequency in the late afternoon and evening. The timing of attacks, therefore, may seem to differ slightly from that in cluster headache (see Episodic Cluster Headache. Nocturnal Attacks. Is there a Nocturnal Preponderance of Attacks?). In some patients there was a tendency for the attacks to accumulate at the end of the night. In one patient, 17 of a total of 18 nocturnal attacks started during the rapid eye movement (REM) sleep phase (Sjaastad *et al.*, 1977; Kayed *et al.*, 1978). While in

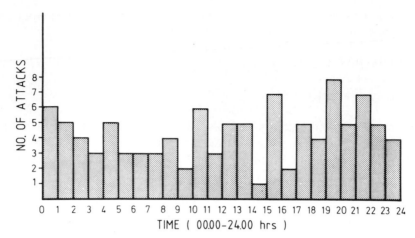

Figure 4.1   The temporal distribution of onset of attacks (total of 105 attacks) in patients with chronic paroxysmal hemicrania ($n = 5$). (From Russell (1984). Courtesy of *Cephalalgia*.)

some patients there may be a connection with the REM phase, this tendency may not be that marked in other cases (see Relationship of Attacks to Sleep Stages).

Frequency of attacks

The frequency of attacks is a characteristic trait in CPH. In our earlier investigations (Sjaastad *et al.*, 1980), we found the mean attack frequency to be 22 per 24 h when based on individual *maximum frequencies* (range 15–30 attacks). The minimum individual attack frequency ranged from 1 to 20 attacks per 24 h, with a mean of 7 attacks per 24 h. There may thus be only a few (1–2) just bearly discernible attacks per 24 h in mild periods.

In Russell's (1984) study, the patients triggered a marking system whenever they had an attack. In this way, the errors due to the patient's own memory of events were more or less eliminated. Five patients were followed for 24–48 h each, and a total of 105 attacks were recorded. The attack frequency ranged from 4 to 38 per 24 h, with a mean of 13.6 per 24 h. This frequency is statistically clearly different from that in cluster headache (mean 1.67; range <1–4 attacks per 24 h). Russell also found a clear relationship between the severity and the frequency of attacks. With mild or moderate attacks, the attack frequency ranged from 4 to 8 (mean 6.5) attacks per 24 h. With severe or extremely severe attacks, the frequency was 13–38 (mean 21.8) attacks per 24 h.

In an entire series of CPH patients ($n = 84$), the mean number of attacks was 10.8 ± 5.0 per 24 h (Antonaci and Sjaastad, 1989). The mean minimum attack frequency was 8 ± 4 (range 2–14), and the mean maximum frequency was 15 ± 7 (range 6–40) attacks per 24 h.

An important diagnostic factor (e.g. in the differential diagnosis versus cluster headache) is the maximum number of attacks in an individual. In all our first cases, this was >15 per 24 h. With more information available, this number has had to be reduced quite considerably. At the stage when the diagnosis is made, the number of attacks may, for example, never exceed 6–8 per 24 h. In order to be able to pick up all CPH cases, we have for years adopted the policy of giving an indomethacin course to all cases with an attack frequency exceeding 4 attacks per 24 h. It is noteworthy that Bogucki and co-workers (Bogucki and Niewodniczy, 1984; Bogucki and Kozubski, 1987) have described a male patient apparently suffering from cluster headache with an attack frequency of up to 30 attacks per 24 h. Overlapping between cluster headache and CPH with regard to attack frequency may thus appear.

Long-term pattern: 'modified cluster pattern'

A typical trait in the chronic form is that headache is present every day, but another almost as typical trait is that the intraindividual attack frequency varies widely, thus in one single patient it may vary from 1 or 2 attacks to 30 attacks per 24 h. During the worst periods, the pain is usually excruciatingly severe and the attacks become somewhat more long-lasting. A soreness persists in the painful area after each attack, so that the patient hardly recuperates before the next attack begins. A mild pain at the peak of the curve may not be consistent with a diagnosis of fully developed CPH. Admittedly, however, our information concerning this specific factor may be too scarce. With a low attack frequency, the attack pattern is at times barely discernible, and there may be a more or less continuous, low-grade headache. This transient, vaguely outlined attack/pain pattern, even in the non-remitting stage of CPH, may probably lead to a mix-up of this stage with the remitting form of CPH, if an exact case history is not obtained.

A constant shift between excruciatingly severe and mild phases takes place, the transition between the two phases usually taking some days. Exacerbations usually last between a couple of weeks and 3–4 months; the remissions last for one to some weeks. It is emphasized that even in the 'severe' period not all attacks are of maximum severity (Russell, 1984). The fluctuation in attack severity as experienced by one patient over half a year is shown in Figure 4.2.

It may be that the 'modified cluster pattern' as seen in CPH (Sjaastad and Dale, 1976) is not only similar to the clustering of attacks in cluster headache from a phenomenological point of view, but is really an expression of a similar mechanism. The curve is set at a slightly higher level in CPH than in cluster headache (Russell and Sjaastad, 1985), so that in CPH (i.e. the chronic form), it actually never quite reaches down to the baseline (Figure 4.3). This difference does not necessarily imply that the attacks are worse in CPH than in cluster headache; it may only indicate that the mechanism behind CPH attacks is more easily triggered. Headache is not always entirely absent in the remission phase of episodic cluster headache; the remission may be punctuated with abortive

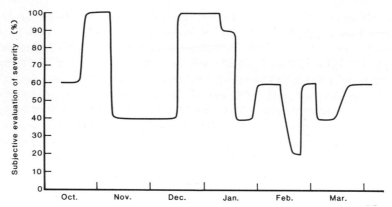

Figure 4.2 Continuous changes of the severity (frequency and intensity) of attacks in a female chronic paroxysmal hemicrania patient over 6 months. Only occasional indomethacin medication was given so that pain parameters could be assessed. The severity may in some cases be even much closer to the baseline, so that it may be difficult to decipher the chronic and non-continuous forms of CPH (see Figure 4.3).

attacks. This accentuates the similarity between the two forms of the cluster headache syndrome. There may also be some fluctuation along the time axis in *chronic* cluster headache. This very aspect of chronic cluster headache has probably so far not been looked into carefully enough.

Over time, the relentless course of CPH continues. We know of a few factors that can interrupt the monotonous rhythm: on a short-term basis, looking forward to an event may increase the attack frequency, whereas worrying may curb the tendency to attacks. On a long-term basis, pregnancy may do away

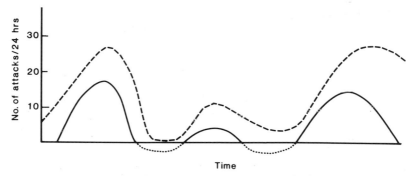

Figure 4.3 Temporal patterns in the non-continuous and continuous forms ('remitting' and 'non-remitting' forms, respectively) of chronic paroxysmal hemicrania. Note that the difference from the baseline may be almost non-existent in the chronic form! (——) Non-continuous form ('remitting' form; 'pre-CPH' stage); (– – – –) chronic or continuous form (or stage).

with attacks more or less completely (in 9 of 10 cases where this type of information was available (Antonaci and Sjaastad, 1989)).

Since CPH is a 'female' disease to some extent, with dependence upon the female life-cycle becomes important. With regard to pregnancy, the headache started again immediately upon delivery in five cases, and it may also start *de novo* right after delivery. Birth-control pills had no influence on the tendency to attacks. Menstruation seemed to have a negative or a positive influence upon the tendency to attacks. We do not have sufficient information to form an opinion about the influence of menopause. In a number of patients at least, the attacks continue with unabated fierceness after the menopause.

DIFFERENTIAL DIAGNOSIS

Cluster headache, particularly the chronic variety, may be so similar to chronic paroxysmal hemicrania (CPH) as to create differential diagnostic problems (see Figure 4.4). Otherwise, the differential diagnostic alternatives in CPH are, generally speaking, similar to those in cluster headache. Such differential diagnostic possibilities include migraine, cervicogenic headache (Figure 4.4) and atypical facial neuralgia. In particular differential diagnostic difficulties arise versus the other hemicranial disorders, e.g. the early stages of the newly discovered 'hemicrania continua', another headache totally responsive to indomethacin (Sjaastad and Spierings, 1984; Sjaastad *et al.*, 1984c; Sjaastad, 1987d). Also, the 'jabs and jolts' syndrome (Sjaastad, 1979; Sjaastad *et al.*, 1979) has caused some differential diagnostic problems due to a partial responsiveness to indomethacin (see below). There are still other hemicranial headaches, reminiscent of CPH, but with lack of indomethacin effect (e.g. Sjaastad *et al.*, 1979; Sjaastad, 1987b). Since so many CPH patients have previously received psychiatric diagnoses, these aspects will also be dealt with. For a more detailed account of the differential diagnostic possibilities, the reader is referred to the section on cluster headache.

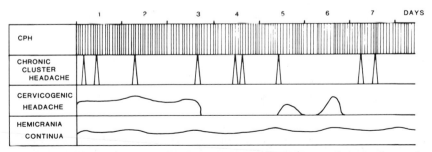

Figure 4.4 Attack patterns in chronic paroxysmal hemicrania, chronic cluster headache, and clinically related unilateral headaches. (From Sjaastad and Spierings (1984). Courtesy of *Cephalalgia*.)

Table 4.7 Comparison of some autonomic features (symptomatic side, during pain phase) of chronic paroxysmal hemicrania (CPH), hemicrania continua and cluster headache

	CPH	Hemicrania continua	Cluster headache
Sweating	±	−	+
Rhinorrhoea	+	−	+
Lacrimation	+	∓	+
Salivation	0	0	0
Corneal indentation pulse amplitudes	+ +	0	+
Pupillometry			
Asymmetry with tyramine ocular drops	−	±	+
Pilocarpine supersensitivity	−	−[a]	+

[a] Only the test on our first patient is reported (Sjaastad and Spierings, 1984).

HEMICRANIA CONTINUA

Hemicrania continua is a unilateral headache that may start rather suddenly, may reach its full strength right away, and then continue 'indefinitely' (primary chronic form, see Figure 4.4). There may be fluctuations in severity, but generally the severity of the headache in hemicrania continua seems to be at a considerably lower level than that in CPH. In the chronic cases first observed, there was never freedom from headache; in other words, there were no attacks. The temporal pattern thus differed widely from that in CPH (Sjaastad and Spierings, 1984; Sjaastad, 1987d). There is, however, some recent evidence to show that, prior to the chronic stage, there is a non-continuous stage, like in CPH. In this stage, the differential diagnosis may be somewhat more difficult (Centonze *et al.*, 1987; Sjaastad and Tjørstad, 1987). The first case diagnosed at this stage was recently reported (Iordanidis and Sjaastad, 1989). Attack frequency and duration will, however, usually differ widely even when the more similar forms of the two headaches are present. The autonomic engagement in hemicrania continua seems to be at a lower level than in CPH and cluster headache (Sjaastad *et al.*, 1984c) (Table 4.7). Salicylates may improve, and indomethacin definitely abolishes the headache in hemicrania continua as well as in CPH, so they have the absolute indomethacin response in common (Bordini *et al.*, 1991).

'JABS AND JOLTS SYNDROME'

This headache has apparently caused some differential diagnostic problems. This phenomenon was described by us in 1979 (Sjaastad, 1979; Sjaastad *et al.*, 1979). The *term* 'jabs and jolts syndrome' (according to the Headache Classification Committee of the International Headache Society (1988) terminology, probably: 'idiopathic stabbing headache') was coined in June, 1979 when Drs Hørven and Sjaastad visited several centres in the USA, in search of new CPH patients. In Chicago, patients suspected of having CPH (but complaining of *short-lasting* attacks with which we were well acquainted from e.g. the CPH patients) during personal interviews told us that they suffered from 'the jabs' and 'the jolts'. So, it was decided to term this headache the 'jabs and jolts syndrome'.

This syndrome consists of short-lasting (usually <1 min duration, and frequently of only a few seconds duration), knife-like head pains, mostly of moderate severity. In the occasional case, they may have a rather fixed location. In other cases, they may for some time be localized in one area, only to be located in another area at another time. The attacks may appear during a circumscribed period, and the frequency of attacks may vary immensely; sometimes they occur in a more isolated fashion and sometimes in groups (Sjaastad *et al.*, 1980; Sjaastad and Hørven, 1982). Some patients experience only a few such episodes altogether; others may experience as many as 50 attacks or more a day for prolonged periods (Table 4.8). Usually, there is no residual pain once the paroxysm is over. In a few cases, there seems to be some interictal soreness of very moderate degree. This type of pain seems frequently to be associated with another headache of some kind, e.g. 'tension headache', migraine, or cluster headache. This pain also seems to appear in individuals otherwise not suffering from headache. It is in all probability the same type of pain attacks that Raskin and Schwartz (1980) later described in migraine, under the designation 'ice-pick-like pain'. In CPH, the pain may appear prior to the chronic stage, and even on the non-symptomatic side. The response to indomethacin is 'partial' or lacking. Despite some clinical similarity with CPH, the mechanism behind the pain may prove different.

We feel that it is important to stick strictly to the diagnostic criteria for the 'jabs and jolts syndrome'. The pain frequently changes location, sometimes within a bout, but more often from one bout to another. The time aspect is probably of utmost importance in the differential diagnosis: the jabs and jolts paroxysms are ultra-short, i.e. usually of only a few seconds duration; they may last up to 1 min. Although the lower margin has not been clearly defined, the duration of CPH attacks in Russell's (1984) series was as low as 3 min. *Severe* attacks of CPH (and these are the ones that should be paid heed to diagnostically) are usually of considerably longer duration. In other words, attacks of 1 min duration at the maximum of pain is *probably* not compatible with a diagnosis of CPH, as far as the present information shows. The duration and localization of pain may seem to be of considerable importance in consolidating the diagnosis. The sex of the patient cannot be used in differential diagnosis.

A similar picture (Averianov *et al.*, 1983) with an absolute indomethacin effect has recently been described (Table 4.8). We have recently described cases with unilateral, ultra- to medium-short attacks, an explosive conjunctival injection, and massive lacrimation at the onset of pain (Table 4.8), but without any indomethacin effect at all (Sjaastad *et al.*, 1978, 1989b).

Table 4.8 Ultra-short and relatively short-lasting headache attacks: some differential diagnostic criteria

Category	Authors	No. of patients	Unilateral pain	Same-sided pain	Cluster pattern: real (+) or modified (M)	Duration of attacks	Indomethacin response	Sex
CPH	Sjaastad and Dale (1974)	84[a]	+	+	M	10–30 min (5–45)	+++	F > M
'Jabs and jolts' syndrome	Sjaastad et al. (1979), Sjaastad (1979)	Multiple	±	∓	?	A few seconds, usually <1 min	++	?
Short-lived; with conjunctival injection, lacrimation, etc. (Sunct)	Sjaastad et al. (1978, 1989b)	Originally:1 Presently: 3	+	+	+ or M	20 s to 2–3 min	–	M
Short-lived; unilateral with cluster phenomenon	Aver'ianov et al. (1983)	1	+	+	+	Around 10 s	+++	

[a] Antonaci and Sjaastad (1989).

DOES CHRONIC PAROXYSMAL HEMICRANIA HAVE A PSYCHOGENIC BACKGROUND?

'Psychogenic headache' according to the Ad hoc Committee on Classification of Headache (1962) can refer to both 'muscle contraction headache' and headache of delusional, conversional, or hypochondriacal states. For the latter headaches it is stated that 'a peripheral pain mechanism is non-existent'. The headache pattern with such headache is not described. Only faint ideas seem to have existed as to *how* such headaches materialize clinically.

Our first patients had previously, among other diagnoses, been given psychiatric diagnoses; it was said that they were neurotic, hysterical, centred on their own condition, and even that they had invented the headache. A full psychiatric/psychological exploration was carried out in our first two patients which failed to demonstrate any psychopathology. Admittedly, 'emotional' symptoms were part of the picture in many patients. Small wonder that this was the situation — the constant flow of attacks in the worst periods, with only a short time to recuperate between attacks, naturally represents a heavy strain on the patients. It takes a strong personality with both stamina and resilience to endure the hardships connected with this condition over the years. Some of our early patients were greatly helped in their struggle by a strong religious conviction. Several of our first patients had contemplated suicide, and some of them claim that if they had not got any relief at the time they would have committed suicide. It is certainly easy to mix up cause and effect in this situation. The presence of 'emotional' symptoms in such a group of patients cannot be taken as an indication that the mentioned symptoms are primary ones.

Needless to say, headache in general, and probably without exception, is influenced by psychogenic factors. This goes for migraine as well as for toothache (and for chronic paroxysmal hemicrania (CPH)). Of course, such views do not affect my firm belief that there is an organic basis for CPH. We have a strong feeling that a strictly *unilateral* headache, with *ipsilateral* autonomic phenomena, and with attacks strictly limited in time, is *a priori* most unlikely to be of purely psychiatric origin. Furthermore, there is a striking discrepancy between the generally absolute ineffectiveness of drugs in this condition and the dramatic effect of indomethacin (and to a lesser extent of other anti-inflammatory agents). Only small amounts of orally administered indomethacin can be retrieved from the spinal fluid. This may be of relevance for its site of action. Indomethacin is, furthermore, not known to have a stabilizing influence on the mind. The entirely rational behaviour of CPH patients as soon as their headache attacks have been alleviated by the administration of indomethacin also attests to the view of a general equilibrium of mind in these individuals. The fact that this headache is vastly or even entirely relieved during pregnancy adds further weight to this view (Sjaastad *et al.*, 1980).

Psychogenic headache should be a headache caused by a *primary* psychiatric illness, i.e. by an intrapsychic conflict—'headache from an idea' (Merskey, 1981). The very existence of such a headache is debatable. If it exists at all, it may be a vague, ill-defined headache. The typical traits of such headache have, in some headache circles, been said to be a non-fluctuating, non-treatable, global headache. If this is true, it will readily be appreciated that none of these three criteria pertain to CPH.

Nevertheless, in various contexts it has been contended that there are underlying psychogenic mechanisms in CPH (e.g. Stein and Rogado, 1980). If psychogenic symptoms and mechanisms were of decisive importance in CPH then, as far as I am concerned, they would have to be present in every case.

There is little reason to believe that in the *do novo* onset of this headache, psychodynamic factors or stress play a role. Furthermore, once the chronic pattern has been established, the attacks seem to continue in their own rhythm (Sjaastad, 1987a). Exacerbations can appear at any time, apparently largely unassociated with external, stressful stimuli. However, that there is an interplay between the psyche and soma even in this, as far as we are concerned, clearly organic condition is illustrated by the experience of some CPH patients. If the patient looks forward to a particular event, attacks are apt to increase appreciably in frequency as well as in severity. Apprehension, on the other hand, may markedly slow down the tendency to attacks.

At the present stage of knowledge, psychogenic mechanisms seem unacceptable as primary steps in the chain of events leading to attacks. Another possibility of course also exists as far as the simultaneous occurrence of psychiatric symptoms and CPH is concerned, such as in some of the American cases (e.g. Stein and Rogado, 1980): CPH cannot be assumed to hit only mentally robust persons. Psychiatrically stigmatized individuals may also be victims of CPH, and *then* the symptoms may be atypical.

THE LINK TO CLUSTER HEADACHE

In the classification (see Tables 1.1 and 4.3), chronic paroxysmal hemicrania (CPH) and cluster headache have been put as subgroups under the same heading, i.e. cluster headache syndrome. What is then the basis for the link to cluster headache? The two headaches mainly have four clinical traits in common:

1. the unilaterality of the pain;
2. the intensity of the pain;
3. the localization of the pain; and
4. the accompanying autonomic phenomena.

Both CPH and cluster headache have a cyclic and a chronic stage, although the cyclic stage is more common in cluster headache than in CPH (Antonaci and Sjaastad, 1989) and both seem to have disordered body chrono-organization (Micieli *et al.*, 1989). Finally, even in the chronic stage of CPH there is a waxing and waning of symptoms ('modified cluster pattern'), reminiscent of the typical cycling of attacks in cluster headache.

As far as the supplementary tests are concerned, there are also similarities (see under the specific sections): the corneal indentation pulse amplitudes (Hørven and Sjaastad, 1977) and the intraocular pressure are increased on the symptomatic side during attacks in both disorders. (It is noteworthy though, that the changes observed in CPH are more marked and clear-cut than those in cluster headache). Quantitation of lacrimation and nasal secretion during attacks (Saunte, 1983, 1984b,c) have shown a similar increase on the symptomatic side in both types of headache. Increased sweating on the symptomatic side has also been found during attack in both conditions, although less regularly in CPH (Sjaastad *et al.*, 1983a). Once an attack is established it is next to impossible outwardly to distinguish between a CPH and a cluster headache attack. This has made us wonder whether there is a final common pathway to attack in the two disorders (Sjaastad, 1978).

However, there are a number of features separating the two headaches:

1. sex preponderance;
2. headache frequency;
3. temporal pattern;
4. duration of attacks;
5. night preponderance;
6. indomethacin effect;
7. ergotamine effect; and
8. other drug effects (lithium, etc.).

It may appear that the difference as for sex, temporal pattern, frequency of attacks and, last but not least, the drug effects are rather crucial factors. It cannot be merely an accidental and trivial feature that in the one disorder there is a clear male preponderance, whereas this is not the case in the other. The same goes for the striking indomethacin effect and lack of ergotamine effect in CPH.

Are then these differences of such magnitude that they substantially and definitely separate CPH from cluster headache? This brings us to the crucial question: What is a disease by definition? The following points of view may be advanced with regard to this topic. In all patients fully affected by a given disease, the aetiology, pathogenesis, pathophysiological and biochemical findings, pathological–anatomical findings, clinical manifestations, and therapy should be more or less identical. If only minute differences exist between two clinical pictures, be it in aetiology, pathogenesis, etc., it may not be practical to give the two conditions different names, although this may be justified from a theoretical point of view. If, however, a more profound deviation from the 'core' symptomatology is encountered in one, or preferably more, of the main parameters, one may be faced with another disorder; it will then be practical to use another term for it.

The present status of CPH can be evaluated on this basis. First, the *clinical* appearance of the two headaches differs to some extent, as outlined above. Next, the striking influence of indomethacin seems to be a decisive feature of CPH, where as far as we know this effect is invariably present (admittedly, since the indomethacin effect is an inclusion criterion, one may to some extent become involved in a circular argument at this point). The indomethacin effect in these cases does not seem to pertain to underlying rheumatic disturbances in the usual sense of the term (Sjaastad and Dale, 1976). Since there is an obvious discrepancy between the indomethacin effect in regular cluster headache and CPH, it is felt that one fundamental step in the chain of events leading to an attack is different in these two disorders. A further indication that the thera-peutic aspects differ is the fact that lithium, one of the front-line drugs in cluster headache, is of no avail in CPH; as a matter of fact it may worsen the suffering.

The discrepancy between the sex distribution in the two headaches adds weight to the view that they differ fundamentally. This together with other features (e.g. lack of typical pupillometric changes in CPH), indicates that the *pathophysiological* characteristics of the disease differ in the two disorders.

Whereas in cluster headache there are some signs of a sympathetic super-sensitivity, such definite signs have not been found in CPH, either pupillome-trically or with regard to the forehead-sweating pattern. On the contrary, there is some evidence for some sort of direct stimulation in CPH, at least in cases of mechanically precipitated attacks (Sjaastad *et al.*, 1983b).

In my opinion the demonstrated differences between the two headache types are so fundamental that they probably are *two different diseases* (Sjaastad, 1987c). However, not only do the two headaches belong to the unilateral headaches category; they also both seem to be ferocious headaches of a 'clustering' type, with an inherent propensity to chronicity. It would, therefore, be most correct to group CPH not as a subgroup under 'cluster headache', but under the 'cluster headache syndrome', at an even level with cluster headache (Sjaastad, 1986a) (see Tables 1.1 and 4.3). The difference in prevalence of the two different headaches is of no significance in this context. This view has recently been accepted by the Headache Classification Committee of the IHS (1988). A consequence of this view is that the pathogenesis of CPH will have to be worked out independently of that of cluster headache.

MECHANICAL PRECIPITATION OF ATTACKS

Four of the 11 chronic paroxysmal hemicrania (CPH) cases that we have studied in detail display an ability to precipitate attacks mechanically, to a greater or lesser degree (Sjaastad *et al.*, 1979, 1982, 1984a). Attacks may be precipitated in these cases either by movements in the neck or by exerting pressure on certain tender spots in the neck. In one particular patient, attacks can be precipitated readily at will at any time when she is in a bad period. The

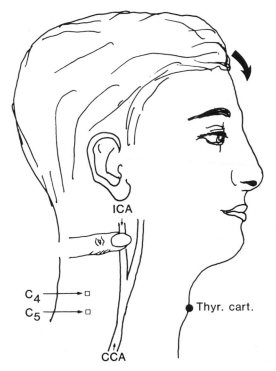

Figure 4.5 A patient with a marked tendency to precipitate attacks of chronic paroxysmal hemicrania. External compression of the internal carotid artery *per se* does not lead to attack, whereas head flexion under such circumstances leads to an attack. Common carotid artery compression alone does not precipitate attack. Forward head movements *alone*, however, precipitate attack. Head flexion *per se*, therefore, seems to be the decisive factor.

attacks are most easily and regularly precipitated by bending the head forwards in this patient, but the attacks can also be provoked by rotating the head towards the symptomatic side. In the other three patients, attacks can only sometimes be precipitated in these ways, but can usually be precipitated by external, mechanical procedures (Figure 4.5).

Attacks precipitated in this way outwardly seem to be very similar or identical to spontaneously occurring attacks. Even supplementary tests seem to give similar results in the two types of attacks: both corneal indentation pulse amplitudes and the intraocular pressure increase, and to a larger degree on the symptomatic side, as do lacrimation and nasal secretion (and, in some instances, forehead sweating).

The tenderness (and the putative locus of precipitation = trigger points) was originally considered to be along the carotid artery on the symptomatic side (Sjaastad *et al.*, 1979). It was, therefore, first thought that we were perhaps faced with a condition like 'carotidynia' (Figure 4.5). In the long run, however, we

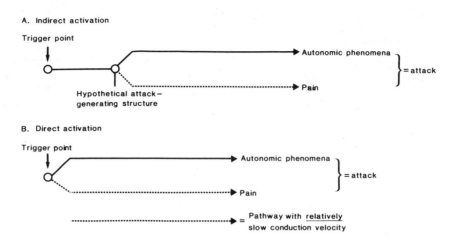

Figure 4.6 Possible explanations for the discrepancy in the latency of pain and the various autonomic phenomena in chronic paroxysmal hemicrania.

were not convinced that we were able to precipitate any attacks from that area. Over time, it was ascertained that the points of excessive tenderness were the anterior aspects of the transverse processes of C_4/C_5, and even the posterior aspects of these processes were tender. Tenderness was as marked over the C_2 root (i.e. posterior to the mastoid process) and over the greater occipital nerve. From these zones, attacks could be precipitated by firm external pressure, and attacks or a relatively short-lasting pain episode sometimes started almost immediately. This is in contradistinction to the case of neck flexion or rotation, where it takes a varying amount of time (5–60 s) to produce the pain. The sequence of pain/autonomic phenomena also differs somewhat with the two precipitation procedures. With neck flexion the autonomic phenomena such as lacrimation (and sweating) may appear many seconds ahead of the pain (see later), thus clearly indicating that these phenomena are not due to the pain *per se* (Sjaastad *et al.*, 1986). With external pressure, the pain and autonomic phenomena seem to develop in parallel.

The reason why the autonomic phenomena appear first may be that they are easier to provoke than the pain. The theoretical models that have been proposed to explain the delay in pain production are presented in Figure 4.6. The activation of the autonomic functions (like lacrimation and sweating) is not a prerequisite for the generation of pain in such experiments; these functions can be more or less abolished by pre-administration of atropine (Sjaastad *et al.*, 1979), while atropine does not influence the tendency to precipitation of attacks. The autonomic phenomena and the pain seem to be parallel features, secondary to a common activation, which presumably takes place at one single spot. This spot is possibly in the neck (in the cases of mechanical precipitation of attacks; see Significance of Trigger Mechanisms, and Pathogenesis).

A 'central' factor can still be assumed to play a not insignificant part in this type of attack.

SIGNIFICANCE OF TRIGGER MECHANISMS

The statements in this section are based on the observation of several hundred attack precipitations, mostly in one patient who can readily precipitate attacks, but also in three of the other patients that we have seen.

One of our patients is able to precipitate attacks readily upon rotation of the head towards the symptomatic side and upon flexion of the head (Sjaastad *et al.*, 1979, 1984a). The precipitation mechanism in this patient is apparently more easily triggered than in the other chronic paroxysmal hemicrania (CPH) cases with a mechanical precipitation mechanism. This patient may be unique and, in other words, may not be representative of CPH patients as such, although she has typical CPH traits otherwise and responds in an absolute fashion to indomethacin. Approximately 10% of patients are able to precipitate attacks themselves (Antonaci and Sjaastad, 1989).

There is a marked intraindividual difference in latency between the initiation of stimulus and the attack onset during neck movements. In the most studied patients, this latency may be from 5 s up to 1 min or more. This variation apparently depends to a large extent on the state of the patient, i.e. the severity of spontaneous attacks at the time, the interval since the last attack, the interval since indomethacin treatment, etc. It is noteworthy that, with neck movements, the first macroscopically observable sign of an oncoming attack is usually lacrimation on the symptomatic side. Sweating on the forehead may appear just as early as lacrimation, but is usually at a subclinical level (see Sweating on the Forehead). If the pain is late in appearing (as during mild attacks), the interval between the onset of homolateral lacrimation/sweating and pain may be 30–40 s or more (see Figure 4.6). In this patient it can, therefore, be ruled out that lacrimation and sweating are secondary to the pain (Figure 4.7(a)). From these observations, it does not seem unreasonable to state that the

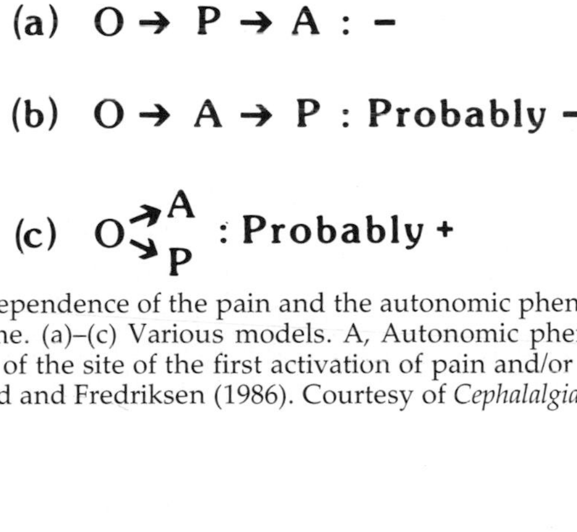

(a) $O \rightarrow P \rightarrow A : -$

(b) $O \rightarrow A \rightarrow P :$ Probably $-$

(c) $O \overset{\rightarrow A}{\underset{\rightarrow P}{}}$: Probably $+$

Figure 4.7 Interdependence of the pain and the autonomic phenomena in the cluster headache syndrome. (a)–(c) Various models. A, Autonomic phenomena; P, pain; O, 'origo' — a concept of the site of the first activation of pain and/or autonomic phenomena. (From Sjaastad and Fredriksen (1986). Courtesy of *Cephalalgia*.)

pain and the autonomic phenomena may operate independently (Sjaastad and Fredriksen, 1986).

During the precipitation procedure, it is possible to predict whether a full attack will appear or not by monitoring forehead sweating, since pain attacks are preceded by forehead sweating (see Sweating on the Forehead) (Sjaastad *et al.*, 1986). Sweating and the other autonomic phenomena are, nevertheless, not necessary factors for the attack, since as demonstrated elsewhere (see Salivation), both atropine and stellate ganglion blockade may annul some autonomic phenomena (e.g. lacrimation and sweating) but not the pain (Sjaastad *et al.*, 1979; Sjaastad, 1986b).

Attacks may also be precipitated by external digital pressure, towards the area immediately behind the mastoid process (over the C_2 root?), over the greater occipital nerve, or over the transverse processes of the C_4–C_5 vertebrae, on the symptomatic side. It was initially felt that the tender points in the anterior aspects of the neck were over the carotid artery. Over time, it was ascertained that it was the transverse processes, and not the artery, that were particularly tender.

This experimental model may explain other aspects of the inter-relationship between the pain and the autonomic phenomena. In attacks triggered by a direct pressure against, for example, C_2, the pain starts immediately. This immediate triggering of attacks may indicate that the actual points are close to the points of significance for the generation of the pain in the attacks precipitated by, for example, neck movements, without necessarily being identical with these points. The reason why the triggering seems to take longer with head bending than with pressure exerted against a manifest trigger point may be that the triggering in the former case is weaker, or that the triggering takes place further away from one source of pain. The pain elicited by direct-pressure procedures is difficult to differentiate from the pain of the attack *per se*; in other words, the transition from the pain due to the exerted pressure and that of the attack *per se* is hard to delineate. For these reasons, it is difficult to distinguish whether in the direct-pressure experiments there is a parallel triggering of pain and autonomic phenomena or whether the autonomic response comes first (see Figure 4.6). A pressure of only a few seconds duration may, under certain circumstances, give rise to an attack, which is accompanied by autonomic phenomena in the usual way.

Theoretically it is still possible that the pain really is triggered by the autonomic impulses (Sjaastad and Fredriksen, 1986). In our trials only a few autonomic impulses have been blocked, i.e. by atropine, stellate ganglion blockades, etc. (Figure 4.8). There may be other, autonomic impulses of importance in this context which may be uninhibited by these measures (Figure 4.7(b)). It is remarkable that, when on indomethacin, the special patient in whom attacks can readily be precipitated is protected against mechanical precipitation of attacks (both by head movements and by external pressure) (Figure 4.8). The tender spots in the neck are also far less tender during

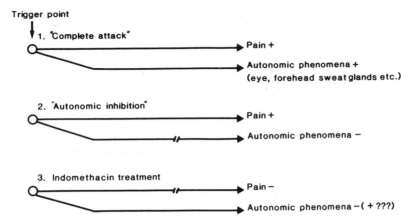

Figure 4.8 Chronic paroxysmal hemicrania: (1) 'Complete attack' with both pain and autonomic phenomena and 'partial' attacks with inhibition of either the autonomic phenomena (2) or the pain (3).

treatment (and, accordingly, during attack-free periods) than in the symptomatic periods.

The occasionally ultra-short latency between the initiation of a mechanical stimulus and the onset of the autonomic phenomena suggests that positive and not negative phenomena, i.e. *stimulation* and not a *deficiency*, underlie the symptom production. The normal functioning of autonomically innervated organs depends, among other things, on a balance between the tone of each of the two main autonomic systems. The possibility cannot be totally rejected that a hypothetical, rather abrupt reduction—or discontinuation—of the tone in one of the systems should create immediate, massive autonomic symptoms, although this possibility seems far-fetched. For example, *a priori* a sympathetic stimulation in functionally intact fibres seems to be a more likely possibility of symptom production than is a sympathetic deficiency in the mechanically precipitated attacks of CPH (Sjaastad *et al.*, 1983b). A stimulation would imply direct production of symptoms in functionally intact nerves, or symptom production through a supersensitivity mechanism in functionally deficient nerves, the end-result being the same, i.e. generation of phenomena characterizing the normal function of the nerves.

The signal from the neck to, for example, the ocular region (lacrimation/conjunctival injection, increased intraocular pressure and increased corneal indentation pulse amplitudes) will have to reach its destination within a few seconds. The number of alternative theoretical explanations for this phenomenon is, therefore, limited. The following possibilities exist with regard to the nature of the signal.

1. autonomic impulses.
2. vascular factors:

(a) occlusion of arterial flow;
(b) vasoactive substance
    (i) primarily mediated through veins,
    (ii) primarily mediated through arteries.

The most likely signal paths from the neck to the eye in precipitated attacks in the patient who can readily precipitate attacks (and in CPH in general?) are the autonomic ones, for the following reasons: This patient is suitable for studies aimed at disentangling the mechanism underlying the generation of attacks in this way. The influence of vascular factors has accordingly been explored in this patient (Figure 4.5) (Sjaastad *et al.*, 1982). All these procedures were carried out when the patient was in a period of a constant flow of attacks, and accordingly attacks could readily be precipitated. Rubbing of the artery as well as manual external flow obstruction were carried out on the common and internal carotid arteries on the symptomatic side. None of these procedures led to any attacks. There is, in other words, no positive evidence for the release theory. In addition, this rules out an anoxia theory based on circulation disturbances in carotid artery flow. In previous years, some migrainologists were of the strong opinion that a release of vasoactive substances might be the cause of the local vascular/autonomic phenomena in the face during the precipitated attack in CPH.

Flexion of the head, whether or not combined with simultaneous external obstruction of the carotid flow, invariably led to attacks. Even in the state of 'no-flow' in the ipsilateral carotid system the signal is mediated from the neck to the eye, forehead sweat glands, etc., when the head is bent forwards. The important feature in attack precipitation, therefore, seems to be neck flexion. This is strong evidence that the signal to the secretory glands is neurogenic in nature.

Could altered flow—or liberation of neurovasoactive substances—in the vertebral artery be the cause for the mediation of the signal from the neck to the face? The vertebral artery is closely linked to cervical spine and could thus be vulnerable during the precipitation procedures. Autonomic nerves in the vicinity of the artery, or even within the arterial wall, could mediate the signal. It has been shown that the vertebral artery lumen can be obliterated at the atlantoaxial point during neck rotation (Barton and Margolis, 1975). Anoxia could therefore be an attack-producing factor. For the unravelling of the mechanism involved, the temporal aspects of the single attack then become important: it may take only a couple of seconds from the start of neck flexion until lacrimation is first observed. The vertebral artery does not furnish the eye with blood directly. If anoxia or liberated vasoneuroactive substances produce the attack, there must, therefore, be at least a two-step reaction to accomplish an ocular effect: first, a vascular influence (on the brain stem) and then, secondarily, an autonomic signal to the eye and then (the production and) the expulsion of tears. Necessarily, these steps must be time-consuming and can hardly take place in the course of a couple of seconds. Moreover, there would be no direct influence on the vertebral artery when attacks are precipitated by direct pressure against trigger points, such as the occipital major nerve.

The possibility of attack mediation via the *venous* system (liberation of vasoneuroactive substances) seems highly unlikely for the reason that the precipitation would necessarily take time. Furthermore, if liberated into venous blood, one would imagine that a substance would be distributed evenly to the two sides with the blood, and not every time to a higher extent to the symptomatic side.

Therefore, the evidence is rather strong that the signal from the neck to the eye, etc., in this particular patient is neurogenic, and there is some indirect, clinical evidence that there may be a 'barrage' along autonomic (sympathetic?) pathways in connection with the precipitation procedure. What happens locally in the eye when the signal has reached the eye is another story: What kind of local actions are taking place in the eye itself, and to what extent do they contribute to the symptomatology of the attack? *Locally* there may be *vascular* reactions or vasoneurogenic reactions.

In conclusion, it seems highly unlikely that the autonomic phenomena are secondary to the pain in such attacks. It seems unlikely, although the possibility cannot be totally rejected, that the pain is secondary to some autonomic phenomenon. The most likely possibility seems to be that pain and autonomic phenomena are triggered in parallel (Figure 4.7(c)) (Sjaastad and Fredriksen, 1986).

TESTS AND STUDIES CARRIED OUT IN CHRONIC PAROXYSMAL HEMICRANIA

It goes without saying that the number of test individuals available for study has been limited in many studies. This applies particularly to the first period when only two patients were known. The *nature* of the studies was also partly such that the number of cases had to be limited: only two cases were studied with regard to histamine catabolism, and only one for electromagnetic flow-metry. The number of cases is given for each of the studies detailed below. The results reported should be viewed in this light. For the same reason, statistical analyses were not employed in the early studies. In more recent studies, however, it has usually been possible to study larger groups of individuals, and comparison with control subjects has been possible in several contexts. The patients usually served as their own controls, attacks being compared with attack-free periods.

VARIOUS SUPPLEMENTARY TESTS

The following supplementary laboratory investigations were carried out with normal or negative results in our two first patients: haemoglobin, erythrocyte sedimentation rate, white cells (count with differential count), red cells, routine urinalysis, serum aspartate aminotransferase, serum alanine aminotransferase, creatine kinase, and ornithine carbamyl transferase, alkaline phosphatase, cholesterol, serum total protein with electrophoretic pattern, quantitation of serum immunoglobulins, fibrinogen, triglycerides, urinary porphyrins, serum iron, iron binding capacity, protein bound iodine, serum creatinine, serum electrolytes, serum vitamin A, vitamin B_{12}, folic acid, antistreptolysin O-test (ASO-test) and antibodies against α-staphylolysin (ASTA). All were within normal limits. Coomb's reaction, Rose–Waaler test and tests for thyroid antibodies, antinuclear factor, and lupus erythematosus cells were negative.

The following clinical tests were carried out with negative results in our first two patients: X-ray of the skull and sacroiliac joints. In our first patient, the urinary excretion of vanylglycolic acid, vanylacetic acid, adrenaline, noradrenaline, 17-ketosteroids, as well as 17-hydroxysteroids were within control limits in the non-medicated, symptomatic period.

HISTAMINE STUDIES

Since cluster headache and chronic paroxysmal hemicrania (CPH) appear to have rather similar clinical manifestations and since histamine originally has been considered to be of importance in the pathogenesis of cluster headache, histamine parameters have also been studied in CPH.

Urinary excretion of histamine

Dunér and Pernow's (1956, 1958) method or Wetterquist and White's method (1970) were employed. Our two first cases were studied. Patient 1 excreted increased quantities of histamine-like activity in urine on most test days (Figure 4.9, Table 4.9), whereas the excretion in patient 2 was mostly within normal limits. There did not seem to be any good correlation between the degree of histamine excretion and the severity of attacks in case 1, slight attacks at times

Table 4.9 Urinary excretion of free histamine[a] in chronic paroxysmal hemicrania

		During exacerbations			During remission	
Patient No.	No. of tests	Histamine excretion (μg base per 24 h) Range	Mean	No. tests with increased excretion	No. of tests	Histamine excretion (μg base per 24 h)
1	17	10–67	40	11	1	15[b]
2	5	5–48	15	1	1	12[b]

[a]Upper control 24 h excretion: 31 μg histamine base in our material (Sjaastad, 1966a).
[b]On indomethacin.

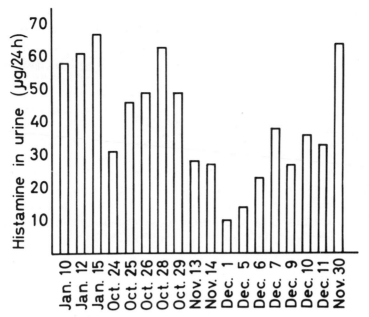

Figure 4.9 Urinary excretion of free histamine in our first chronic paroxysmal hemicrania patient. The upper control limit in our own study was 31 μg base per 24 h (Dunér and Pernow's (1956) method). (From Sjaastad and Sjaastad (1970). Courtesy of *Acta Neurologica Scandinavica (Copenhagen)*.)

being associated with definitely increased excretion, and severe attacks being associated with only slightly increased or even normal histamine (=free histamine) excretion. Salicylates seemed to reduce the urinary excretion of histamine appreciably, and withdrawal of salicylates was followed by an increase in urinary histamine output during periods with pronounced attacks in patient 1 (Sjaastad and Sjaastad, 1964, 1965, 1970, 1977b).

The urinary excretion of conjugated histamine (partly or entirely identical with N-acetylhistamine) was within the normal range.

Histamine catabolism

Also studied in the first two patients was the catabolic pattern of [14C]histamine, 0.075–0.1 mci of which was given either orally or subcutaneously in each experiment (one oral and two subcutaneous tests in patient 1, and one subcutaneous test in patient 2). No drugs were allowed during or just prior to study. The total radioactivity was determined in urine (0–6 h and 6–24 h portions) and faeces. Also examined was the exhaled CO_2, as described by Sjaastad and Sjaastad (1971, 1974). Furthermore, [14C]histamine and its metabolites in urine were determined with both autoradiography and Schayer's

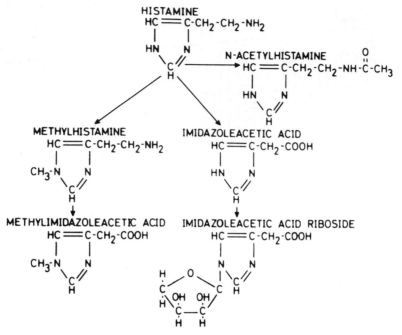

Figure 4.10   The major metabolic pathways of histamine in man.

isotope dilution technique (Schayer and Cooper, 1956). The catabolic pathways are shown in Figure 4.10 (for further details see Cluster Headache).

The urinary, faecal, as well as the expiratory air excretion of radioactivity were within control limits after both oral and subcutaneous administration of the histamine. However, the patient with partly increased urinary histamine output showed a dramatic change in the catabolic pattern, whereas in the other patient the findings were within control limits (Table 4.10; for comparison with cluster headache, see also Tables 2.27 and 2.28). Imidazole acetic acid (ImAA) is the end product of oxidative deamination of histamine (see Figures 4.10 to 4.12), and it is subsequently linked to a riboside (ImAA-R). In this case, there was a strikingly small proportion of ImAA-R compared with ImAA, both during the 0–6 h interval (2% versus 54%, respectively) and during the 6–24 h interval (11% versus 30%, respectively) in one of the experiments. This test was carried out when the patient was suffering from severe paroxysms. Even a second test in the same patient, carried out when she was much less severely afflicted, showed a preponderance of ImAA relative to ImAA-R (i.e. 29% versus 21%). However, a third (oral) test in the same patient showed no deviation from normal (Table 4.10). It should be emphasized that this patient had only scarcely discernible attacks during the oral study. Ordinarily, ImAA-R seems to outweigh ImAA on subcutaneous administration of [^{14}C]histamine. The inverse ImAA-R/ImAA ratio on subcutaneous histamine application in this patient is remarkable.

Table 4.10 The fate of [14C]histamine in chronic paroxysmal hemicrania patients: the figures are percentages of the sum of the three actual main metabolites[a]

Patient No.[b]	Time after [14C]histamine administration (h)											
	0–6				6–24				0–24			
	ImAA-R	ImAA	ImAA-R + ImAA	MelmAA	ImAA-R	ImAA	ImAA-R + ImAA	MelmAA	ImAA-R	ImAA	ImAA-R + ImAA	MelmAA
Subcutaneous administration[c]												
1	28	10	38	62	–	–	–	–	–	–	–	–
2a	21	29	50	50	–	–	–	–	–	–	–	–
2b	2	54	56	44	11	30	41	59	6	47	53	47
Oral administration[d]												
2c	27	12	39	61	50	5	55	45	34	10	44	56
Range, healthy controls	34–50	6–13		41–57	55–75	3–7		23–45	43–60	4–11		34–48

ImAA-R, imidazole acetic acid riboside; ImAA, imidazole acetic acid; MelmAA, methylimidazole acetic acid.
[a] Data from Sjaastad and Sjaastad (1977a). Courtesy of the *Journal of Neurology*.
[b] Patient 1: patient with chronic paroxysmal hemicrania during symptomatic period. Tests 2a–2c were carried out in another patient with chronic paroxysmal hemicrania. Test 2a was carried out 12 days after discontinuing indomethacin treatment, the attack pattern just starting, but still with only very moderate pain. Test 2b was carried out on a day with severe attacks. Test 2c was carried out 5 days after discontinuation of indomethacin, during a relatively symptom-free period.
[c] Determined by autoradiography and the isotope dilution technique.
[d] Determined by autoradiography.

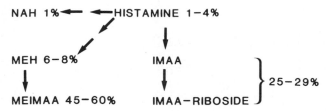

Figure 4.11 The relative significance of the major catabolic pathways of histamine in man ([^{14}C]histamine administered parenterally). NAH, *N*-acetylhistamine; MEH, methylhistamine; MeImAA, methylimidazole acetic acid; ImAA, imidazole acetic acid. See also Figure 4.10. According to Schayer and Cooper (1956), Kobayashi and Freeman (1961), and Lindell and Westling (1966).

In males, the ImAA-R/ImAA ratio seems to be higher than 1.0, frequently rather markedly so, with oral loading (a mean 0–6 h ratio of 4.6 (Sjaastad and Sjaastad, 1974)), as well as with subcutaneous loading (Kobayashi and Freeman, 1961), i.e. a mean 0–6 h ratio of 1.4 and a lowest observed ratio of 1.0. In migraine, a mean 0–6 h ratio of 2.25 was found on subcutaneous [^{14}C]histamine administration (Sjaastad and Sjaastad, 1977a). However, our patient was female, and the catabolic pattern in females seems to differ somewhat from that in men (Nilsson *et al.*, 1959). The free ImAA fraction seemed to constitute the major part of the total ImAA when [^{14}C]histamine was given parenterally to two females in the fertile age group. Our patient, however, was far beyond the fertile age (58 years old and bilateral ovariectomy had been performed when she was 47 years old).

It is difficult to interpret the demonstrated abnormality. It does not appear to result from a primary defect of oxidative deamination since the 0–6 h total ImAA fraction (sum of ImAA-R and free ImAA) was in fact higher in this patient than in other experiments with subcutaneous application of [^{14}C]histamine (one patient with cluster headache and one with CPH). ImAA is the precursor of ImAA-R, and what constitutes the abnormality in this patient could just be that the ImAA-R formation lags behind. However, the fact that the level of ImAA by far exceeds that of ImAA-R even between 6 and 24 h, hardly fits with this explanation—by this time, ImAA-R ought to have been the predominant catabolic product.

On a day with severe paroxysms of headache, a markedly pathological ImAA-R/ImAA ratio was found, i.e. 0.04, whereas on a day with moderate attacks the ratio was 0.7. Even the latter, minor reduction in the ratio may be significant, since during a period of minimal symptoms the ratio was 2.3. A clearly reduced ImAA-R fraction was, as already mentioned, found only on subcutaneous and not on oral loading of [^{14}C]histamine in this particular patient. The difference in mode of administration could, therefore, possibly be the cause of this discrepancy. A more likely explanation, however, is that the conversion of ImAA to ImAA-R is inadequate during severe attacks: full-scale attacks seem to have as their counterpart a markedly reduced ImAA-R, whereas the complete absence of headache attacks annuls the biochemical

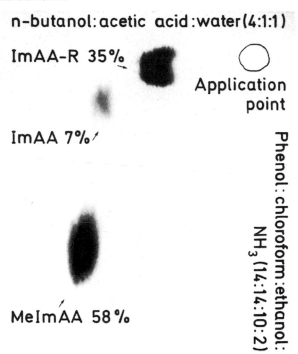

n-butanol:acetic acid:water(4:1:1)

ImAA-R 35%

Application point

ImAA 7%

Phenol:chloroform:ethanol: NH₃ (14:14:10:2)

MeImAA 58%

Figure 4.12 Separation of the three major urinary histamine metabolites. The separation was done using descending paper chromatography with: (1) n-butanol:acetic acid:H₂O (4:1:1); and (2) phenol:chloroform:ethanol:NH₃ (14:14:10:2). (From Sjaastad and Sjaastad (1977). Courtesy of the *Journal of Neurology*.)

abnormality, irrespective of the mode of histamine administration. For most of the time this patient exhibited increased urinary excretion of histamine. A possible connection between the increased free histamine output in urine in this patient and the aberration in ImAA-R formation is intriguing.

However, the inactivation of [^{14}C]histamine seemed as complete in this patient as in the other experiments, and the total ImAA fraction did not seem to be reduced. Thus the possibility that the aberration observed is causally linked to the increase in histamine output seems, at this stage, somewhat unlikely.

The following points of view should, however, be appreciated in this context. The mean (corrected) urinary output of histamine base in man may seem to be around $18\,\mu$g base per 24 h (e.g. Sjaastad, 1966a). Down to 1% of intravenously infused histamine (see Lindell and Westling, 1966) may be excreted unmetabolized in the urine. If, therefore, only an additional 1–2% of the histamine is not catabolized, this will result in a borderline high or increased histamine level in the urine. Viewed from this point of view, it is still possible that there may be some connection between the moderately increased histamine output (i.e. up to $67\,\mu$g per 24 h) in this patient and the decreased ImAA-R fraction.

The fact that the anomaly was found only in one patient makes it unlikely that this anomaly is of consequence for the CPH *as such*. In addition, it is unlikely that there is any causal relationship between the total histamine turnover in the body, as reflected by the histaminuria, and the headache. The reason for this is that the fairly constantly increased histamine output was found only in one patient and even then did not correspond to the headache intensity. The possibility remains that the histaminuria reflects the disease process, in other words it is a secondary phenomenon.

To establish beyond doubt whether or not there is a causal connection between the histamine abnormality and a given headache, *in casu* CPH, is a formidable task. To obtain more definite evidence for a cause-and-effect relationship would, as a minimum, necessitate further studies, including the study of the entire spectrum of endogenous histamine metabolites. The results obtained so far do not seem promising enough to justify any such further investigations.

PROSTAGLANDINS

Prostaglandin E_2 was determined in blood as described by Unger *et al.* (1971) in our two first patients. In accordance with a suggestion of Sandler (1972), arterial samples were used, and sampling was carried out before, during, and after attacks. Multiple samples were frozen immediately upon blood withdrawal. No consistent attack-induced trend in prostaglandin blood levels was found (Bennett *et al.*, 1974). It should be noted that these studies were carried out with the rather crude methods of the time. This type of study should, therefore, be repeated.

KININ STUDIES

Blood kinin-like activity, kininase, as well as kininogen were determined in our first two patients. The methods used in these studies are, in essence, the same as those used by Ofstad (1970).

The mean kininase level seemed to be somewhat lower in patient 1 than in controls, but with no definite changes related to attacks (Table 4.11). The kinin levels were found to be clearly elevated during one single attack in each of the two patients (8 and 10 ng ml^{-1}, respectively), but also between and immediately after attacks a minor elevation was occasionally encountered. Kininogen, determined by means of the trypsin method (Dinitz *et al.*, 1961), seemed to be lower in patient 1 than in controls; an obvious trend relating to the course of the headache was, however, absent (Table 4.11). It is stressed that these studies were done using the admittedly rather coarse methods of the time. The results must, therefore, be viewed with caution.

Table 4.11 CPH. Kinin-like activity (ng ml^{-1}), kininogen (μg ml^{-1}), and kininase (in Rugstad units (Rugstad, 1966)) in our first two patients[a]

	Kinin-like activity			Kininogen			Kininase		
	Mean	Range	No. tests	Mean	Range	No. tests	Mean	Range	No. tests
Patient 1									
Attack	4.2	2–8	4	3.1	2.4–3.8	4	8	6–9	3
Atack-free interval	2.6	1.3–4	4	3.3	3.2–3.5	5	7	6–9	4
Patient 2									
Attack	4.0	1.6–10	6				10	8–12	5
Attack-free interval	3.1	1–6	7				10	8–11	11
Controls	2.5	1.5–4.0	7	5.8	5.0–7.5	7	13	8–14	7

[a]Data from Sjaastad and Dale (1976). Courtesy of *Acta Neurol Scand*.

COAGULATION FACTORS

These were determined several times during and between attacks in our two first patients, since in Egeberg's (1970) study of families with a partial factor XII deficiency and bleeding tendency some of the affected individuals seemed to suffer from somewhat atypical headaches. A classification of these atypical headaches was not attempted at the time. No significant alterations were, however, detected for factors V, VII, VIII, IX, XI, XII or II + X in our patients. I am indebted to Dr O. Egeberg for having carried out these studies.

MUSCLE BIOPSY AND IMMUNOLOGICAL INVESTIGATIONS

Routine histological examination of tibialis anterior musculature revealed no abnormality whatsoever (two first patients). Muscle tissue was also treated with fluorescine tagged antisera against IgG, IgA, IgM and complement. Specific fluorescence could not be detected with these sera (Prof. G. Husby, at the time working at Rheumatological Research Institute, Oslo).

ELECTROMAGNETIC FLOWMETRY

This technique has been used to study the flow in the main arteries of the neck (Hardesty *et al.*, 1961; Kristiansen and Krog, 1962). This method was used on our first patient (Broch *et al.*, 1970). Under general anaesthesia the implantable flow probes were placed around the exposed, but intact internal carotid arteries, approximately 1 cm cranially to the unexposed carotid sinus. Care was taken not to damage the sinus and the sinus nerve. The size of the probes

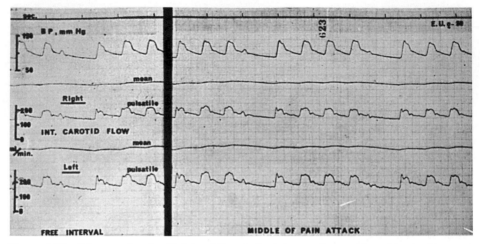

Figure 4.13   Mean and pulsatile blood flow in both internal carotid arteries in the pain-free interval and during the middle part of a pain attack (15 February 1967). The femoral blood pressure was monitored continuously during the registration. Note the extrasystoles and their effect on blood flow. (From Broch *et al.* (1970). Courtesy of *Cephalalgia*.)

(5 mm) was chosen to ensure a tight fit between probe and artery, in order to obtain an adequate flow signal.

Pulsatile and mean blood flow in both internal carotid arteries was monitored continuously during four subsequent attacks, and during two of them blood pressure was measured intra-arterially in the femoral artery with a Statham transducer (Figure 4.13). Spinal fluid pressure was also partly monitored continuously (see Cerebrospinal Fluid Pressure).

Evidently, the onset of headache attack was not accompanied by any definite change in intra-arterial blood pressure (see Intraarterial Blood Pressure During Attacks) or mean or pulsatile carotid artery blood flow on either side (Figure 4.13). Neither was there any definite alteration in the shape of the pulsewave tracings. A difference in pulsatile amplitudes between the two sides persisted throughout the second day of registration (Figure 4.14). The most plausible reason for this difference is a change in the probe/artery relationship.

A decrease in cerebrospinal fluid pressure was observed between the fourth and eighth minutes of the attack. The patient, who had a continuous flow of attacks at the time of study, remained free of attacks for the 5 days following removal of the equipment.

Continuous monitoring during several attacks revealed no alterations in blood flow through the internal carotid arteries. If circumscribed areas of vasodilatation were present within the brain, these would appear to be well compensated for by other areas of vasoconstriction, since the total flow was unchanged. These findings consequently do not provide any evidence for a generalized vasodilatation within the internal carotid vascular bed during the pain phase.

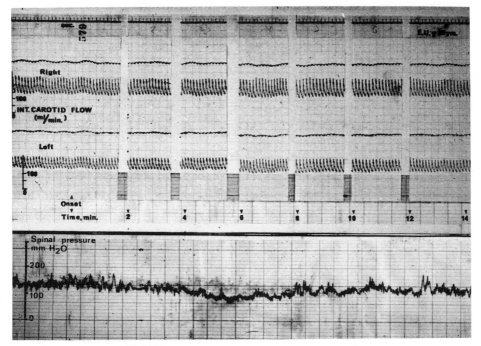

Figure 4.14 CPH. Electromagnetic flowmetry of internal carotid artery mean and pulsatile flow bilaterally, between attacks and during a spontaneously occurring attack. Lower tracing: simultaneous monitoring of intrathecal pressure. (From Broch *et al.* (1970). Courtesy of *Headache*.)

Furthermore, there may seem to be a marked discrepancy between the ocular findings (see later) on the one hand and the internal carotid artery blood flow on the other.

REGIONAL CEREBRAL BLOOD FLOW MEASUREMENTS

With electromagnetic flowmetry, the total carotid flow is estimated, but possible regional differences in flow cannot be elucidated in this way. Attack and attack-free-interval rCBF measurements were, therefore, carried out on the symptomatic side in two of our first patients, using a ^{133}Xe clearance technique. In the first patient, the regional cerebral blood flow (rCBF) study was done in the carotid artery distribution area, whereas in the other patient it was measured after selective catheterization of the vertebral artery via a transfemoral approach (Sjaastad *et al.*, 1977). The tracer was injected approximately 2 min after the onset of a typical attack, and the clearance curves were registered for 10 min, the attack still being present at the end of the recording. All flow parameters were calculated using a computer and the equations of Sveinsdottir *et al.* (1971).

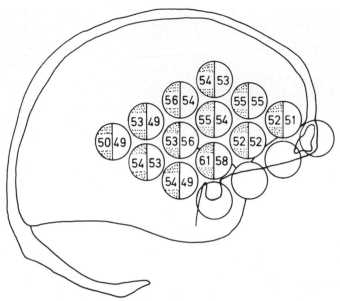

Figure 4.15   Mean blood flow pattern (in ml/100 g/min) in the right (symptomatic side) carotid artery distribution area during (left half of circles) and after (right half of circles) a pain attack. (From Sjaastad *et al.* (1977). Courtesy of the Biomedical Press.)

Figure 4.15 shows the position of the 16 detectors over the right hemisphere during the carotid artery flow study. No appreciable differences were observed between the slopes of the initial 2 min of the original clearance curves for attack and the attack-free interval in patient 1, most of the slopes being quite normal (Figure 4.16). All flow values, i.e. the mean values for rCBF, and flow fast and flow slow within the carotid artery perfusion area were within the normal range; there were no inter-regional differences in flow outside the error limits of the method, nor were there any significant differences between flow values obtained during and after a pain attack (Figure 4.15, Table 4.12).

In the second patient, rCBF was measured before and during an attack provoked by bending the head forwards. Corrected overall mean blood flow in the vertebral artery distribution area was 62.5 before and 66.5 ml/100 g/min during the pain attack, the increase being insignificant (Figure 4.17). The apparently significant increase in three detector areas was considered to be of doubtful importance since the *patient hyperventilated strongly during the attack* ($apCO_2$ = 24.6 mmHg). This may create false inter-regional flow differences since the obtained values had to be converted to an arterial pCO_2 of 40 mmHg based on correction formula, taking into account the mean and not the regional flow or the individual reactivity of cerebral vasculature to pCO_2. The areas with the possible increase in flow were at the base of the brain. It may thus be that the flow in the basal, posterior areas is slightly increased during the provoked (as well as the spontaneous) attack of CPH.

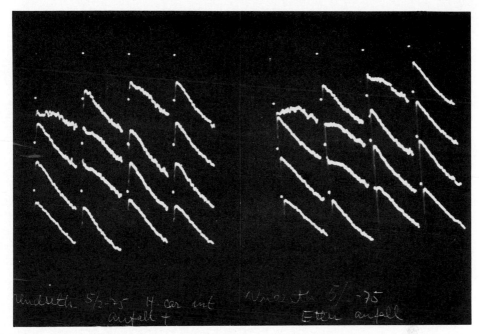

Figure 4.16 Cerebral blood flow in the right carotid artery distribution area of a patient with chronic paroxysmal hemicrania. Two-minute semilogarithmic recordings of cerebral blood flow during (left) and after (right) a right-sided pain attack. There is no appreciable change in the initial slopes. The four channels with irregular clearance curves were positioned over the orbit. (From Sjaastad *et al*. (1977). Courtesy of the Biomedical Press.)

Table 4.12 Mean rCBF values during and after attack, on the symptomatic side in the carotid artery distribution area of chronic paroxysmal hemicrania patients[a]

	After attack	During attack	Difference
rCBF mean[b]	51	52.2	+2.3%
rCBF mean[c]	55.4	56	+1.1%
rCBF initial	51.3	53.6	+4.3%
Flow fast	81.1	87.3	+7%
Flow slow	26	27.6	+5.8%
Relative weight grey	0.47	0.43	−0.04
Relative weight white	0.53	0.57	+0.04
$apCO_2$	41	37.5	−3.5

[a]From Sjaastad *et al*. (1977). Courtesy of the Biomedical Press.
[b]Biexponential.
[c]Height/area.

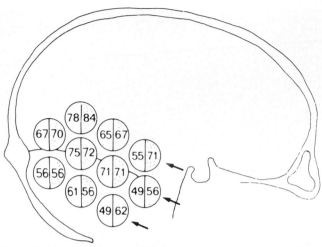

Figure 4.17 Second chronic paroxysmal hemicrania patient. Mean blood flow pattern in the vertebral artery distribution area before (left half of circles) and during (right half of circles) an attack of pain provoked by bending the head. Note the three detector areas with an apparently significant increase in mean blood flow (arrows). (From Sjaastad *et al.* (1977). Courtesy of the Biomedical Press.)

Electromagnetic flowmetry showed that there is no total flow change of functional significance in the total internal carotid artery perfusion area during attacks. This finding was corroborated by means of the xenon method which showed that there are no definite signs of distribution changes during attacks, within the same area. There may, however, be distribution changes in basal, posterior parts of the brain.

INTRA-ARTERIAL BLOOD PRESSURE DURING ATTACKS

Such studies were carried out with a Statham transducer in two patients, and two attacks were studied in each of them. No definite changes were discovered when the attack and attack-free periods were compared (see also Figures 4.13 and 4.18).

CEREBROSPINAL FLUID PRESSURE

This was monitored continuously during one spontaneous attack in our first patient (Broch *et al.*, 1970). During a 20 min attack, an even curve was obtained except for a drop in cerebrospinal fluid (CSF) pressure between the fourth and eighth minutes of the attack (Figure 4.14). Mean and pulsatile blood flow in the internal carotid arteries were monitored simultaneously by electromagnetic flowmetry and, as usual, showed no definite changes. The reduction in CSF pressure could *a priori* be caused by hyperventilation. Routine pCO_2 analyses carried out during the test did not reveal any marked deviations from normal

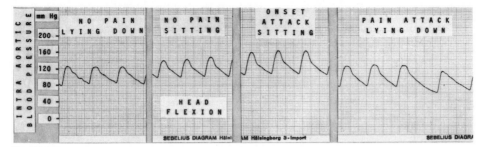

Figure 4.18 Intra-aortic pressure monitoring during a moderate chronic paroxysmal hemicrania pain attack precipitated by head flexion. No change in pressure was observed during the attack, as compared to the pre-onset supine level. Note the slight bradycardia during attack. (From Sjaastad *et al.* (1979). Courtesy of *Headache.*)

resting values. It has been observed clinically over the years that some patients with CPH hyperventilate during attacks; the patient studied here belongs to this category. This clinical impression of attack-related hyperventilation in CPH has been substantiated by end-tidal CO_2 measurements (Sulg and Sjaastad, 1983). Although the mechanism behind the reduction in CSF pressure in this special case remains somewhat obscure, hyperventilation may have played a role, in that individual sensitivity to CO_2 changes may also differ.

RELATIONSHIP OF ATTACKS TO SLEEP STAGES

A sleep laboratory registration of all night sleep was carried out in three of our first patients, according to the standard techniques of Rechtschaffen and Kales (1968). Analysis of the sleep parameters was done as described by Williams *et al.* (1974). The sleep quality was poor, as demonstrated by the low sleep-efficiency index and the marked increase in the number and duration of awakenings (see Table 4.13). The most characteristic finding in all three patients was a marked reduction of the rapid eye movement (REM) stage. Two main patterns were identified with regard to the time of nocturnal attacks and the REM stage. In one patient, there was a marked 'timelocked' relation of attacks to the REM stage (Figure 4.19). One single attack (out of a total of 18 attacks) occurred outside the REM stage. It is emphasized that this patient possesses an extraordinary ability to generate attacks mechanically (Sjaastad *et al.*, 1979). The other two patients did not exhibit attacks time-locked to the stage REM (Figure 4.20). This difference in the association of attacks with REM sleep is surprising. It may point to an inhomogeneity of the CPH syndrome. Bono *et al.* (1985) demonstrated a normalization of sleep abnormalities and an annulment of nocturnal attacks after intravenous indomethacin (50 mg) administration. However, in this patient also only one of five attacks during the test night was related to REM sleep.

Table 4.13 Various sleep parameters in three patients with chronic paroxysmal hemicrania

Parameter	Mean values for patients			Values for control females[b]	
	1 (age 58 years)	2 (age 60 years)	3 (age 38 years)	20–39 years	50–59 years
Total sleep time	338	245	311		
Time in bed	458	410	406	429.2 ± 21.7	430.8 ± 34.9
% SPT (sleep period time)					
Awake[a]	25.2	27.6	9.9	0.5 ± 0.5	4.9 ± 6.5
I	4.4	6.4	5.2	4.2 ± 2.4	4.9 ± 2.2
II	49.1	38.7	50.7	52.4 ± 5.9	57.8 ± 6.5
III[a]	7.3	9.2	13.0	5.3 ± 1.9	6.5 ± 2.4
IV	8.4	8.3	11.9	12.4 ± 6.2	4.1 ± 5.3
III + IV	15.7	17.4	24.9	17.7 ± 6.7	10.6 ± 6.1
Sleep efficiency index[a]	0.74	0.64	0.77	0.96 ± 0.02	0.93 ± 0.07
No. of awakenings[a]	7	8	6.5	1.1 ± 0.8	4.6 ± 2.1
No. of REM periods	3	3	5	4.2 ± 0.9	4.3 ± 0.9
REM[a]	5.5	9.9	9.3	25.2 ± 3.6	21.8 ± 3.3
No. of awakenings with headache (total)	6	8	18		
Headache in REM periods	—	1	17		
Headache <3 min after REM	—	—	—		
Headache 3–9 min after REM	—	1	—		
Headache >10 min after REM	6	6	1		
No. of nights	1	2	4		

REM, rapid eye movement.
[a]Significant difference.
[b]According to Williams *et al.* (1974).

PUPILLOMETRY: HORNER'S SYNDROME?

In some of our first patients, we suspected Horner-like changes on the symptomatic side (e.g. Sjaastad *et al.*, 1979). One reason for this assumption was that the pupil on the symptomatic side might be clinically slightly smaller than the other. In three of 11 patients studied by us there was a tendency to drooping of the eyelid on the symptomatic side during periods of severe attacks. In the patient studied in most detail (the patient with the marked ability to precipitate attacks), the tendency to a drooping upper eyelid was not much more pronounced during attack than between attacks. In another patient observed during multiple spontaneously occurring attacks, the drooping of the eyelid was combined with a rather clear upper eyelid oedema, the ptosis probably being secondary to this. Forehead sweating is dealt with in detail elsewhere (see Sweating on the Forehead). Suffice it to say in this context that there does not seem to be any anhidrosis in CPH. The facial temperature was

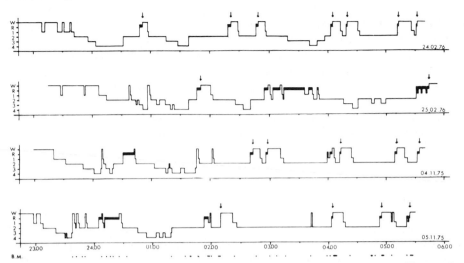

Figure 4.19 Four 1-night polygraphic sleep profiles in the same patient. The vertical axis indicates the sleep stages. The arrows indicate onset of headache attacks. BM, Body movements. Note the different tendency to attacks early and late during the night in this patient (patient with a marked ability to precipitate attacks): midnight–2 a.m., two attacks; 4–6 a.m., 11 attacks. (From Kayed *et al.* (1978). Courtesy of *Sleep*.)

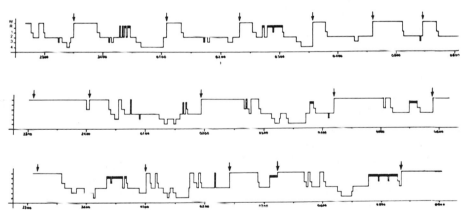

Figure 4.20 Polysomnographic sleep profiles in two female chronic paroxysmal hemicrania patients (6 and 10 attacks, respectively). Note that, although the attacks in the upper tracing appear rather regularly, the interval between attacks varies considerably (patient 1, Sjaastad and Dale, 1976). (From Kayed and Sjaastad, unpublished observations.)

paid heed to by Horner (1869), and he ascribed the facial temperature increase on the symptomatic side to an underlying vasodilatation. Corneal temperature has been measured between attacks of CPH (see elsewhere), and an asymmetry has been found with the higher temperature being on the symptomatic side. This is *per se* consistent with Horner's syndrome, but may certainly be due to other underlying mechanisms as well (e.g. liberation of vasoactive peptides). Drummond (1985) described a forehead temperature asymmetry in one case, the symptomatic side being the warmer one; the asymmetry increased during attacks. Sjaastad *et al.* (1986) did not always find this pattern (see Corneal and Forehead Temperature).

Light reflexes, hydroxyamphetamine, and phenylephrine tests were carried out using a binocular, infra-red television pupillometer (Whittaker Corp.); with this instrument events can be monitored in true time; the instrument has a resolution power of 0.05 mm. Pupillometry during the basal condition and during attacks ($n = 2$) showed a slight tendency to miosis on the symptomatic side (Sjaastad *et al.*, 1979; Smith, Smith and Sjaastad, 1979, unpublished data). Drummond (1985) found a slight miosis on the symptomatic side during attack ($n = 1$). Later on, de Souza Carvalho *et al.* (1988) carried out pharmacopupillometry in six patients, and obtained normal and borderline results in all.

There are thus no definite signs of a Horner's syndrome, not even a latent one, in CPH, despite the fact that several of the solitary factors making up a Horner's syndrome occasionally seem to exist: a miosis, a tendency to a drooping eyelid (oedema), and vasodilatation.

DYNAMIC TONOMETRY

Dynamic tonometry (Hørven, 1968) was originally carried out in two patients during and between attacks (Sjaastad and Dale, 1976). Later (Hørven *et al.*, 1989), we studied a total of seven patients (for details of the technique, see Cluster Headache).

Intraocular pressure

During the pain-free interval, the average intraocular pressure (IOP) was 15.2 and 14.7 mmHg on the symptomatic and non-symptomatic sides, respectively, versus a mean control value of 14.4 ± 2.38 (mean $\pm$ SD) mmHg (Hørven *et al.*, 1989). The average IOP was markedly increased on the symptomatic side during pain attacks, i.e. 19.4 mmHg, both when compared to the pre-attack level and when compared with the non-symptomatic side during attack, i.e. 17.3 mmHg. There was thus a clear-cut, but less marked increment in IOP on the non-symptomatic side during attack. Due to the frequency of attacks, eye tension could be recorded both before and just after onset of pain in two of the patients. The time between headache onset and IOP measurement was much less than 1 min (20–30 s or less) (Broch *et al.*, 1970; Sjaastad *et al.*, 1977). The results obtained for the patient with the pronounced ability to precipitate attacks are shown in Figure 4.21. A marked rise in IOP was also observed in the other case, amounting to 5–6 mmHg on the symptomatic and 2.5–3 mmHg on the non-symptomatic side (Table 4.14).

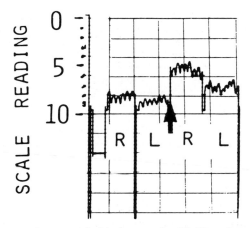

Figure 4.21 Eye tension recorded before and *c.* 20–30 s after onset of pain (arrow) in a chronic paroxysmal hemicrania patient with attacks on the right side. R, Right eye; L, left eye. A right-sided eye tension increase from 8 to 5.5 is observed (5.5 g plunger load), which corresponds to an increase in intraocular pressure of 10.2–15.9 mmHg. (From Hørven and Sjaastad (1977). Courtesy of *Acta Ophthalmologica* (*Copenhagen*).)

Table 4.14 Intraocular pressure (mmHg)[a] before and <0.5–1 min after onset of attack in chronic paroxysmal hemicrania[b]

Case No.	Symptomatic side			Non-symptomatic side		
	Pain free	Pain	Difference	Pain free	Pain	Difference
1a	12.2	17.3	5.1	13.4	15.9	2.5
1b	11.2	17.3	6.1	12.2	17.3	5.1
3	10.2	15.9	5.7	9.4	12.2	2.8

[a]Friedenwald's 1955 converting table (Friedenwald, 1957).
[b]From Sjaastad *et al.* (1977). Courtesy of the Biomedical Press.

In order to create an increment in IOP of 5–6 mmHg, an increase of about 12 mm³ in intraocular volume is necessary (Hørven, 1970a). Normally, approximately 3 mm³ aqueous humour is formed per minute, and a similar amount of fluid leaves the eye per minute. A blocked drainage of aqueous humour can, therefore, *not* explain this abnormality. The formation of aqueous humour during attack would have to be drastically increased to account for these findings. Changes in aqueous humour turnover can thus hardly be the mechanism underlying the observed increment in IOP. Measurable changes in ocular rigidity were not found. Since the changes in IOP were so marked and appeared so rapidly, the most likely explanation for this sudden increment in IOP during the attack is an acute vasodilatation with a corresponding, increased volume of the intraocular vascular bed.

Table 4.15 Pupillary dilatation on tyramine (ocular) application and attack-induced increase in intraocular pressure (IOP): comparison of chronic paroxysmal hemicrania (CPH) and 'hemicrania continua' (symptomatic side)

	Reduced tyramine response	IOP increase
CPH	−	+
Hemicrania continua	±	−

The increase in IOP during attack may be of differential diagnostic significance versus hemicrania continua (Table 4.15).

In CPH patients, the IOP seems to decrease slowly with time after having reached a peak in the early phase of the attack, until a more or less equilibrium situation is established between the two sides after 15–20 min (*pari passu* with the decrease of pain?). Sometimes, after an attack, the IOP on the symptomatic side might even be lower than that on the other side. Thus, an effect similar to that seen during tonography occurs, although the initial IOP rise is not induced by an external force such as the tonometer weight, but by an intrinsic factor in the eye. The level of IOP induced during the attack is not so high that it seems likely that the pain is caused by it. On the other hand, such a possibility is hard to refute for the following reason: the decisive factor may not so much be the *absolute* level of the pressure. The very abruptness of the attack, i.e. the speed with which the pressure is augmented (without possibilities for immediate adjustments) may be of major importance for the creation of pain.

Corneal indentation pulse amplitudes

For definitions of and techniques used to measure corneal indentation pulse (CIP) amplitudes, see Cluster Headache. The mean CIP amplitudes were of equal height on the symptomatic and non-symptomatic sides outside attacks, i.e. 33.4 and 31.3 μm, respectively (mean control value = 30.6 ± 9.8 (mean $\pm$ SD)). CIP amplitudes increased clearly during attacks ($n = 7$), most markedly so on the symptomatic side, but also on the non-symptomatic side, the mean values being 54.6 and 33.4, respectively (Hørven *et al.*, 1989). The increase was even more marked in our first patient (Table 4.16). Generally, CIP amplitudes during attack tended to be >50% larger in CPH than in cluster headache (Hørven *et al.*, 1989) (Figure 4.22). Thus, the CIP amplitude pattern during attack seems to some extent to distinguish CPH patients from cluster headache patients, the mean values on the symptomatic side differing significantly ($p < 0.01$). The larger CIP amplitudes in CPH both between and during attacks suggest either a larger intraocular vascular bed in these patients or a true difference in the pathogenesis of these disorders.

With regard to the volume change (ΔV) per minute, a significant side difference was present during attacks with the larger values being on the

Table 4.16 Mean attack-induced increment in CIP amplitudes as a percentage of the amplitude between attacks (taken as 100% for each eye)[a]

Patient No.	No. of attacks observed	CIP on non-symptomatic side (%)	No. of attacks observed	CIP on symptomatic side (%)
1	4	130	4	200
2	2	111	2	132

[a]From Sjaastad and Dale (1976). Courtesy of *Acta Neurologica Scandinavica (Copenhagen)*.

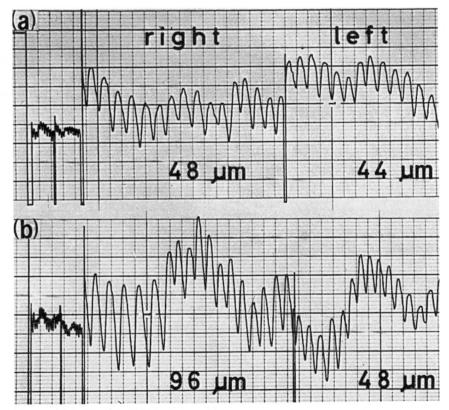

Figure 4.22 Dynamic tonometry results obtained (a) just prior to and (b) 11 min later during pain attack in a patient with chronic paroxysmal hemicrania. Note the marked attack-induced increment in CIP amplitudes from 48 to 96 μm on the symptomatic (i.e. right) side. Low and medium sensitivity was employed for registration. (From Broch *et al*. (1970). Courtesy of *Headache*.)

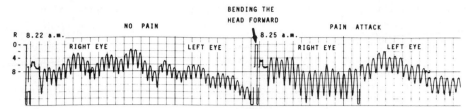

Figure 4.23   Corneal indentation pulse (CIP) measured during a moderate precipitated right-sided attack in chronic paroxysmal hemicrania. Symptomatic side increase in CIP amplitudes (ΔV per minute, before attack 246, during attack 361) and intraocular pressure, i.e. from 17.3 to 18.9 mmHg. (From Sjaastad *et al.* (1979). Courtesy of *Headache*.)

affected side (Figure 4.23), i.e. 380 and 275 mm^3 min^{-1}, respectively, versus 222 and 206 mm^3 min^{-1}, respectively, in the attack-free period (mean control value 203 ± 53.2 (mean $\pm$ SD) mm^3 min^{-1}). The results obtained between attacks were significantly lower than those obtained during attacks, the difference being most pronounced on the symptomatic side (Hørven *et al.*, 1989). If bradycardia should occur, the CIP amplitudes would increase correspondingly, the product (CIP amplitudes × pulse rate) being fairly constant (Hørven and Gjønnæss, 1974). The increased ΔV per minute during the pain attack clearly demonstrates that the CIP amplitude increment by far outweighs the influence of the bradycardia effect during attacks. The increment in amplitudes thus cannot be explained on the basis of bradycardia alone, a factor which, moreover, should affect the non-symptomatic to the same degree as the symptomatic side.

Atropine (0.6 mg) was administered subcutaneously to the patient with the marked ability to precipitate attacks. There was no tendency to diminished, attack-related CIP amplitudes on the symptomatic side as a consequence of atropine medication (on the contrary, there was increased asymmetry, if anything: the mean non-symptomatic/symptomatic side CIP amplitudes before and during attacks (given as ΔV min^{-1}) were 270/325 before atropine versus 264/372 after atropine (Sjaastad *et al.*, 1979)). That there really was a systemic effect of atropine at the time of attack precipitation was made likely by the fact that attack-related lacrimation and nasal secretion were clearly diminished.

It is emphasized that the *phase* during which these parameters are measured may be of decisive importance for the magnitude of the pathological findings. If the pain is fading away and the attack is about to stop, a situation for assessing the abnormal findings may no longer exist. If measurements are carried out in the later part of the attack, therefore, the findings may not be representative of the pathology characteristic of the attack. These parameters should be assessed when the pain is maximal or close to maximal. Intraocular pressure (IOP) and CIP have invariably been found to increase during attacks in our cases. Increased IOP and CIP amplitudes, therefore, seem to be characteristic, integral features of CPH attack. Whether there are exceptions to the rule of increased values during attacks, is not known. We suspect that if the pain is maximal, increased values will be obtained. Milder cases of CPH, the existence of which we have become aware of more recently, may not invariably have augmented IOP/CIP values during attack. IOP and CIP may also be valuable parameters in understanding the pathogenesis of CPH (see Pathogenesis).

CORNEAL AND FOREHEAD TEMPERATURE

The *corneal temperature* was recorded using a specially constructed thermometer probe (Hørven and Larsen, 1975) and a Brush Mark 220 recorder. (For details of the technique see Cluster Headache).

Corneal temperature was measured in two of our early patients (Hørven and Sjaastad, 1977). Contrary to what was found in ordinary cluster headache, a raised corneal temperature was observed on the symptomatic side also in the headache-free phase in CPH (mean symptomatic side 34.6°C; non-symptomatic side 33.9, as compared with a control average of 33.7) (Figure 4.24). This side difference increased two-fold during attack, and averaged 1.55°C (Table 4.17). The temperature on the non-symptomatic side did not increase during attacks. For interpretation of these data, see Cluster Headache.

Cutaneous temperature registrations have also been performed by using fast transducers during and between attacks of CPH (for details regarding the recording equipment and technique, see Sjaastad *et al.* (1986), and also the corresponding section under Episodic Cluster Headache). The points where temperature was measured correspond to the points in the forehead measured during sweat estimations (see Cluster Headache).

Sjaastad *et al.* (1986) found that the forehead temperature might show various patterns during precipitated attacks: there may be a dissociation

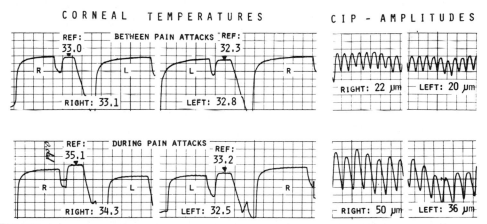

Figure 4.24 Increase in corneal temperature (+°C) and corneal indentation pulse (CIP) amplitudes during a pain attack of chronic paroxysmal hemicrania (right side). REF, reference temperature. (From Hørven and Sjaastad (1977). Courtesy of *Acta Ophthalmologica (Copenhagen)*.)

Table 4.17   Corneal temperature (in +°C) in chronic paroxysmal hemicrania

	Between attacks			During attacks		
Patient	Symptomatic side	Non-symptomatic side	Difference	Symptomatic side	Non-symptomatic side	Difference
1	34.5	33.8	0.7	35.4	33.4	2.0
2	34.75	34.0	0.75	35.0	33.9	1.1
Average	34.63	33.9	0.73	35.2	33.65	1.55

between forehead sweating and temperature, or there may be a synchronous increase in both (number of patients studied = 2). No definite temperature increment was found prior to sweat increase in this type of experiment.

There may be an acute intraocular vasodilatation during attack. The most likely explanation for the observed rise in corneal temperature during attacks of CPH seems to be an increased ocular pulsatile blood flow through the eye; this tends to reduce the temperature gradient between the posterior and anterior parts of the eye. The frequency of attacks in CPH may possibly explain the fact that the cornea is warmer on the symptomatic side, even between attacks (Table 4.17). The discrepancy between CPH and cluster headache in this respect may be due to a difference in the duration of the attack-free periods. In cluster headache, there may be 12 hours or more between attacks.

SWEATING ON THE FOREHEAD

Evaporimeter measurements of forehead sweating (in $g\,m^{-2}\,h^{-1}$) during and between attacks were carried out in six female patients, the patients serving as their own controls (Sjaastad *et al.*, 1983a). The results obtained were also compared with those in a control group ($n = 5$). For details of the equipment and techniques used, the reader is referred to the corresponding section under Cluster Headache.

Increased sweating on the symptomatic side during attacks was observed in two patients, both when compared with the non-symptomatic side during attack and when compared with the symptomatic side outside of attack (Figure 4.25). In addition, the levels were increased compared to sweating in controls. Three patients, two of whom only had mild attacks at the time of study, showed slightly higher sweat values on the symptomatic than on the non-symptomatic side, but generally within the control range. In one patient, the obtained values were within the normal range. These results show that increased, attack-related forehead sweating does not seem to be a necessary condition for CPH.

In the patient in whom attacks can readily be precipitated by head flexion and by pressure against certain circumscribed points in the neck (mechanically precipitated attacks (Sjaastad *et al.*, 1979)), sweating was invariably increased

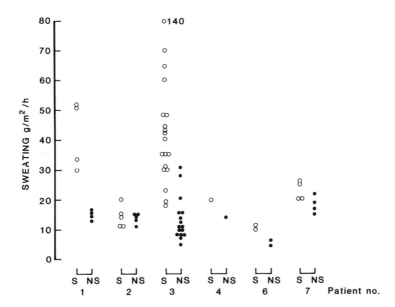

Figure 4.25 Sweating during spontaneous chronic paroxysmal hemicrania attacks on symptomatic (S) and non-symptomatic (NS) sides (middle part of the forehead, position I). Pain severity and the interval between onset of attack and measurement have not been taken into consideration. (From Sjaastad *et al.* (1983a). Courtesy of *Cephalalgia*.)

on the symptomatic side during severe attacks (Figure 4.26). Sweating was also increased on the non-symptomatic side in approximately 50% of the attacks in this patient, but generally to a lesser extent than on the symptomatic side. If no pain ensued during precipitation manoeuvres, sweating would not increase. Sometimes, a transitory pain (lasting a few seconds), but no real attack, followed attempted precipitation, and only occasionally was the pain then associated with a very moderate sweat increase. If a real attack ensued, marked sweating (as well as lacrimation) appeared 15–30 s ahead of the pain (Figures 4.6 and 4.27). The level of sweating attained during the first seconds of head flexion in the patient in whom attacks can easily be precipitated thus gives a good indication as to whether or not the pain part of the attack is going to follow suit. The level of sweating thus has *predictive value* in such experiments. There is a clear relationship between the autonomic (e.g. the sweating) activation and pain generation, since with all real attacks sweating was pronounced. A schematic drawing of this situation is shown in Figure 4.28.

Furthermore, there is a temporal dichotomy between pain and these autonomic phenomena in these experiments, the sweating appearing far ahead of the pain. The sweating is accordingly not due to the pain. The needlessness of peripheral autonomic phenomena for the development of the pain part of the attack is also demonstrated by the atropine experiments ($n = 5$). As also dealt with elsewhere (see The Atropine Effect on Sweating, Lacrimation and Nasal

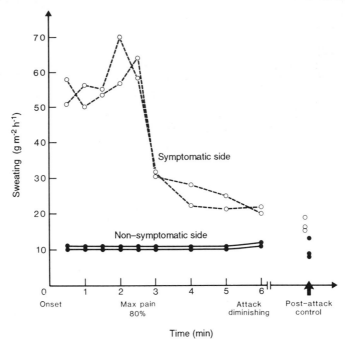

Figure 4.26 Two precipitated attacks (by bending the head forwards) in a chronic paroxysmal hemicrania patient (female, 33 years old). Note the preponderance of sweating in the medial part of the forehead on the symptomatic side. Sweating is maximal at 2–3 min after pain onset. (From Sjaastad *et al.* (1983a). Courtesy of *Cephalalgia*.)

Secretion), systemically administered atropine more or less abolished sweating, lacrimation and nasal secretion, but was of no importance in the development of the pain part of the attack (Sjaastad *et al.*, 1986). However, the corneal indentation pulse amplitudes seemed not to be influenced by systematically administered atropine (Sjaastad *et al.*, 1979).

   In an attempt to disentangle the mechanism underlying the increased sweating occasionally seen in CPH, forehead sweating was measured after various provocation tests, i.e. body heating, exercise, and subcutaneous pilocarpine administration (0.1 mg/kg body weight) in eight patients (Saunte *et al.*, 1983a). There was no definite deficit in heat-induced or exercise-induced sweating on the symptomatic side of the forehead; the right/left and symptomatic/non-symptomatic side ratios in controls and patients, respectively, were around 1.0 (Figure 4.29). Pilocarpine did not lead to any marked, initial, temporary predominance of sweating on the symptomatic side either (Figure 4.30). Thus, the hypersensitivity phenomena which could explain the ipsilateral forehead sweating increase during attacks were not found. This is contrary to the findings in cluster headache. The localized sweating increase observed in the forehead during attacks in some patients with CPH does thus not seem to be due to a sympathetic deficit with superimposed hypersensitivity

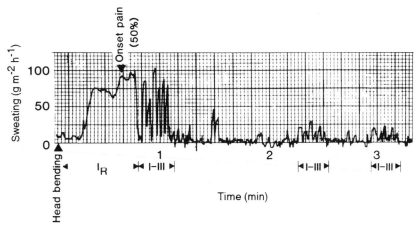

Figure 4.27 Temporal inter-relationship between forehead sweating and pain in a chronic paroxysmal hemicrania patient (female, 33 years old). IR, Site I on right (symptomatic) side; sites I–III (see Figure 2.30). Attack induced by head flexion. Note that the forehead sweating starts clearly before the onset of pain. The pain continued for several minutes. Lacrimation and conjunctival injection may occur simultaneously with the sweating in such experiments. (From Sjaastad *et al.* (1986). Courtesy of *Cephalalgia*.)

phenomena. The increased sweating may possibly be a result of a direct sympathetic stimulation. Admittedly, many other possibilities exist, due to the putative complex innervation of the sweat glands (see Pathogenesis).

The evaporimetric (and pupillometric) characteristics of headache patients may, in addition to being of pathophysiological significance, aid in distinguishing between the different unilateral headaches (Table 4.18).

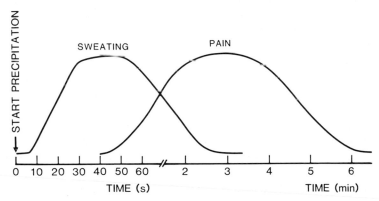

Figure 4.28 The sequence of sweating and pain in a chronic paroxysmal hemicrania attack precipitated by head flexion. (From Sjaastad *et al.* (1986). Courtesy of *Cephalalgia*.)

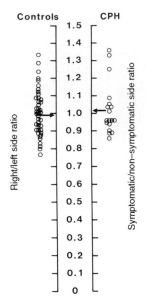

Figure 4.29 Heat-induced forehead sweating (weighted values, position I; see Figure 2.30) in chronic paroxysmal hemicrania (CPH) patients (seven patients, 18 tests) and controls (*n* = 42). Arrows indicate mean values. (From Saunte *et al.* (1983a). Courtesy of *Cephalalgia*.)

Table 4.18 Forehead sweating and pupillometry in various types of unilateral headache

	Symptomatic/non-symptomatic side ratio		
	Cluster headache	Chronic paroxysmal hemicrania	Cervicogenic headache[a]
Forehead sweating			
Attack	>1	(≥)1	=1
Heating	<1	(≤)1	=1
Pilocarpine	>1	(≥)1	=1
Pupillometry			
Basal	≤1	≤1	=1
Indirectly acting sympathicomimetic agents	<1	=1	=1
Directly acting sympathicomimetic agents	>1	=1	=1

[a]Fredriksen *et al.* (1988).

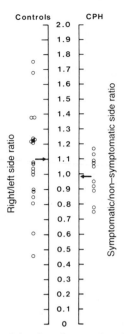

Figure 4.30 Pilocarpine-induced forehead sweating (weighted values, position I; see Figure 2.30) in chronic paroxysmal hemicrania patients (seven patients, 10 tests) and controls ($n = 20$). Arrows indicate mean values. (From Saunte *et al.* (1983a). Courtesy of *Cephalalgia*.)

HEAT-INDUCED 'SWEATING TIME'

The time it takes for forehead sweating to reach a level of $>75 \, \text{g m}^{-2} \text{h}^{-1}$ continuously for >2 min upon body heating was measured in eight patients (18 tests), not treated with indomethacin at the time (Stocchi *et al.*, unpublished data). In healthy controls (11 females and 11 males), the mean delay was 2.1 min in males and 12.3 min in females. In CPH (only females) the mean delay was 38 min; the corresponding figure in cluster headache ($n = 27$) was 26 min.

It thus seems that it takes longer to provoke sweating by heating in CPH patients than in controls. Some CPH patients complain that they 'never sweat'. A piece of additional information evolved from these experiments: in a couple of cases, it took a long time to reach the $75 \, \text{g m}^{-2} \text{h}^{-1}$ level and there was a marked fluctuation in sweating after this level had been reached. This tendency was most marked in the patient with the pronounced ability to precipitate attacks mechanically (see Figure 4.31). In controls, there are only small 'dips' in the curve. Heating studies should, therefore, be conducted over an extended period of time and not just for a couple of minutes. If this tendency is confirmed in larger series, it may indicate that the feed-back system for forehead sweating in these cases does not operate properly.

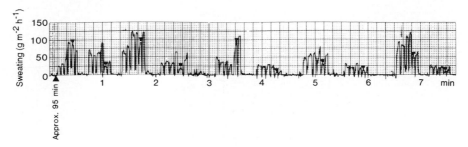

Figure 4.31   Irregularity of forehead sweating in chronic paroxysmal hemicrania. Heat-induced sweating (in g/m²/h). (▼) The point on the forehead directly above the external canthus on the symptomatic side (position III, see Figure 2.30). Sweating at this site is followed for approximately 7 min from the 95th minute of the test onwards. Note the marked fluctuation in sweating at this point with five 'dips' on the curve. (From Sjaastad *et al.* (1986). Courtesy of *Cephalalgia*.)

QUANTIFICATION OF VARIOUS AUTONOMIC FUNCTIONS

Various autonomic functions in CPH have been quantified by Saunte (1983, 1984c). Lacrimation and nasal secretion were quantified using Schirmer's test tapes, and salivation was quantified using a special suction technique. It was documented that the saliva collected from the two sides of the mouth floor truly reflects the combined secretion of the submandibular and sublingual glands on the two sides separately (see also Cluster Headache).

Lacrimation

Lacrimation during the basal condition ($n = 7$) did not differ appreciably from that in controls, and there was no definite asymmetry. During the attack, lacrimation increased clearly on both sides in all patients (eight attacks in four patients), but predominantly on the symptomatic side, so that the mean symptomatic/non-symptomatic side ratio during attacks was 2.7. The mean attack-induced/basal secretion ratio on the non-symptomatic side was 1.6. Atropine administration (0.6–1.5 mg) abolished attack-related lacrimation. This indicates that transmission mediated by acetylcholine may play a role in the lacrimation. Pilocarpine stimulation (10 experiments in seven patients) increased the secretion on the symptomatic side relatively more than on the non-symptomatic side, but the level on the symptomatic side did not quite reach the attack level (Figure 4.32).

Nasal secretion

Nasal secretion during the basal condition (10 studies in seven patients) probably did not differ from that of controls, and the secretion was symmetrical

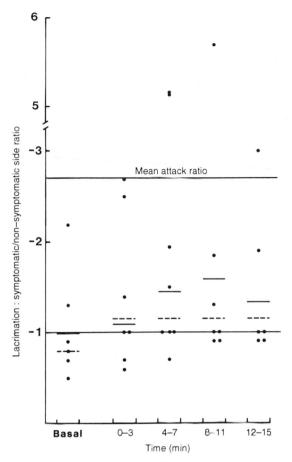

Figure 4.32 Lacrimation in the basal condition and as provoked by pilocarpine (0.1 mg/kg body weight, subcutaneously) in chronic paroxysmal hemicrania. Pilocarpine was administered to seven patients. (————) The unweighted mean ratio for each time interval. One patient had an exceptionally high ratio during attacks (n = 5), i.e. 5.5. (– – – –) The mean ratio for the remaining patients (except patient 7) during the pilocarpine test. The mean ratio during attack (four patients, eight attacks) is also indicated (mean ratio 2.69). (From Saunte (1984b). Courtesy of *Cephalalgia*.)

(Figure 4.33). During attacks (nine studies in three patients), a *bilateral* increase in secretion was demonstrated, but it was most marked on the symptomatic side. The mean symptomatic/non-symptomatic side ratio during attack was 1.3 (Figures 4.33 and 4.34). The mean ratio of attack to basal secretion was 1.9 on the non-symptomatic side. Parenteral atropine administration seemed to reduce nasal secretion during attacks. Pilocarpine stimulation (10 tests in seven patients) produced a clear increase (more than two-fold) in nasal secretion, but

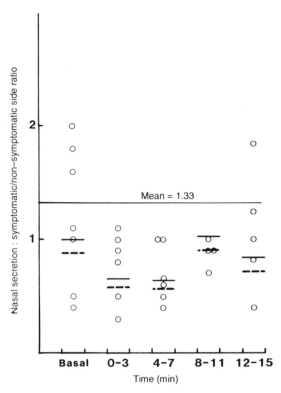

Figure 4.33 Nasal secretion in the basal condition and provoked by pilocarpine (0.1 mg/kg body weight, subcutaneously) in chronic paroxysmal hemicrania (seven patients, nine attacks). Patient No. 7 invariably had the highest ratios and for that reason, the ratios also were calculated excluding this patient: (———) means including patient 7; (– – – –) means excluding patient 7. The mean symptomatic/non-symptomatic side ratio during attacks was 1.33. (From Saunte (1984b). Courtesy of *Cephalalgia*.)

did not produce a side preponderance (Figure 4.33). One patient studied both during and outside attacks showed no cell increase or preferential increase in basophils in nasal smear preparations (Selmaj and Pruszcynski, 1984).

Salivation

Salivation (11 tests in seven patients) was low during the basal state, i.e. mean 0.13 ml min^{-1}, which is within the control range, and it was fairly even on the two sides. During attack (nine tests in four patients) the quantities were generally below the sensitivity of the method. Pilocarpine (11 tests in seven patients), however, produced profuse salivation (increased by a factor of 10.8 on the non-symptomatic side) and of a similar magnitude in patients and controls (Figure 4.35), and there was no significant side asymmetry.

Pilocarpine thus increased all three types of secretion and sweating in CPH, but particularly salivation and sweating, as was the case in control individuals.

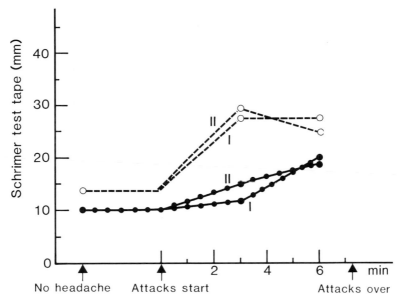

Figure 4.34 Nasal secretion in two chronic paroxysmal hemicrania attacks (approximately 50% of maximum pain) provoked by bending neck forwards (female patient, 33 years old). Note the moderate increment in nasal secretion on the non-symptomatic side. (○) Symptomatic side; (●) non-symptomatic side). (Courtesy of C. Saunte, unpublished data.)

The pattern as far as salivation is concerned differs completely from that during attack (where no increase in salivation is found). This suggests that during attacks the salivary glands are not under the influence of the mechanisms which underlie pilocarpine-mediated secretion. In other words, the mechanism underlying the autonomic manifestations during attacks of CPH seem to differ fundamentally from a pure parasympathetic stimulation pattern, despite the fact that some functions, such as lacrimation and nasal secretion, are massively influenced by atropine during attacks of CPH. It should be noted at this point that the action of pilocarpine may differ from that of the parasympathetic transmitter.

The tendency to inverse patterns as for salivation during attack and pilocarpine stimulation may possibly fit with the idea that CPH attacks are associated with increased sympathetic activity. Sympathetic stimulation in man is known to be associated with dryness of the mouth. Admittedly, there may be other conceivable explanations for the observed phenomena. The innervation/transmitter patterns of these glands may be much more complex than is presently known.

The atropine effect on sweating, lacrimation and nasal secretion was examined in other experiments, the dosage of atropine varying from 0.6 to 1.5 mg, subcutaneously. Attacks were precipitated >0.5 h after atropine administration (on the patient with the marked ability to precipitate attacks mechanically;

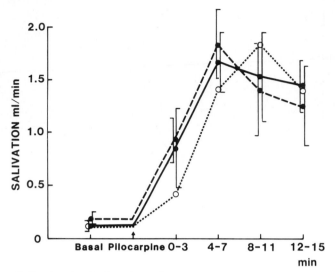

Figure 4.35   Salivation in the basal condition and provoked by pilocarpine (0.1 mg/kg body weight, subcutaneously) in seven chronic paroxysmal hemicrania patients outside attack, and 20 controls. Each point represents the mean ± 1 SD. (●——●) Patients, symptomatic side; (●–––●) patients, non-symptomatic side; (○–––○) controls, mean of left and right sides. (From Saunte (1984b). Courtesy of *Cephalalgia*.)

number of studies = 5). In general, there was no increase in sweating during attack in the presence of atropine, whereas this patient in the absence of atropine usually showed a clear increase in sweating, mostly on the symptomatic side (Sjaastad *et al.*, 1986). Likewise, the usual attack-related increment in lacrimation and nasal secretion, which mostly occurred on the symptomatic side, did not occur in the presence of atropine. We, therefore, seem to be faced with two different patterns in such experiments: (1) the corneal indentation pulse amplitudes which were uninfluenced by atropine; (2) lacrimation/ rhinorrhoea/sweating, where a clear reduction in secretion was found.

AUDIOLOGICAL PARAMETERS

During attacks of headache, some patients reported a hearing loss and a sensation of increased pressure in the ear on the symptomatic side, whereas the hearing in the contralateral ear was experienced as normal. Furthermore, during vocalization, three of six patients had a 'closed box' sensation on the symptomatic side (Sjaastad *et al.*, 1977, 1980). Some patients experienced hypersensitivity to sounds but no change in hearing during headache.

Audiological parameters were studied in three of our first patients (Sjaastad *et al.*, 1977). The hearing threshold was measured during and after attacks in a soundproof chamber, using a calibrated (International Organization of Standardization standard) pure-tone audiometer. The threshold level for the acoustic stapedius reflex was tested as was the middle-ear function, using

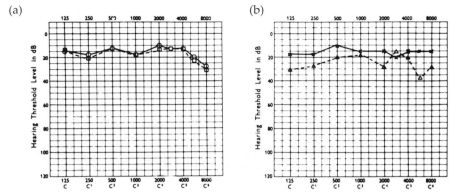

Figure 4.36 Hearing thresholds (means of four measurements) in a chronic paroxysmal hemicrania patient (female, 61 years old) during and outside left-sided attacks. (a) Right ear: (□) during attack; (○) outside attack. (b) Left ear: (▲) during attack; (×) outside attack. (From Sjaastad *et al.* (1977). Courtesy of the Biomedical Press.)

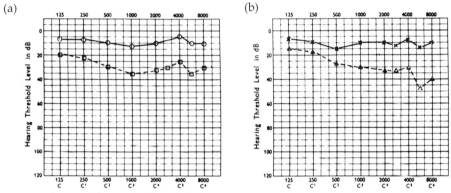

Figure 4.37 Hearing thresholds (arithmetic means of five measurements) before and after treatment with indomethacin in a chronic paroxysmal hemicrania patient (female, 62 years old). Indomethacin eliminated the headache. (a) Right ear: (○) during treatment; (□) before treatment. (b) Left ear: (×) during treatment; (△) before treatment. (From Sjaastad *et al.* (1977). Courtesy of the Biomedical Press.)

tympanometry and observation of impedance changes elicited by tactile and acoustic stimulation (Djupesland, 1975). The reflex test was used to differentiate between sensorial hearing loss of cochlear and retrocochlear type. In our first patient, the hearing threshold level was also measured before and after treatment with indomethacin.

In two patients, who had the feeling of an altered hearing threshold during attack, a moderate hearing loss was measured on the symptomatic side during attack, whereas no change in the hearing threshold was observed on the non-symptomatic side (Figure 4.36). In the third patient, with no subjective symptoms, no such difference was found. Indomethacin therapy in the one patient tested seemed to improve the hearing bilaterally (Figure 4.37). The unilaterality of the transient pathological phenomena makes it unlikely that they can be ascribed to reduced vigilance during severe pain attacks.

Middle-ear pressure and middle-ear function were invariably normal both during and after attacks, as were the acoustic stapedius reflex thresholds. This suggests that the demonstrated sensorineural hearing loss is of cochlear type. Hypersensitivity to sounds and the 'closed box' sensation also indicate a transitory cochlear dysfunction.

The mechanism behind the sensorineural hearing loss in two of our three patients is unknown. Since our findings indicate that the hearing loss is both temporary and cochlear in origin, the hearing loss may possibly be produced by cochlear vascular changes similar to those observed in the eye during attacks.

HEART-RHYTHM DISTURBANCES

In the early days of the CPH story, it was noted that patients could get multiple extrasystoles during attack (Sjaastad and Dale, 1976; Christoffersen, 1979) and also bradycardia (Hørven and Sjaastad, 1977).

Russell and Storstein (1984) used continuous electrocardiogram recording to monitor 105 spontaneously occurring attacks in five female patients, who had not taken any medication for at least 24 h prior to study. The patients triggered a marking system when they got the attacks and when the attacks ended, and noted the severity of the pain on a diary card. Heart rhythm was calculated at regular intervals prior to, during, and after attacks. There was a slight increase in heart rate (± 2.5 beats min^{-1}) at the onset of attacks ($p < 0.05$), a change seemingly not dependent upon the severity of attack or upon the absolute level of heart rate prior to attack. A slight decrease in pulse rate then frequently occurred at the height of attack, but this did not occur in approximately 50% of attacks. Two of the five patients developed arrhythmias during the attack: sinoatrial block with escape beats, atrial fibrillation, as well as bundle branch block. The abnormalities were most pronounced at the height of attack.

A tendency to rapid and pronounced changes in heart rate was a conspicuous finding. These spectacular changes did not occur at any set period of attack, so the occurrence was completely unpredictable. The pattern in provoked attacks seemed to be the same as in spontaneously occurring attacks. The pulse rate pattern in CPH differs significantly from that in cluster headache, in that the increase in pulse rate at onset is significantly higher and the subsequent fall significantly more marked in cluster headache than in CPH ($p < 0.0001$ and <0.005, respectively).

These findings are not readily understandable. Parasympathetic overactivity has been shown to induce as well as maintain auricular fibrillation (Loomis *et al.*, 1955; Burn, 1957; Alessi *et al.*, 1958). Centrally caused arrhythmias mostly seem to reflect the net sum of parasympathetic and sympathetic activity (Wallace *et al.*, 1967). In the presence of simultaneous sympathetic stimulation, parasympathetic impulses may in various ways cause instability of the predominant pacemaker region.

PNEUMOENCEPHALOGRAPHY

Pneumoencephalography has to our knowledge been carried out in only one patient, i.e. in our first patient, in whom it was carried out twice with a 7 year interval. The lateral ventricles seemed to have increased by 2–4 mm over the course of that period and were of borderline dimensions at the last examination.

COMPUTED-TOMOGRAPHY SCANS OF THE BRAIN

Computed-tomography scans have been carried out in 28 cases. No systematic changes have been found (Antonaci and Sjaastad, 1989).

NUCLEAR MAGNETIC RESONANCE SCANNING OF THE BRAIN

Two of our cases were submitted to nuclear magnetic resonance (NMR) scanning of the brain. Normal results were obtained.

X-RAY EXAMINATION OF THE CERVICAL SPINE

Such investigations were carried out in our first cases ($n = 5$) and rendered normal results except in the patient with the excessive propensity to attack precipitation, in whom a spina bifida of C_1 was detected.

ELECTROENCEPHALOGRAPHY

Electroencephalography (EEG) recordings were made in 31 cases reported in the literature; they were mostly normal. In one patient, θ activity and even focal, sharp activity as well as $6 \, s^{-1}$ positive spikes were found on the standard recording on the symptomatic side outside attacks. These changes persisted during attacks. Both hyperventilation and compression of the carotid artery on the symptomatic side produced more slow waves in this case than is usually seen (Hasan *et al.*, 1976).

CEREBRAL ANGIOGRAPHY

Cerebral angiography has been carried out in two of our patients. In one patient, it was done in a pain-free period (carotid angiography on the symptomatic side) and demonstrated a small, berry aneurysm of the medial cerebral artery on the symptomatic side. This was believed to be merely an incidental finding of no significance with regard to the attacks. This patient has been asymptomatic for more than 12 years on indomethacin, provided the dosage is adequate. In our patient with the marked ability to attack precipitation, cerebral angiography showed no localized or generalized changes in arterial diameter either in the free interval or during a moderately severe, precipitated attack. Selective carotid and vertebral artery angiographies were also carried out when the patient's head was rotated maximally to the right (i.e. symptomatic side; this usually precipitates attack), but no attack ensued at this time. There was normal vertebral artery contrast filling on this occasion. The right carotid artery showed an irregular ('stationary-wave' like) appearance during rotation to the right, which was absent during the following contrast injection (carried out without turning the head). The significance of this finding is uncertain. It is noteworthy, however, that similar findings have been made in Tolosa–Hunt syndrome (Kettler and Martin, 1975). On a worldwide basis (Antonaci and Sjaastad, 1989), angiography has been performed in 16 cases. In two cases, small aneurysms were detected: in addition to our own case, there was one case showing a small anterior communicating artery aneurysm.

TESTOSTERONE

Serum testosterone has partly been found to be reduced in cluster headache. It was, therefore, natural to estimate levels of testosterone in CPH as well. Testosterone was measured during the attack in four female CPH patients. The values varied from 70–90 ng/100 ml (mean 80 ng/100 ml), and were slightly higher than in four females with various headaches other than cluster head-ache (mean 67.5 ng/100 ml) (Romiti *et al.*, 1983). The mean age in these two groups was 46 and 37 years, respectively. The values in the CPH group were, however, well within the normal range for females (100–50 ng/100 ml).

PSYCHOLOGICAL/PSYCHIATRIC EXAMINATIONS

Such exploration in our first two patients showed no signs of primary emotion-al disturbances. In our first patient, a verbal IQ of 105 was found; there was evidence of higher pre-morbid intelligence (Sjaastad and Dale, 1976).

FLUORESCEIN APPEARANCE TIME

Fluorescein (5 ml of 10% fluorescein sodium) was injected into the arm vein during attack in our first patient, and the time for its appearance in both eye grounds was determined accurately (Broch *et al.*, 1970). The latency was of the same order of magnitude on the two sides, i.e. 13.3 and 13.6 s, respectively. The blood velocity thus seems to be at the same level on the symptomatic and non-symptomatic sides. The changes in the eye, as demonstrated by dynamic tonometry, are rather marked. The lack of signs of changes on the symptomatic side with the fluorescein test during attack suggests, but does not prove, that *local ocular factors* underlie the ocular-attack-related changes.

THYMOXAMINE EXPERIMENTS

Thymoxamine, an α-receptor blocking agent (Turner and Sneddon, 1968), was administered locally in the palpebral cleft (0.1% solution, two drops) on both sides, in the patient who could readily precipitate attacks mechanically (Sjaastad *et al.*, 1986). Intraocular pressure was measured prior to thymoxamine administration, 30–60 min after the administration, and at various stages of precipitated attacks. Two different methods of intraocular pressure measurement were used, i.e. applanation tonometry (two different attacks) and dynamic tonometry (one attack). While a distinct intraocular pressure increment invariably accompanies the attack on the symptomatic side in this patient, no such definite pressure increase was observed during attacks after thymoxamine application (see Figure 4.38). There was no influence of thymoxamine on the pain component of the attacks.

These experiments show that the impulses leading to the attack-related increase in intraocular pressure may in some way be mediated through a stimulation of α-receptors. Of course it is also possible that the mechanism of action of thymoxamine is not as specific as claimed (e.g. Day, 1979). There may

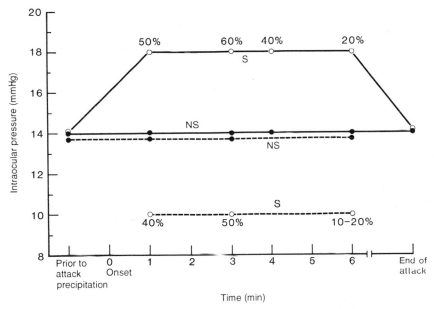

Figure 4.38 The results of applanation tonometry before and during precipitated attacks in a chronic paroxysmal hemicrania patient (female, 33 years old). (———) Attack without thymoxamine. (– – – –) Attack approximately 40 min after bilateral thymoxamine instillation into the conjunctival sac. (○) Symptomatic (S) side; (●) nonsymptomatic (NS) side. The severity of pain is given as a percentage along the time axis for both attacks. Note the lack of pressure increment on the symptomatic side after thymoxamine. A second test in the same patient showed principally the same pattern. (From Sjaastad *et al.* (1986). Courtesy of *Cephalalgia*.)

be another explanation for the lack of intraocular pressure increase during the thymoxamine experiments: thymoxamine may lead to an intraocular vasodilatation of such magnitude that, when the vasodilatory impulses associated with the attack are transmitted, the vessels cannot be dilated any further. However, the dynamic tonometry recordings made in these experiments (see Sjaastad *et al.*, 1986) do not give the impression that this is the case.

These experiments also show that the pain during CPH attacks is not caused by an increase in intraocular pressure *per se*. Another inference that can be drawn from this type of experiment is that the pain part of the attack evolves separately and independently of at least one type of autonomic phenomenon. In other words, there seems to be at least a partial dichotomy between the pain and the autonomic phenomena in CPH.

STELLATE GANGLION BLOCKADE

Bupivacain blockade was carried out in the patient who can precipitate attacks readily mechanically. Whereas this patient shows a marked increase in sweating during usual attacks, there was no or only a minimal increase in forehead sweating during precipitated attacks ($n = 2$) during the blockade. The pain part of the attack was unaffected by the procedure (Sjaastad *et al.*, 1986). This type of experiment also seems to show that there is a dichotomy between the pain and certain autonomic components of the attack. Furthermore, the fact that sweating can be more or less abolished by sympathetic blockade adds weight to the view that sweating during attacks may be caused by impulses mediated through the cervical sympathetic fibres or fibres that run together with them (although it does not render any definite evidence as to the *nature* of the *transmitter*).

ORBITAL PHLEBOGRAPHY

An intriguing new challenge is the possible connection between CPH and the Tolosa–Hunt syndrome, as proposed by Hannerz *et al.* (1987b). They described a patient with CPH in whom a supraorbital vein phlebography showed the characteristic findings of the Tolosa–Hunt syndrome (see Cluster Headache).

The authors speculate that the demonstrated venographic abnormalities underlie the headache of three different headache types: the Tolosa–Hunt syndrome (and similar cases), cluster headache, and CPH (Hannerz *et al.*, 1984, 1987a,b). It is admittedly difficult to refute this hypothesis. There may, however, possibly be other explanations for their findings. First of all, although the diagnosis in the patient in question may seem to be consistent with CPH, the case is not necessarily a straight-forward one. The patient had had ankylosing spondylitis for years and later iritis, first on one and later on the other side. The use of a drug like phenylbutazone (as a test) would, therefore, have been indicated in a case like this. The apparent superiority of steroids versus indomethacin in this patient could possibly be viewed in this light. Further-more, the most marked venographic abnormalities were observed on the non-symptomatic side. The pathogenetic significance of the phlebographic findings may, therefore, to some extent be questioned. Supraorbital venography aids in localizing the pathological process; it is probably not as sensitive in decipher-ing the nature of the various pathological processes in this topographical area. Theoretically, the underlying pathology impinging upon the vein wall and deforming the lumen may vary, e.g. processes in the bony structures, in the dura and in the vessel wall itself; and within these structures there may be various pathological processes, e.g. an inflammatory or autoimmune process and malformations. Therefore, a positive orbital phlebography in two clinical pictures like CPH and the Tolosa–Hunt syndrome does not prove that the processes involved are one and the same. There is a requirement for this test to be undertaken on a larger series of subjects.

STATUS AND FUTURE

PREVALENCE OF CHRONIC PAROXYSMAL HEMICRANIA

Chronic paroxysmal hemicrania (CPH) is, in all probability, a rare headache. The number of cases is increasing fast, to a large extent due to the propagation of the knowledge that this headache exists. However, this process is probably still only in its beginning. We presently have rather detailed information on 84 cases of CPH (Antonaci and Sjaastad, 1989). In many other cases there is only fragmentary information, mostly obtained on the basis of hearsay. In the early phase, solitary cases were published. There were case reports on the first case from such and such country; *male* cases were reported, since these were supposed to be rare. Cases in whom the disorder seemed to stop after a short course of indomethacin were also reported separately. Reports on such cases are not usually published any more. At present, information on CPH may be hidden in articles on quite different subjects (Romiti *et al.*, 1983; Watson *et al.*, 1983; Devoize *et al.*, 1986). Since some cases are not published at all, the number of publications is, therefore, not an adequate index of the real number of cases diagnosed and treated.

Some idea of the relative frequency of CPH and cluster headache may be gained from series that cover both disorders. In the series studied by Manzoni *et al.* (1983b), there were 180 cases of cluster headache, versus four cases of CPH. Our own series consists of approximately 280 cluster headache patients, and we presently have nine Norwegian CPH patients (Table 4.19). Such figures must of course be regarded with great caution at present.

In any event, the prevalence of CPH seems to be much lower than that of cluster headache. The recent awareness of CPH cases with a more moderate

Table 4.19   The relative frequency of chronic and remitting forms of cluster headache and chronic paroxysmal hemicrania (CPH) in various series

| Source | Cluster headache | | CPH | | Chronic CPH (% of cluster headache) |
	Total	Ratio of episodic to chronic form	CPH total	Ratio of remitting to chronic form	
Manzoni *et al.* (1983b)	180	8.5:1	4	0:4	2.2
Our series	280	—	9	2:7	2.5
Kudrow (personal communication, 1987)	960	5:1	9	7:2	0.2

symptomatology may to some extent modify this view. Furthermore, it may be that the prevalence of the pre-chronic stage (the 'remitting form' (Sjaastad, 1989)) is higher than what we suspect today. Some (many?) cases may be 'arrested' at that stage.

The importance of making the correct diagnosis even in such a rare disease is first and foremost due to the therapeutic alternative at hand.

RELATIVE FREQUENCY OF THE CHRONIC AND REMITTING ('PRE-CHRONIC') FORMS

In cluster headache, the prominent form, quantitatively speaking, is the episodic one, the chronic form being a rare variant; in the series studied by Manzoni *et al.* (1983b) the ratio of episodic to chronic cases was 8.5:1 (Table 4.19). In some cases an evolution from the episodic to the chronic form takes place (so-called secondary chronic cases).

The two first CPH cases that were observed belong to the *primary chronic* category (Sjaastad and Dale, 1974). The information given in 1980 (Sjaastad *et al.*, 1980) on our first case (Sjaastad and Dale, 1976) is *a posteriori* incorrect, the original information (that the headache was primary chronic in this case) being the correct one. The first described picture thus represents CPH without a pre-CPH stage, corresponding to the *primary form of chronic cluster headache* (see Table 4.20). Opposite to what was the case in ordinary cluster headache, the chronic form was thus discovered first in CPH (in 1974).

Since the chronic stage of CPH was discovered first, attention has naturally been focused mostly on this form. Unless one had tried to assume prophetic powers, it would at that time have been impossible to foresee that a non-continuous, pre-stage would antedate the continuous stage. The existence of a non-continuous pre-stage was brought to light when the case histories of the first eight cases of definite CPH were scrutinized (Sjaastad, 1979; Sjaastad *et al.*,

Table 4.20 The various stages or forms of the two varieties of cluster headache syndrome

Chronic paroxysmal hemicrania	Cluster headache
Remitting form	*Ordinary episodic form*
Non-continuous, 'non-chronic' form ('pre-CPH')	
Unremitting form	*Chronic form*
1. With previous pre-CPH stage ('evolved from the remitting form') 2. Without an antecedent, 'remitting' stage[a] (ordinary, 'original' CPH), ('unremitting from onset')	Secondary chronic form ('evolved from episodic' form) Primary chronic form ('unremitting from onset')

[a] Only form accepted by the Headache Classification Committee of the IHS (1988) (see also Table 4.3).

1980). CPH with a pre-stage, characterized by non-daily headache, corresponds to the *secondary chronic form of cluster headache* (Table 4.20).

As a result of another development, cases have for many years been diagnosed while in the non-chronic stage. Thus, Stein and Rogado (1980) described two cases with a non-continuous headache. We (Russell and Sjaastad) have followed up one patient since 1979, but have never reported the case *in extenso*, but have only alluded to it. Jensen *et al.* (1982) also reported a case, and Pelz and Merskey (1982) reported another. Furthermore, yet another possible case was reported in this early period but, unfortunately, under the designation of cluster headache (Geaney, 1983). In addition, there are several published or still unpublished cases from recent years. Kudrow *et al.* (1987) have recently added some cases. None of these cases have yet, as far as we know, reached the chronic stage. There has thus for years been an increasing awareness of the significance of the partly long-lasting, non-continuous stage in CPH (Sjaastad, 1987c); we indicated, in 1986 (Sjaastad, 1986b) that: 'The pre-chronic CPH may prove to be more frequent than we recognize', ... 'the chronic (stage) being the end stage in only a few cases'. The headache at this stage of CPH seems to correspond to the ordinary, *episodic ('cyclic') cluster headache* (Table 4.20).

It has not been proven that any of the cases diagnosed in the chronic stage had attacks with the typical autonomic findings in the non-chronic stage, nor that they responded to indomethacin in this stage.

Real *proof* that such cases belong to the CPH cycle will be at hand when a headache in this category can be demonstrated to be transformed to a chronic one. Nevertheless, existing evidence suggests that the patients detected in the chronic stage and with an antecedent, non-continuous pre-stage really have had the same disorder all the time, only with moderately different manifestations. The knowledge that many cases of CPH have been through a non-continuous pre-stage, the complete indomethacin effect in those cases that are presently diagnosed as being in the pre-stage, and the marked changes observed in the ocular autonomic variables (intraocular pressure and corneal indentation pulse amplitudes) in one of our own cases in this stage make a close relationship likely. Basal values for intraocular pressure were 12.2 mmHg on both sides in one of our patients. During attack, the corresponding values were 13.4 and 11.2 mmHg on the symptomatic and non-symptomatic sides, respectively. The corresponding corneal indentation pulse amplitudes in the basal state were 24 and 23 μm, respectively, and during attacks 56 and 38 μm.

Until recently, we have admittedly had only vague ideas about the relative frequency of the chronic and remitting forms of CPH (Table 4.19). Opposite to the case in cluster headache, the chronic stage seemed to be the dominating one, quantitatively speaking. In the series studied by Kudrow *et al.* (1987), there appears to be a relatively higher proportion of cases in the remitting (pre-continuous) stage than in other series. The ratio of remitting to chronic cases of CPH in the series of Kudrow *et al.* was 3.5 (i.e. seven and two cases, respectively). In the Norwegian series, the ratio was 0.29 (two and seven cases, respectively) (Table 4.19). Although the figures are small, this 10-fold difference is striking. This discrepancy in the relative occurrence of the two stages of CPH could be due to under-diagnosing of the remitting stage in our own series or to an under-diagnosing of the chronic variety in Kudrow's series. In order to make a rough estimation of which these under-/over-estimations could have been made, the prevalence of chronic CPH cases versus the total number of cluster headache cases can be used as an indicator. In Kudrow's series, this ratio is only approximately one tenth of the ratio in the other two series (Table 4.19). The relatively *low* prevalence of chronic CPH cases in Kudrow's material is striking.

As a matter of fact, the relative frequencies of remitting CPH and cluster headache do not seem to differ greatly between our series (i.e. two out of 280 cases; 0.7%) and Kudrow's series (i.e. seven out of 960 cases; about 0.7%). In other words, the striking difference concerns the prevalence of chronic cases. These by far insufficient epidemiological data do, however, not enable us to draw any definite conclusions as to the relative importance of the pre-continuous and continuous stages of CPH. Recently, however, we have obtained some more firm evidence for the relative frequency of the remitting and non-remitting forms.

In a recent review of known cases of CPH (Antonaci and Sjaastad, 1989), 49 of 84 cases (58%) were primary chronic cases. If the cases that have made the transition from the remitting to the chronic stage are added (18% or 22%), the group presently exhibiting a chronic pattern would be 67 cases or 80% of the known cases. Only 17 cases were known to be in the remitting stage. The ratio between the remitting and chronic stage in the entire material is, therefore, 17/67 = 0.25, which corresponds fairly well to the ratio given by us in 1987 (Sjaastad, 1987), i.e. 0.29 (Table 4.19).

As more information is accumulated, a more concrete basis for our view of the relative prevalence of the various clinical forms of CPH may be obtained. The remitting form may still be relatively under-represented at the present time because the diagnosis of this form may be relatively difficult. Some adjustments to the relative importance of the two stages of CPH may, therefore, still be necessary. At present, the chronic form is the dominating one. These observations tend to show that the term *'chronic* paroxysmal hemicrania' is justified as the name for the whole CPH group. There seem to be parallel stages of cluster headache and CPH, as depicted in Table 4.20.

THE NON-CONTINUOUS STAGE OF CPH: WHICH APPELLATION SHOULD BE USED FOR IT?

The term 'cluster headache' was coined by Kunkle *et al.* in 1952. The term is a suitable designation for a disease in which the substrate is unknown since, in an almost metaphorical way, it explains an essential feature of this disease. This term deserves to be used at least until the aetiology and pathogenesis of cluster headache are unravelled.

The first descriptions of the chronic form of cluster headache appeared later. At the time when the name 'cluster headache' was invented, the existence of a chronic form of the headache was, therefore, unknown. Because the episodic form was discovered first, the intention was to give a descriptive designation focusing the 'episodicity'. Since both a chronic and a non-chronic stage of cluster headache existed, one is bound to be faced with some difficulty. This situation could have been prevented if *non-descriptive terms* had been used. To speak of a chronic cluster headache is a contradiction in terms: How can a headache that is supposed to be intermittent ('clustering') be chronic? Particularly meaningless is the expression 'primary type of chronic cluster headache'. If the headache has never 'clustered'; why on earth use the term 'cluster headache' then? This term should, nevertheless, be kept, not only because of tradition, but because the link to cluster headache as such must be retained!

The parallelism to CPH is obvious. However, in CPH the sequence of discoveries was diametrically opposite, the chronic form being discovered first. The terminology is readily explicable on the basis of this development. The terminology is 'opposite' that of cluster headache, since in CPH a *descriptive* term was also used: the 'chronic' nature of the headache was focused on and not the 'cyclic' nature. If the 'pre-chronic stage' had been discovered first, the disorder would have been given another name; and in its turn the continuous, chronic form would have been designated 'the chronic variety of this headache'.

A weakness similar to that in cluster headache terminology has been obvious in CPH terminology, at least since 1979, when a non-continuous (non-chronic) stage in CPH was discovered (Sjaastad *et al.*, 1980). How can a headache that is 'chronic' be 'non-chronic'? This shortcoming may partly be solved by terming the pre-stage 'pre-chronic' or 'non-continuous'. The term 'pre-chronic' implies that the headache will, sooner or later, become chronic. The possibility remains, however, that the non-continuous stage may be permanent. So, there will still be inconsistencies, as in cluster headache, and these inconcistencies will have to be lived with, since a term describing temporal aspects was originally introduced.

If we believe that there is a link between the non-chronic and the chronic forms of CPH, then this should be apparent from the designations used for the two varieties. This is the core of nomenclature and classification. If these rules are not implemented, confusion will arise on the part of users. As discussed in the previous section, there is ample evidence to show that the two headaches are two facets of the same disease process.

'Cluster headache' is a term consisting of two words and, therefore, descriptive terms (adjectives) further characterizing the headache can only be added to the *whole* expression, and not to part of it. One can add 'chronic' to 'cluster headache', but one cannot add 'chronic' to only 'cluster' or to only 'headache'. 'Chronic headache' would be completely meaningless, as would 'chronic cluster', which, furthermore, would be medical slang.

The above viewpoints have a clear bearing on CPH. The complete term 'chronic paroxysmal hemicrania' consists of three words that must be compared with the two words 'cluster headache'. The complete term cannot be split up or divided, because the identity of the term is then lost. Any descriptive adjectives would have to be *attached to the entire term, and not just to part of it* (Sjaastad, 1987b). Thus, 'pre-chronic CPH' or 'pre-chronic stage of CPH', or 'non-continuous stage of CPH' or 'non-chronic paroxysmal hemicrania' would be acceptable terms from *this* point of view. Terms like 'CPH, non-chronic stage' or 'CPH, non-continuous stage or form' are more neutral and palatable. '"Episodic" paroxysmal hemicrania' (Kudrow *et al.*, 1987), however, is not acceptable, in accordance with the aforementioned criteria, because 'chronic', which is part of the term, has been deleted. The link to CPH is no longer evident from this term. The ratio between continuous and non-continuous cases of CPH seems clearly to be in favour of the former (see the preceding section). The ratio between chronic and non-continuous cases should, however, not be decisive for the nomenclature.

We will have to live with the mentioned inconsistencies in terminology, both for CPH and cluster headache, until the aetiology and pathogenesis of these headaches are known. Then, and only then, can these terms be changed; the original terms mentioned are already part of common usage, and should be retained until then. It is my feeling (Sjaastad, 1989) that the 'non-continuous' stage would be best termed the 'remitting stage'—the secondary chronic form (i.e. with a 'pre-CPH stage' would then accordingly be CPH: 'unremitting form, evolved from the remitting form' (see Table 4.20).

CHRONIC PAROXYSMAL HEMICRANIA IN OTHER RACES

Up to 1987, CPH had only been reported in Caucasians. Joubert *et al.* (1987) have described CPH in an African black, and the picture, clinically speaking, seems very much the same as in the original description.

THE SO-CALLED INDOMETHACIN-RESPONSIVE HEADACHE

This term has recently been introduced in the headache literature (Diamond *et al.*, 1982; Medina and Diamond, 1981). It seems to be an unfortunate term, and the reasons why are discussed below.

If the words of this term are analysed, they should be taken to convey two types of information.

1. The patients in this group do invariably respond to indomethacin; this ought to be a requirement—a 'must' (otherwise why 'indomethacin-responsive'?)
2. We are dealing with one type of headache and one type only ('headache'). In other words, all headache forms where indomethacin is effective are more or less identical and only represent facets or nuances in a continuum of related headaches.

It is, therefore, rather surprising when one discovers that not all patients in the described material respond to indomethacin. Furthermore, we are, in all probability, dealing with *different types of headache*, not *one* headache.

It is clear from the original source (Diamond *et al.*, 1982) that it is by no means mandatory that all patients respond to indomethacin (nine out of 54 patients did *not* respond, and only 50% responded in a complete way; moreover, 'complete' was defined by the author as 90–100% response). We, therefore, are faced with a situation where we are invited to accept that there are non-indomethacin responsive 'indomethacin-responders'. This is the actual situation. Put in this way, it is rather obvious that 'something is rotten in the state of Denmark'. To me, it seems as though, in this context, premises and findings have been mixed up, in addition to a failure to *define* 'a headache'.

There is good reason to believe that indomethacin may be effective in various, probably distinct headaches. As far as I am concerned, it is important to distinguish between a *complete* and a *partial* effect of indomethacin. The absolute effect, as observed in CPH, is a dramatic and flabbergasting event, to the extent that it seems unbelievable to both the patient and the physician. This effect is probably a *sine qua non*. Such an effect may be indicative of a specific (or rather specific) pathophysiological or metabolic aberration. Indomethacin in CPH may 'hit the nail on the head'. A partial effect, however, may be shared by many of different disorders and may not be a sufficiently sound foundation for any classification to be made. The effect that indomethacin exerts in CPH is rather specific, in that other non-steroidal anti-inflammatory drugs (NSAIDs) probably do not exert an influence near this level. Indomethacin eliminates the headache in two headache forms, i.e. in CPH and in another recently described and possibly distinct headache form 'hemicrania continua' (Sjaastad and Spierings, 1984). In other headaches with a *partial* indomethacin effect, various NSAIDs have a beneficial influence on the pain. This partial effect may be an example of a pharmaceutical approach that does not hit the nail on its head.

Indomethacin has a *partial*, beneficial influence in the 'jabs and jolts' syndrome. A moderate effect has also been observed in 'benign exertional headache' (Diamond and Medina, 1979; Mathew, 1981; Diamond, 1982). These terms may represent distinct headache entities. Indomethacin may have a *moderate* effect in some cases of cluster headache (Sicuteri, 1965; Mathew, 1981), although this observation has not been corroborated by others as far as I am aware. Even 'cervicogenic' headache is occasionally partly influenced by indomethacin and other NSAIDs.

The similarity of CPH and some of the other headache groups in the 'indomethacin responsive headache' is only superficial, the similarity possibly even consisting of one solitary feature, i.e. the response to indomethacin. A comparison between CPH and benign exertional headache thus brings out several distinguishing points. First of all, although attacks can be precipitated also in CPH, the modes of precipitation are different in these two clinical headache forms. In CPH, the precipitation mechanism is linked to movements of the neck or direct pressure on certain pressure-sensitive points in the neck, whereas in cough headache/exertional headache, the main precipitating mechanism is apparently mostly the Valsalva manoeuvre (Rooke, 1968). (In 'cervicogenic' headache' (Sjaastad *et al.*, 1983c), however, both types of precipitation mechanism occasionally seem to co-exist, so there may be a fleeting transition between these forms of precipitation). The degree of sensitivity of the sensitive structures may explain why one or the other or both mechanisms of precipitation prevail. It may, therefore, be that cervicogenic and benign exertional headaches are not widely different as far as the basic mechanisms for precipitation are concerned. The attacks in most CPH patients, however, seem to start spontaneously without being precipitated.

The type of attack that ensues may be more important in distinguishing between the two types of headache. In benign exertional headache, precipitated attacks seem to be the only ones; they are usually relatively short-lasting (seconds to minutes) — fading away after the end of the stimulus — and the headache is mostly bilateral, only approximately one-third of the cases being unilateral (see Table 4.21). The pain is usually of moderate severity (Rooke, 1968). These features seem to differ clearly from those in CPH.

Another point seems to be crucial as far as differences between these two disorders are concerned: CPH mainly seems to be a female disorder (Vincent, 1988; Antonaci and Sjaastad, 1989), whereas in exertional headache there is a

Table 4.21 A comparison of the clinical symptoms of chronic paroxysmal hemicrania and 'benign exertional headache'

	Chronic paroxysmal hemicrania	Benign exertional headache
Sex	Female preponderance	Male preponderance
Location of pain	Unilateral	Bilateral (unilateral 1/3)
Degree of pain	Severe	Moderate (usually)
Duration of pain attacks	10–30 min	A few minutes[a]
Lacrimation/rhinorrhoea	Present	None
Prognosis	Probably few cases with remission	Rather good

[a] A more long-lasting variety has also been reported.

clear male preponderance (thus, according to Rooke (1968), the male-to-female ratio is 4:1). These two headaches, therefore, seem to be distinct headaches.

Hemicrania continua (Sjaastad and Spierings, 1984; Spierings *et al.*, 1985) also may be different from CPH. The clinical appearance of the fully developed forms of these headaches differ completely. In the fullblown form of hemicrania continua there is a low-grade, totally continuous headache, with few or no autonomic accompaniments. The feeling that several hemicrania continua patients have, i.e. that there is something wrong with the eye itself, may also be important from a differential diagnostic/pathogenetic point of view. The pupillographic findings in the two headaches also seem to differ slightly (Sjaastad *et al.*, 1984c).

The discrepancy between the attack-related increase in intraocular pressure in hemicrania continua and CPH may not in itself necessarily indicate a difference in pathogenesis: a difference in the degree of abruptness of the onset of pain in the two headache types may explain this discrepancy. In hemicrania continua, the headache is low-grade and continuous, so that adaptive mechanisms may be able to cope with the tendency to pressure increase. When, however, an attack starts with lightning rapidity, as in CPH, the pressure-regulating mechanisms may not be able to cope with the situation, due to the abruptness and fierceness of the attack. Whether these discrepancies signify a real difference between the two headaches is still debatable.

There is another point that is critical as far as the classification system is concerned. Let us just for a moment seriously consider the possibility that 'indomethacin responsive headache' is an acceptable term. There is a clear clinical link between cluster headache and CPH (see The Link to Cluster Headache), although pathogenetically they are probably different at some stage. In the present book, CPH is categorized as a subgroup of the cluster headache syndrome, on an equal footing with cluster headache. If CPH were to be included in the 'indomethacin-responsive headache', what then is the linkage of the latter *whole group* to cluster headache? Should the cluster headache syndrome be split and should only one fraction (CPH) be taken away? Such a splitting should not be allowed to take place. Mathew (1981) has described cases of cluster headache that show some response to indomethacin. If these really are cases of true cluster headache, should they then be categorized under indomethacin-responsive headache and *not* under cluster headache? Such headaches, if they exist, will of course still have to be categorized under cluster headache. So, there is no need for the term 'indomethacin-responsive headache', even from this angle. The opposite solution would naturally lead to an intolerable situation.

The term 'indomethacin-responsive headache' may be as meaningless as lumping together all diseases responsive to penicillin or cortisone, terming them 'the penicillin responsive disorder' and 'the cortisone responsive disorder'. These examples are actually not too far fetched! The absurdness of the situation is, however, easier to recognize with these two remedies than with indomethacin, because in the former case so many different disorders pertaining to so many different organs are encompassed. Basically, however, the situation is probably the same in the headache field, the difference being that the scope of disease conglomerate is less.

There are in all probability *various* headaches that respond to indomethacin. Sometimes a single letter makes all the difference. Much could have been saved if an 's' had been added at the end! The correct terminology could be 'indomethacin responsive headaches' or, as proposed by Mathew (1981), 'indomethacin-responsive-headache syndromes'. All these headaches should not be given an all-inclusive designation (Diamond *et al.*, 1982): '. . . a **new** headache **syndrome** responsive to indomethacin' (the emphasis in bold type is mine). The novelty of the so-called syndrome is also illusive; it was established since 1974 (Sjaastad and Dale, 1974) that headache cases having an absolute indomethacin response exist. The introduction and uncritical use of this term has caused confusion and disorientation in a difficult terrain, a terrain which is certainly intricate enough in its own right without the addition of extra difficulties. The term, as far as I am concerned, is a misnomer, for which reason it should be abandoned. Graham (1988) has also voiced scepticism about accepting this syndrome.

The moral that can be drawn from this situation is that the response to a single drug is not sufficient evidence on which to base any classification. The response is one of the features characterizing the headache (and, in particular, clearly so if the response is dramatic and absolute). But, the other typical features of the disorder are also important—and a classification or categorization should only be made on the basis of the total picture.

WAS CHRONIC PAROXYSMAL HEMICRANIA DESCRIBED PRIOR TO 1974?

Isler (1986) has retrieved an old German article concerning 'hemicrania horologica' written by Iohannes Christoph. Ulrich Oppermann (in Latin, 1747). To be certain about the details in this report, we have had a translation of the original Latin text made directly into Norwegian. No major discrepancy was observed between Isler's own English and the Norwegian translation of the Latin text.

The report deals with a 35-year-old German woman, who has apparently continuously had severe headache attacks exactly on the hour, day and night, in recent years, except during a pregnancy. This timing was so exact that when there was a discrepancy in the timing between the headache and the town clock, the latter proved to be off, and not the other way around. There is no mention of associated autonomic disturbances.

Several characteristics seem to emerge from Oppermann's account:

1. the patient was a woman;
2. the attacks were vehement;
3. the attacks were frequent, rather short-lasting, and also nocturnal;
4. the attacks were accurately timed (exactly on the hour);
5. the attacks had been going on for several years; and
6. the headache was termed a 'hemicrania'.

Admittedly, some of these traits are reminiscent of chronic paroxysmal hemicrania (CPH). Isler apparently feels that a diagnosis of CPH generally can be established on the basis of the temporal pattern, the frequency of attack and, above all, the regularity of attacks. Isler seems to be of the opinion that this case represents an early description of CPH; later (Isler, 1987) his conviction seems to have increased: '"Hemicrania horologica" is hardly different from a rare variant of cluster headache, namely, chronic paroxysmal hemicrania . . .'.

Does this way of arguing stand up to reason? Some pertinent differential diagnostic traits count against a CPH diagnosis in the German case.

1. 'Unilaterality' may be of various kinds: a 'side-locked' unilaterality and a unilaterality that shifts side (Sjaastad and Saunte, 1985; Sjaastad *et al.*, 1989a). In Isler's summary report (1986), Oppermann's original description of the location of the headache was left out. The statement, however short it may be, runs as follows: *'more on the left than on the right side'*. In CPH, the headache is, almost without exception at least as far as we know at present, strictly unilateral and without bilaterality or side-shift (Antonaci and Sjaastad, 1989). In the German case, the headache was apparently not strictly unilateral. This is, in fact, a rather heavy counter-argument against a CPH diagnosis in the German case.
2. As far as we are concerned, a regularity in timing like that recorded in the German case is not a typical trait of CPH. To the best of our knowledge, none of the cases hitherto described in detail has exhibited a regularity of this degree. Our first patients (Sjaastad and Dale, 1974, 1976) showed a *rather strict* timing *at times*, and when the attack frequency for a limited time was around 24 per 24 h, the mean interval between attacks amounted to around 60 min. When we stated that there was 'almost

clockwork regularity', this was meant to indicate that there were not, *with the given frequency*, sometimes 2–3 attacks per hour, the interval between attacks at other times being 2–3 h. The 24-h time-span was punctuated with attacks at rather regular intervals ('the patients can foretell almost exactly when the next attack is going to start' (Sjaastad and Dale, 1974)). But the interval between attacks was not exactly 60 min on such occasions—it could be 55 min; it could be 65 or even 75 min. The lack of *absolute* clockwork regularity in our cases is evident from the following statement: 'The attacks appear with intervals of approximately 1–3 h around the clock' (Sjaastad and Dale, 1976).

3. The impression one gets from the German report is that of a *constant timing*. In CPH, however, the *variability in attack frequency* seems to be the typical trait (Sjaastad and Dale, 1974, 1976) and not a steadily high attack frequency. As early as 1976 we stated that: 'In periods with severe attacks, the attacks also become more frequent and somewhat more long-lasting'. 'In the best periods, the attack pattern might at times be less pronounced, even only vaguely outlined . . .'. The fluctuation of the attack frequency may be a reflection of the cycling in the other headache in the cluster headache syndrome, the cluster headache. For that reason, the term: 'modified cluster pattern' was introduced for the pattern observed in CPH. The lack of (or rather the lack of a description of) a phenomenon similar to 'the modified cluster pattern' of CPH, as well as the constancy of the headache timing, count rather clearly against the presence of CPH in Oppermann's case.

4. The severity of headache *per se* is difficult to assess in the German case, since the patient apparently also had terrible toothaches, and these seem to have concurred with the headache. To assess the severity of a headache in the presence of a *severe* toothache is a tough task, regardless of the fact that the attacks were regular in timing.

There is another strong counter-argument against accepting a diagnosis of CPH in the Oppermann case. In general, the definition of a disorder is not, and should not be, linked to the effect of a drug. There may, however, seem to be exceptions to this rule. Thus, in CPH, the diagnostic link to NSAIDs and, in particular, to indomethacin (*absolute* effect), is so firm that, without a positive therapeutic trial with this drug, it is presently thought that a diagnosis cannot be made. This test may continue to be a diagnostic *sine qua non* for all practical purposes, even when the substrate of this headache has been identified.

Indomethacin was made available approximately 200 years after Oppermann's description. It will therefore, in essence, be impossible to identify CPH cases in the older literature, i.e. before the NSAIDs era. If typical case histories from older times should exist, one may *suspect* that they contain CPH elements, but firm conclusions with regard to identity can and should not be made. This view is especially important since patients ($n = 3$; one case seen with J. R. Graham and two from our clinic) have been observed with as frequent and short-lasting,unilateral attacks as in CPH, and with other headache character-istics most similar to those of CPH, but diagnostically in all probability at variance with CPH, since the indomethacin effect is completely absent. It is also noteworthy that Bogucki and Niewodniczy (1984) have described a 'cluster headache patient' with an attack frequency of up to 30 attacks per 24 h.

An interesting feature, possibly of some etiological significance, is that the German patient suffered from smallpox in the first year of her life, 'from which she not only had many marks in her face, but she also sustained such a lesion in her left eye from them, that she nearly lost its sight'. I do not specifically know about any such reported sequella of smallpox as headache. It is worthy of note, however, that the left eye was affected, i.e. the eye on the side which was principally affected by the later developing headache. Bizarre headache may follow in the wake of various lesions and traumas to the forehead/face, as we ourselves also have witnessed several times (Sjaastad, 1989b). (For further details, the reader is referred to: Sjaastad (1987b)).

In summary, a diagnosis of CPH cannot be established in Oppermann's case with a reasonable degree of certainty. The diagnosis in Oppermann's case is not known and probably will never be definitely known. It certainly sounds like an interesting case that we would have loved to study.

TREATMENT

Since the frequency of attacks is so high and since each paroxysm of head pain is of relatively short duration, prophylaxis is the only natural approach to drug therapy in CPH. This goes for the chronic stage with its fluctuations, as well as for the 'pre-chronic stage' ('remitting form') where each bout has to be treated, provided the stage is of some length.

ANTI-INFLAMMATORY AGENTS

Indomethacin

Indomethacin is the drug of choice in chronic paroxysmal hemicrania (CPH) and in most cases it should be given continuously. The trial dosage in a suspected case of CPH should be 150 mg or more per 24 h. It will be known within a few days, or even a few hours (depending upon dosage and the stage of disease), whether or not one is faced with a case of absolute indomethacin response. We have extended the trial period to 3–4 days, as a precautionary measure.

The maintenance dosage is usually between 25 and 100 mg day^{-1}. When a high dosage is needed, the dosage should be evenly distributed over the daytime. When night attacks are prominent, the last evening dosage should be given at a late hour and, eventually, another dosage on awakening—or even at a set time during the night. However, due to the fluctuating course ('modified cluster pattern' (Sjaastad and Dale, 1976)), the dosage will have to be adjusted accordingly. There is no such thing as a fixed, permanently adequate dosage of indomethacin in most cases. A streamlined adjustment along the time axis according to the need for the drug is mandatory to keep the patient headache free, and the dosage of indomethacin may actually be titrated.

In a number of patients, the dosage would seem to vary as much intra-individually as interindividually. This means that anywhere from 12.5 to 250 mg day^{-1} may be required in a single patient to keep the attacks away. This is actually what has happened in two of our first four cases. The 'modified cluster pattern' may be a tricky phenomenon for the unexperienced observer. The transition from a period with moderate attacks to one with maximal attacks may occur rather fast (Figure 4.2), and dosage adjustment must then follow suit. Otherwise, a rather pronounced deterioration may be the consequence. It is possible that this very phenomenon may be one reason why the claim has been made that there is not an absolute indomethacin response in all cases. In some patients, the fluctuations in severity seem to be much less marked; accordingly also the drug requirements fluctuate less in such cases. The patients generally adapt easily to the policy of regulating the dosage according to symptoms and become specialists themselves in this field.

We have usually given the drug orally. In a few cases, we have used suppositories, due to dyspeptic trouble. In some cases in the literature, indomethacin has been discontinued due to dyspepsia or ulcer formation. In a couple of our cases, dyspepsia and/or ulcer formation have made transitory discontinuation of indomethacin necessary, but a permanent discontinuation has never been necessary for this reason. We have, under such circumstances, combined indomethacin and histamine H$_2$ blocking agents. In a couple of our cases, we have included gastroscopy on a 1/2–3/4 yearly basis, and on this regime our patients have managed nicely.

As far as we know today, there is invariably an *absolute* effect of indomethacin in CPH. A *partial* effect does not suffice as a diagnostic criterion, as far as we presently know, provided an adequate dosage is given. As far as we can see today, the beneficial effect of indomethacin in CPH is a basic and necessary criterion of the disorder. An indomethacin non-responsive CPH case is prob-ably a *contradictio in adjecto*. My reasoning in this regard is as follows. There are cases showing a symptomatology very similar to that of CPH, but which are absolutely non-responsive to indomethacin. The absolute lack of indomethacin response would indicate that there is probably a crucial difference as to the nature of the head pain in these patients and in CPH. The efficacy of indomethacin in CPH is so fundamental that the drug test probably will remain a diagnostic criterion even after the mechanism underlying CPH has been identified. In the future, indomethacin will probably be substituted by as effective, but less harmful, drugs.

Since the response to indomethacin in our practice has been a diagnostic criterion (a *sine qua non*), we are admittedly in a situation where we may, theoretically speaking, overlook potential cases of CPH. We can at the present time not avoid this special situation, as long as the substrate for this headache is unknown.

The bioavailability of the drug in a given case may come into focus as one possible explanation for a lack of effect. We have also noted that during febrile periods (viral infections?) there may be transitory deteriorations where indomethacin seems to be of less avail. Even following a dosage augmentation to 250–300 mg daily (we have not used higher dosages) there may be reminiscences of attacks or even overt, moderate attacks for a few days in such a situation. A similar deterioration during respiratory infection was noted by Horton (1964) in cluster headache.

In one of our patients (the one who readily can precipitate attacks), a sort of 'CPH-status' has developed a couple of times, with a continuous (for several days), severe headache that otherwise seemed to have the characteristics of CPH. The dosage of indomethacin has been increased to a maximum during these episodes. Whether it was this or the natural course of the headache that brought the 'status' to an end can only be speculated upon.

On discontinuation of indomethacin, symptoms usually reappear within 12 h to a few days, probably depending upon the 'stage' the patient is in. Long-lasting remissions have, however, been observed after indomethacin discontinuation (Jensen *et al.*, 1982; Sjaastad *et al.*, 1983). Even in *chronic* cases, discontinuation of the drug may occasionally lead to a long-lasting freedom of headache (Sjaastad and Antonaci, 1987).

There are no indications of a tachyphylaxis, so the drug requirement does not seem to increase over the years. On the contrary, the drug requirement seems to have diminished over the years in a couple of our cases: in one (Sjaastad and Antonaci, 1987), the indomethacin requirement faded after many years of chronic suffering. There is no definite evidence that the disorder, once it has reached the chronic stage, progresses in any way under the cover of indomethacin. Whether indomethacin given in the remitting stage can obviate the further progression to the chronic stage is not known.

Other anti-inflammatory agents

Before the indomethacin effect in CPH had been discovered, the patients themselves had found out that acetylsalicylic acid was the most effective drug they had been exposed to. They had continued to ingest huge quantities of the drug (6–8 g day^{-1}) for years. In general, the effect of acetylsalicylic acid is mediocre in CPH. In the more moderate periods (see The Modified Cluster Pattern), it might provide relatively good help, in that it alleviates the pain and probably increases the interval between attacks. In the more severe periods, it may take away 'the top of the pain', but usually no more than that (Sjaastad and Dale, 1976). Recently, Kudrow and Kudrow (1989) found that small doses of aspirin (i.e. 15 mg kg^{-1}) caused the attacks to cease in a 9-year-old male. They speculate that there may be a preferential sensitivity to aspirin in children, since aspirin is of only moderate avail in adult CPH patients.

A range of anti-inflammatory and other agents were, originally and at a later stage, tried in the prophylaxis of this disorder; e.g. naproxen (in a dosage of up to 750 mg day^{-1}), ketoprofen (up to 300 mg day^{-1}), brufen, tanderil, butazolidine, and tolfenamic acid (Sjaastad and Dale, 1974, 1976). All these agents seemed to have some effect but, in the dosages employed, the effect seemed to be moderately to clearly less than that of indomethacin. The effect was probably approximately at the level of that of acetylsalicylic acid, or perhaps at a slightly higher level. Later, piroxicam was also tried, with moderate effect.

Cortisone (prednisone, in dosages of 10–40 mg day^{-1}) was given only to our two first patients. It led to the disappearance of attacks for approximately 4 weeks in one patient, after which time the attacks recurred, despite a dosage increase. In the other patient, prednisone was ineffective. In retrospect, a higher dosage of prednisone could have been tried in the latter case. When considering the adverse effects of chronic cortisone treatment, however, its possible effect is of little *practical* consequence, at least in the chronic cases. Theoretically, however, it would have been of considerable interest to have somewhat more definite information as to whether or not cortisone is generally effective in CPH. In a recent case report, Hannerz *et al.* (1987b) have observed a good effect of prednisone in one case (dosage 60 mg day^{-1}, and tapering off over the course of 6 weeks), and the beneficial effect continued after drug discontinuation. In this case, there was apparently also complete indomethacin effect on 75 mg day^{-1}, but only as long as the drug was continued. An increase in indomethacin dosage was not attempted. In an experimental situation like the one described by Hannerz *et al.*, the patient can, unfortunately, not be his own proper control. It may well be that, if indomethacin had been administered *at the time when prednisone was administered*, this would have led to the same results as obtained with prednisone. Hypothetically, there may be many explanations for this observation (see Orbital Phlebography). Anyhow, indomethacin has a time-honoured, absolute effect in CPH if given in adequate dosages, whilst prednisone does not seem to have such an action.

THE EFFECT OF INDOMETHACIN IN CHRONIC PAROXYSMAL HEMICRANIA

Specificity

The demonstrated effect of indomethacin in CPH is striking. It seems to be absolute, but dose-dependent, and the dosage can be titrated in a given situation in a given patient. It may seem incorrect to link the diagnosis of a disorder to the effect of a particular drug, particularly a drug with seemingly a relatively broad spectrum of effects. Admittedly, such a drug may have been substituted by other, better, and more specific drugs within a relatively short time and, sooner or later, it may even have gone into oblivion. CPH may be the exception that proves the rule. As long as we do not have *absolute* criteria for the disorder, and as long as the disease process itself is hidden, it may seem appropriate to link the diagnosis of CPH to indomethacin. The reasons for this are, first and foremost, that the effect is so dramatic and that it seems to be rather specific. For the establishment of a CPH diagnosis, the typical attack pattern, etc., must, of course, also be taken into consideration.

Could the demonstrated indomethacin effect possibly depend on a placebo effect? We think such a possibility can be safely excluded. First, prior to the establishment of a correct diagnosis, most of the patients have been subjected to a variety of drugs, all of which have been ineffective, and many of which made the symptoms worse (except acetylsalicylic acid). Second, double-blind experiments with identically appearing and tasting placebo and indomethacin capsules have been carried out in two of the patients during a phase of frequently occurring attacks (Sjaastad and Dale, 1974, 1976). Later on, similar experiments were carried out in a couple of other patients. These experiments in CPH rendered a clear-cut answer in favour of a real indomethacin effect in CPH. Experiments like these must be designed in a special way, to be meaningful: after indomethacin discontinuation, one must wait until severe attacks have set in and then start indomethacin or indomethacin placebo administration. On discontinuation of the active drug, there may be a period of only very moderate attacks or almost no attacks because the patient is in a 'valley' in the longitudinal curve of development (see Figures 4.2 and 4.3). If indomethacin placebo should happen to be administered during such a time, one might get a false impression of a placebo effect.

How specific is this drug effect in CPH? This question may be divided into two parts:

1. Is indomethacin far superior to other drugs as far as the treatment of CPH is concerned? In other words, is it in a class of its own in CPH?
2. Is indomethacin effective only in CPH of all headaches? Or does it also influence other headaches and even related conditions that can be mixed up with CPH?

For the time being, indomethacin seems to be superior to the other drugs tested in CPH. Such drugs include ketoprofen, naproxen, phenylbutazone and piroxicam. Indomethacin is, nevertheless, not the ideal drug in CPH. The ideal drug would be a specific drug, as potent as, or even more potent than, indomethacin in this respect and with few or none of the adverse effects associated with indomethacin therapy—above all the gastric ones. Therefore, there may in the future be drugs superior to indomethacin in the treatment of CPH.

'Hemicrania continua' (see elsewhere) is so far the only other headache in which an *absolute* indomethacin effect has been demonstrated (Sjaastad and Spierings, 1984). Clinical and, to some extent, pupillographic characteristics seem to separate this headache from CPH (Sjaastad *et al.*, 1984c). The nosological status of this headache is, nevertheless, as yet somewhat uncertain (see also The So-called Indomethacin-responsive Headache).

There are, however, other headaches that show a *partial* indomethacin effect: The 'jabs and jolts' syndrome (Sjaastad, 1979; Sjaastad *et al.*, 1979) is such a syndrome ('idiopathic stabbing headache' (?), Headache Classification Committee of the IHS, 1985). In our experience, the effect of indomethacin in this syndrome is usually moderate, and rarely, if at all, complete. This syndrome has occasionally proved to be a difficult differential diagnosis versus CPH. Therefore, in this book it is dealt with in the section on Differential Diagnosis.

Benign exertional headache (Rooke, 1968; Porter and Jankovic, 1981) is also abated by indomethacin (Mathew, 1981). The characteristics of this headache are a bilateral, short-lasting, usually moderate headache, without accompanying symptoms like nausea, rhinorrhoea, lacrimation, etc. This headache occurs more frequently in males than in females. The clear-cut temporal relationship with exertion or sexual intercourse and a relatively low-grade attack frequency are also typical features (Table 4.21). The response to indomethacin is apparently only *partial* and *varying* in this headache. The dosage used was 75 mg day^{-1} (Lance, 1982).

Since we discovered the indomethacin effect in CPH, we have been searching for headache cases with an indomethacin response. In an occasional case with traumatic 'cervicogenic headache' (Sjaastad *et al.*, 1983c; Pfaffenrath *et al.*, 1984a) we have seen a moderate response to indomethacin or other NSAIDs (in particular piroxicam). We have also recently seen two cases with tumours (in one case an osteosarcoma in the temporal bone; in the other case, a tumour in the nasopharynx, both on the symptomatic side) with a *transitory*, more or less complete effect.

So, the indomethacin effect is not limited to CPH. There may, of course, also be other headaches in the future in addition to CPH and hemicrania continua that will respond completely to indomethacin.

The finding that lithium has a contrary effect in CPH, whereas it is a drug of choice in cluster headache, is a strong argument for a dichotomy between the two disorders. The almost opposite relationship as far as indomethacin is concerned, is another, as depicted in the theoretical model in Figure 4.39.

On the significance of the indomethacin effect

The striking, rapidly occurring, and continuous effect of indomethacin is remarkable. Where and how does indomethacin act in CPH?

Orally administered indomethacin seems to be recovered from the spinal fluid in only small amounts, and indomethacin is not *known* to exert any central effects. This may be of relevance for its site of action in CPH. The striking indomethacin effect and the mechanical precipitation mechanism might point to an arthralgic affection of the cervical spine in these patients. On the other hand, CPH has occasionally begun at an early age, far from the age when degenerative joint disease tends to start. A rheumatoid-arthritis-like effect in

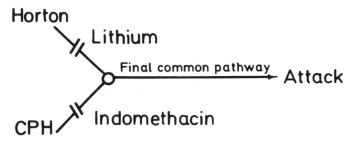

Figure 4.39 Possible inter-relationship between cluster headache (Horton's headache) and chronic paroxysmal hemicrania (CPH). Lithium blocks the tendency to attacks in cluster headache, whilst aggravating attacks of CPH. Indomethacin abolishes attacks of CPH, whereas cluster headache usually is not, or is only very moderately, influenced. The attacks of CPH and cluster headache appear quite similar clinically. There is possibly a 'final common pathway' for the two headaches, as depicted. However, this may not be quite so since, for example, the tendency to sweating seems to differ between the two types of headache. (From Sjaastad (1977). Courtesy of A. P. Friedman and Research and Clinical Studies in Headache.)

the cervical spine seems unlikely, since relevant tests were normal. It is noteworthy that one of our patients had a spina bifida of the C_1 verterbra (the patient who can readily precipitate attacks) (Sjaastad *et al.*, 1979).

The question of the significance of possible, minor neck movements as precipitating factors comes up in cases of CPH in whom attacks cannot readily be precipitated mechanically. A study of the sleep pattern in our patient with CPH who is able to precipitate attacks in constant succession by neck movements, showed that nightly attacks almost invariably occurred without any appreciable neck movements (Kayed *et al.*, 1978). In one of our patients who cannot precipitate attacks, single attacks can start when the patient is lying absolutely still in the supine position, as far as we can judge. So, if neck movements are of significance for the generation of attacks in CPH in general, such movements are probably very minor, possibly on a sub-clinical level.

The pain, also in the mechanically precipitated attacks, does not have the clear, shooting quality of the root pain in, for example, cervical disc protrusions, and it does not last for seconds only. The observed regularity of the attacks in some patients, with 1–2 h intervals, during both the day and the night, also makes it unlikely that a pure radicular lesion is the underlying cause. The pain may last (almost?) as long with a precipitated as with an ordinary spontaneously occurring attack, i.e. 5–15 min. On the other hand, precipitated attacks of CPH generally last for a shorter time than do precipitated attacks of cervicogenic headache. The possibility of a C-fibre pain in these cases of CPH, as proposed by Grønbæk (1982, 1985) in various other connections, should be considered. The rather slow development of pain in some mechanically precipitated attacks may point in this direction.

The beneficial effect of indomethacin seems to appear somewhat faster than would be expected in an ordinary rheumatoid affection. Because of the striking effect of indomethacin, a Bechterew-like affection was also suspected (Sjaastad and Dale, 1976). The sacroiliac joints, however, seemed normal. Nor did the HLA antigen pattern point to a Bechterew-like disorder. Furthermore, phenyl-butazone was of no benefit in our first two patients.

Indomethacin could influence localized painful structures with spatial re-lationship to the spine, thereby also explaining the mechanical precipitation of headache. Indomethacin has various properties that theoretically could be of therapeutic importance:

1. It possesses antibradykinin effect. Nevertheless, its efficacy in combating the pain in our patients is unlikely to be due to this property. Ketoprofen seems to be as potent as, and occasionally up to 10 times more potent than, indomethacin as for the various variables studied, with regard to antibradykinin properties (Julou et al., 1971). Ketoprofen, nevertheless, seems to be far less efficient than indomethacin in reducing the pain in CPH. Ketoprofen does not seem to be more efficient in this respect than salicylates (Sjaastad and Dale 1974, 1976).
2. It has anti-inflammatory properties. This effect of indomethacin is of the same order of magnitude as that of ketoprofen (Julou et al., 1971).
3. It has analgesic effect. This effect seems to be only slightly more marked than that of naproxen (Roszkowski et al., 1971), whereas the therapeutic efficacy of indomethacin (dose 75 mg) far outweighs that of naproxen (dose 750 mg).
4. It has antipyretic effect: ketoprofen is 3–4 times as potent as indometha-cin in this respect (Julou et al., 1971).

Another aspect to consider when comparing the effect of the various NSAIDs is that optimal dosages may not have been given in our trials. Thus, the optimal dosages of naproxen and brufen have been increased during the time that has elapsed since our drug studies were carried out.

A local effect of indomethacin in the eye would also be feasible. A signal from the neck (in, for example, the mechanically precipitated attacks) could in a reflex way be mediated to the ocular area. Whilst corneal indentation pulse increase, lacrimation, etc., would normally ensue, indomethacin might block these events locally. Therefore, indomethacin eyedrops (two drops at a time) were instilled repeatedly into the conjunctival sac on the symptomatic side ($n = 3$). This procedure had no effect on the occurrence or severity of attacks or on the corneal indentation pulse amplitude or the intraocular pressure. This type of procedure does, however, not disprove that indomethacin may have a local effect in the eye, since the penetration of indomethacin through the cornea may be too limited.

The observation that eyedrops of indomethacin seem to be ineffective may, nevertheless, fit in with our general concept of the pathogenesis of CPH. In our view, the ocular symptoms and signs are secondary to impulses reaching the eye, originating elsewhere. The ocular after-effects cannot be mended by the same drug that counteracts the pathological process at the site of origin of the impulses. As stated elsewhere, there is little, if any, reason to believe that pain during the attack is generated through increased intraocular pressure, since in the thymoxamine experiments pain was generated despite a lack of an intraocular-pressure increase. The possibility remains that ocular mechanisms other than an increase in intraocular pressure could underlie the pain. It is our firm belief, however, that enunciation (as proposed by our first patient!) would probably not have led to any improvement in CPH. The local ocular phenomena during attack are probably mediated through various pathways/ transmitters and may be counteracted in other ways. Thus, the lacrimation may be reduced with atropine and the intraocular pressure increase with thymoxamine.

Although their pharmacological profiles differ somewhat, NSAIDs generally inhibit cyclo-oxygenase, the enzyme which converts the precursor arachidonic acid (endoperoxides) to the active substances, the various prostaglandins of the PGE and PGF series. Cortisone exerts its effect at a different step in the process, that is by inhibiting the lipoxygenase. There will thus be differences between the end-result after indomethacin and cortisone treatment as far as prostaglandins are concerned. The various NSAIDs exert different bodily effects. Since the NSAIDs generally inhibit cyclo-oxygenase, even ASA being a potent inhibitor and since indomethacin seems more potent than the other NSAIDs in counteracting the pain attacks, it seems likely that indomethacin exerts its effects via other channels as well.

Other properties of indomethacin, such as the lipophilicity *per se* or in conjunction with the aforementioned effects, may underlie the therapeutic efficacy of indomethacin in CPH. Quite unknown effects of indomethacin may also be important in this respect.

The sensitivity of nuchal trigger points is clearly reduced under the influence of indomethacin. In cases of mechanical precipitation of attacks, indomethacin may exert its influence by desensitizing trigger mechanisms. These may actually be rather widely distributed.

There is no proof at hand to show that cases of mechanical precipitation of attacks are identical to those which do not have this property. However, the similarity of the attack pattern and the accompanying signs in both groups, as well as the indomethacin effect, indicate that they are two manifestations of one and the same disease process. One should, therefore, believe that the same mechanisms as those that apply in the mechanically precipitated attacks also underlie the 'ordinary' CPH cases—that is, those lacking precipitation mechanisms. The possibility exists that in these two patient categories there is a 'final common pathway', but that it is the stimulation mechanism of this pathway that differs. Therefore, the basis for the efficacy of indomethacin in relieving the pain of CPH in general remains obscure.

ANTIHISTAMINICS

Histamine H_1 receptor antagonists are completely ineffective in CPH, and the same goes for the histamine H_2 receptor antagonist cimetidine, at a dosage of 1.6 g day^{-1} (Sjaastad *et al.*, 1977).

BUDIPINE

Budipine (butyldiphenylpiperidine) has been tried as a therapeutic remedy in parkinsonism. In an open study, Krüger *et al.* (1988) treated three CPH patients with budipine. Two of them responded 'substantially' to 60 mg budipine per day. The third, a female, who responded completely to indomethacin, showed only a minor positive response to budipine.

ACUPUNCTURE/TRANSCUTANEOUS NERVE STIMULATION

Acupuncture and/or transcutaneous nerve stimulation (TNS) have been tried as therapeutic measures in five patients with CPH. The TNS was carried out with a 2-Hz stimulation at acupuncture point L 14, i.e. in the first interosseal space on the side ipsi- or contra-lateral to the headache. The other specifications were as follows: stimulus intensity of 30–60 A and 45 min sessions repeated at 4–6 h intervals (Sjaastad *et al.*, submitted). The trial period lasted at least 2–3 weeks. Two patients claimed that during periods with weak attacks there was some effect, but in periods with severe/extremely severe attacks this method was of no avail. The other patients were unable to detect any definite effect even with moderately severe attacks.

PATHOGENESIS

If one is faced with a headache like this, where *pain* is the *major* symptom, it is difficult to know where to start an attempt to unravel the pathogenesis. At the beginning of the 1960s, we decided to start from *two different angles:* chronic paroxysmal hemicrania (CPH) seemed to be rather similar to cluster headache or 'histaminic cephalgia', so it was decided to study *histamine metabolism.* Pain was most marked in the ocular/periocular area; it was, therefore, also decided to study various *ocular* and related variables.

HISTAMINE METABOLISM

Increased urinary excretion of histamine and a low imidazole acetic acid riboside/imidazole acetic acid (ImAA-R/ImAA) ratio were present in only one of the two patients studied. It was, therefore, felt that these changes, though definite enough, probably reflected a peculiarity characterizing just one patient rather than this type of headache (Sjaastad and Sjaastad, 1977a,b) (for details see Histamine Studies). No further studies were therefore carried out on histamine metabolism in CPH.

THE SIGNIFICANCE OF OCULAR VARIABLES

The study of the *ocular parameters* proved more rewarding: Intraocular pressure and the corneal indentation pulse amplitudes were clearly and invariably increased during attacks when compared with the period between attacks ($n = 7$), and significantly more marked on the symptomatic than on the non-symptomatic side (Broch *et al.*, 1970; Hørven *et al.*, 1972, 1989; Hørven and Sjaastad, 1977; Sjaastad *et al.*, 1977).

In CPH, the incessant flow of attacks makes it possible to stand by and be ready to measure the intraocular pressure and corneal indentation pulse amplitude just before and at the beginning of attacks. Measurement of intraocular pressure at the beginning of attack shows that there is a rather abrupt change in intraocular volume. Could an abrupt volume change of this magnitude be due to an increase in aqueous humour production or to a hindrance to its removal? Could it be due to oedema formation? Or is it more likely that it is due to vasodilatation? And in the latter case, is it due to a 'primary' vasodilatation or is it due to an external stimulus, be it neurogenic or transported via the blood?

A priori, a vasodilatation seems to be the most likely explanation for the abrupt and marked intraocular pressure increment at the onset of attack. The possibility of course remains that there is a combination of causes for this increment, e.g. a co-existing vasodilatation and minor oedema formation.

However, the timing of the events indicates more clearly than in cluster headache that vasodilatation is entirely, or almost entirely, responsible for the observed changes in intraocular pressure. The increase in corneal temperature during attacks (Hørven and Sjaastad, 1977) is most probably also caused by intraocular vasodilatation (see elsewhere), although there may be other explanations for it.

Patients with CPH tend to have a relatively small pupil on the symptomatic side (Sjaastad *et al.*, 1979). Pupillometric studies (see elsewhere) did not provide any definite evidence for a sympathetic deficit in CPH (de Souza Carvalho *et al.*, 1988). Cluster headache (Kunkle and Anderson, 1961; Nieman and Hurwitz, 1961; Riley and Moyer, 1971; Fanciullacci *et al.*, 1982; Salvesen *et al.*, 1987a,b) seems to differ from CPH in this respect, since in cluster headache there seems to be a Horner-like picture (see Cluster Headache).

A SEARCH FOR GENERALIZED VASCULAR/AUTONOMIC DISTURBANCES

The question arose whether the attack-related, putatively circulatory changes are restricted to the eyes or are more extensive. In order to explore this question, we have measured the intra-arterial pressure, the cerebrospinal-fluid

Table 4.22   Effect of atropine on the autonomic parameters[a] of chronic
paroxysmal hemicrania attacks

Clear reduction *or removal*	No change
Tearing	Pain
Rhinorrhoea	Corneal indentation pulse amplitude
Sweating	Intraocular pressure

[a]Salivation was not tested, but it is already non-existent.

pressure, the fluorescein appearance time, and we have carried out electro-cardiogram registrations (Russell and Storstein, 1984). Apart from some electrocardiogram changes that were less marked than those in cluster head ache, there were few signs of abnormality with these tests. In other words, there seem to be few systemic autonomic abnormalities during the CPH attack.

In a further search for more extensive autonomic manifestations, a study of sweating (see Sweating on the Forehead) was carried out. Whereas it has been demonstrated in cluster headache that forehead sweat glands on the sympto-matic side behave abnormally, this was not invariably so in CPH: whilst some patients did sweat excessively during attack, others did not. Obvious signs indicative of a sympathetic deficiency have not been found in CPH. This, therefore, also shows another point of considerable interest: the mechanism underlying a so frequently occurring phenomenon of the cluster headache attack as sweating may seem to differ from that underlying sweating in CPH. This observation combined with the observation of a difference in pupillo-metric patterns indicates that the pathogenesis of cluster headache and of CPH may differ.

There seems to be a clear dichotomy between the appearance of sweating and pain in precipitated attacks. The generation of pain is no pre-condition for the appearance of sweating: the sweating is, in other words, not caused by the pain (Figure 4.27). Further elucidation of the interconnection between sweating and pain was made in other experiments: if atropine was administered ahead of attack provocation, no, or only very moderate, sweating (and lacrima-tion) would occur in association with the pain attack. The same goes for anaesthetic blocking of the stellate ganglion (Sjaastad *et al.*, 1986). The pain does thus not seem to depend upon autonomic drive leading to sweating (and lacrimation) (Table 4.22).

The interconnection between pain and autonomic phenomena may be even more sophisticated than outlined above, as demonstrated by precipitation experiments in which it was possible to obtain advance information on pain generation by monitoring forehead sweating (Sjaastad *et al.*, 1986) (Figures 4.27 and 4.28). The situation thus seems to be that, when the mechanism of pain generation is set in operation, a parallel stimulation of the sweat glands takes place. However, the manifestations of sweat-gland stimulation appear ahead of the pain. We have no reason to suspect that the sweat fibres are really irritated in true time prior to eliciting the mechanism that eventually leads to a pain paroxysm. The ultimate difference in timing between the two events probably only means that it takes somewhat longer for the manifestations of the irritation of the pain-provoking mechanism (the pain itself) to appear (Figure 4.6).

Further evidence that these may be correct interpretations and inferences has been obtained through two types of observations: lacrimation, mostly on the symptomatic side is also visible within a short time after the precipitation of an attack (probably at approximately the same time as the sweating, although we have not quantified these two variables in the same experiments). Furthermore, if a pain-producing procedure that is accompanied by a clear increase in sweating is interrupted prior to the onset of pain, the pain may come anyhow after another 10–20 s. This may mean that the mechanisms eventually leading to pain actually have been set off at approximately the same time at which the irritation of the sweat fibres started, and that the process—at least at times—may be irreversible once it has been triggered.

AN ATTEMPT TO INTERPRET THE AUTONOMIC PHENOMENA

The autonomic phenomena in CPH could, according to the traditional view, materialize through the parasympathetic or through the sympathetic system, and they could be related to over- or under-activity of the specific system. A relative over-activity of e.g. the sympathetic system could either be due to a *primary* over-activity of this system, or it could be a *secondary* phenomenon, due to the partial or total discontinuation of parasympathetic activity. Supersensitivity could also be involved. Modern views on autonomic transmission necessitate that transmitters other than the classical ones should also be taken into consideration. When discussing the status of the autonomic involvement in CPH, it is mandatory to separate the autonomic aspects of the attack from the pain part of it. The autonomic phenomena, despite a predominance on the symptomatic side, are bilateral in most instances. Therefore, CPH is a bilateral disorder in this respect.

The autonomic phenomena that occur during attack are manifold. The intraocular pressure increases early in a precipitated attack, in consort with lacrimation, forehead sweating, etc. It seems reasonable to assume that there is a common denominator to all these circumscribed autonomic phenomena. The tempo of the process (e.g. the appearance of lacrimation over the course of a couple of seconds) seems to fit better with a stimulation than with an inhibition process (e.g. the inhibition of a retention mechanism of *pre-produced* tears, if such a process is conceivable).

However, a massive *sympathetic* stimulation alone can hardly explain the entire attack-related autonomic symptomatology, e.g. the lid oedema and the occasionally observed small pupil on the symptomatic side. With a sympathetic stimulation, one would thus have expected a mydriasis. A super-sensitivity reaction to sympathicomimetic agents may be excluded for the same reason, since it would lead to the same signs and, moreover, no definite signs of super-sensitivity have been discovered as regards the sweat glands and iris in CPH.

Additional information may be obtained from the thymoxamine experiments (Figure 4.38) (Sjaastad *et al.*, 1986), in which there was a dichotomy between pain and intraocular-pressure increase, the intraocular pressure being normalized and the *pain* being uninfluenced by thymoxamine. The pain of the attack is, therefore, unlikely to be caused by increased intraocular pressure. The results of the thymoxamine experiment are compatible with a sympathetic stimulation during attack, the mediation possibly being via sympathetic α receptors.

Again, the situation may be much more intricate than that outlined here. The total effect that is observed during an attack may be a result of the initial sympathetic stimulus *and secondary* effects (activation of other vasoactive processes). Atropine minimizes the extra outpouring of sweating and lacrimation during attacks, whereas an α-blocking agent, thymoxamine, seems to block the attack-related, intraocular pressure increase. Although the original stimulus to all the organs involved may have been one and the same, various transmitters and blocking agents may be operative at the peripheral site. It is noteworthy that atropine does not influence the increase in corneal indentation pulse amplitudes during attacks. It should be noted that the action of atropine on the intraocular pressure of the attack has *not* been studied (only its influence on the corneal indentation pulse amplitude). The balance of evidence still counts against a pure sympathetic stimulation during attack, since the pupil does not widen during attack.

How can the lacrimation that occurs in an attack be explained? The parasympathetic supply stems from the facial nerve (Figure 2.48). Parasympathetic stimulation gives rise to a massive outpouring of tears. In the older literature, it was also recorded (e.g. Duke-Elder, 1963) that sympathetic stimulation may occasion lacrimation (mechanism?). Sweat glands are, according to the traditional view, innervated by sympathetic fibres only, although the transmitter at the muscarinic site is acetylcholine. Increased lacrimation and sweating co-exist during the attack, despite the fact that these two autonomic functions are thought to depend on different autonomic innervations.

Could it be that there are 'various types of lacrimation' and that 'the type of lacrimation' connected with CPH attacks has an innervation pattern more like that pertaining to the sweat glands? The mechanisms underlying normal lacrimation—and sweating—may not be quite as well known as is desirable.

Nasal secretion was increased during attack (Saunte, 1984c), whereas salivation (from the sublingual/submandibular glands) was very moderate during attack. The pattern following pilocarpine stimulation, i.e. increased lacrimation, nasal secretion, sweating and salivation, differs clearly at one point from that observed during spontaneous attacks, i.e. with regard to salivation (and partly with regard to sweating). This discrepancy is striking and is also found in cluster headache. It seems unlikely, therefore, that a purely parasympathetic stimulation pattern is consistent with the pattern found during attacks. Reservation is taken from the fact that pilocarpine stimulation is not necessarily identical with acetylcholine stimulation. Acetylcholine as such has not been tried in such studies. This should be done. Atropine does counteract *some* of the accompaniments of the attack, but not all, and clearly not the pain (Table 4.22).

There seems to be a rather *localized* outburst of autonomic activity in CPH cases with a mechanical precipitation mechanism, and the pattern of the phenomena observed does not fit with a mediation by one of the two classic transmitters. Transmitters other than the two traditional ones may, therefore, be of crucial importance in mediating the impulses in CPH. The study of the whole panorama of transmitters in nerves in these areas is well under way (e.g. Tervo and Tervo, 1987; Vecchiet *et al.*, 1987).

There are clear *vascular* phenomena that occur in the ocular/periocular area (conjunctival injection during attacks, permanently widened palpebral vessels, etc.). The regulation of the tone of these vessels may be intricate (e.g. Krog, 1964a,b; Dahl, 1973a,b, 1986; Burnstock, 1985; Edvinsson, 1985; Owman and Hardebo, 1986). The regulation of ocular circulation appears to be complex (e.g. Bill, 1975) and is apparently only partly understood.

Stimulation of other types of autonomic fibres running together with the sympathetic fibres could possibly explain some of the attack-related findings. A model that may fit with this concept is involvement of substance-P fibres in the trigeminovascular system (Moskowitz, 1984). Stimulation of such fibres leads to liberation of substance-P not only at the central end of the neuron, but also, through antidromic stimulation, at the peripheral end of the neuron (Bill *et al.*, 1979). It has been shown that intracameral injection of substance-P causes miosis, protein leakage from the vessels, as well as a reduced functioning of the blood–aqueous barrier. According to Lembeck (Lembeck and Holzer, 1979; Lembeck, 1983), neurogenically caused oedema may be due to extravasation produced by substance-P liberation.

The manifestations of substance-P injection are thus rather similar to the symptomatology of CPH: small pupil, 'extravasation', as well as intraocular pressure increase. Of course, similarity does not mean identity. This striking similarity, however, may definitely be worth looking into more closely, since the miosis observed in CPH (Sjaastad *et al.*, 1979) does not seem to be due to a sympathetic deficiency. Prostaglandin E_1 and E_2 also cause miosis at high concentrations (Bill *et al.*, 1987), possibly through an effect on substance-P containing fibres. The interactions between substance-P and prostaglandins may be interesting from a pathogenetic point of view. Such interactions may also put the indomethacin effect in CPH into perspective. Somatostatin, an inhibitor of substance-P release, should accordingly also be tried in CPH.

According to Bill *et al.* (1987), the variations in response to substance-P in the eye do not so much depend on the extent of the release as on the number of receptors present. Intraocular nerves have also been demonstrated to contain neuropeptides such as calcitonin gene related peptide (CGRP), vasoactive intestinal peptide (VIP), and neuropeptide Y. There is partly a co-existence of two peptides in solitary nerve fibres, for example of CGRP and substance-P. Needless to say, to obtain effect there is a requirement for release and the presence of corresponding receptors.

The question of whether the local ocular vascular phenomena (vasodilatation and possibly also the oedema) are caused by neurogenic or vascular mechanisms is addressed here again. The mediation of the signal from the neck to the eye in patients with mechanical precipitation of attacks is probably neurogenic in nature (see previously). If patients with a marked precipitation capacity are true cases of CPH, then the underlying pathology should be the same as in 'ordinary' cases of CPH. Accordingly, also in patients who are unable to precipitate attacks, the stimulus may be neurogenic in nature. It may be that in mechanically precipitated attacks 'the route' to attack is short-circuited.

The mechanisms outlined above must not be taken to have any bearing on what occurs locally in the neck itself where some of the initial steps of an attack seem to take place. The pathological mechanisms that occur locally in the neck can only be speculated upon. A (slight?) localized oedema formation/vascular reaction may take place. There may be a direct pressure on nerves. Indomethacin most likely brings about its beneficial action at *this level* in CPH cases with mechanical precipitation of attacks.

So, the question of whether the mechanism is 'vascular' or 'neurogenic' can hardly be answered by an 'either'/'or'. The message from the neck to the eye seems to be neurogenic. However, within the globe of the eye, vascular reactions seem to take place, whereas in the sweat glands (in those that exhibit sweating) there may be a more *direct* action on the sudorific apparatus. At present we have only vague ideas about the abnormal reactions taking place in the trigger areas in the neck, antedating the generation of the signal to e.g. the eye.

CONCLUDING REMARKS

In patients in whom mechanical precipitation of attacks is possible, the neck seems to be of fundamental significance for the generation of attacks. If such patients are representative of CPH as such, the neck consequently should be of major importance in CPH generally. Why the 'ordinary' CPH patients cannot precipitate attacks mechanically is an unsolved problem. Of course the possibility remains that CPH with mechanical precipitation of attacks differs essentially from 'ordinary' CPH; at the present time this is not considered very likely.

Another aspect of CPH is as important: CPH is rather similar to cluster headache and is categorized together with it. As clearly expressed in connection with the pathogenesis of cluster headache, we favour 'the midline theory' (Sjaastad, 1988b), with affection of structures in and/or in close connection with the cavernous sinus in cluster headache. If CPH is so closely linked to cluster headache, how then can the pathogenesis of the two headaches appear to be so different—both with regard to localization of the process and the underlying mechanisms?

Is it possible that CPH with mechanical precipitation of attacks and cluster headache have a common denominator? Conceivably, hyper-excitable areas in the neck are activated in cases of CPH with mechanical precipitation. If this assumption is correct, then *reflex mechanisms* might come into play in these attacks, and sensory impulses from the nuchal area may be communicated to the trigeminal system in the brain stem. The signal could then be led to the same area where the autonomic phenomena of cluster headache presumably originate, i.e. the cavernous sinus area. The peripheral autonomic phenomena in the ocular area might be caused by retrograde impulses in the trigeminovascular system. In this way, the mechanism usually leading to attack may be 'short-circuited'. This is an extension of Kerr's principle (Kerr and Olafsen, 1961; Kerr, 1964) according to which nociceptive stimulation in the neck may give rise to *pain* in the trigeminal area. Such an extension does, of course, not have any firm scientific basis. There are, as outlined in the various sections in this book, clear differences between CPH and cluster headache, as far as autonomic features are concerned, i.e. differences between forehead sweating, pupils, and attack-induced intraocular pressure and corneal indentation pulse amplitudes. This probably indicates that the substrate for these manifestations differs somewhat in cluster headache and CPH. Otherwise, the CPH patients with mechanical precipitation of attacks could (would?) have had attacks showing cluster headache characteristics.

It is remarkable that orbital phlebographic changes have been found in various unilateral headaches, i.e. Tolosa–Hunt and Tolosa–Hunt-like disorders, cluster headache, and CPH (Hannerz *et al.*, 1987a). A necessary task in the immediate future will be to extend these investigations to include other unilateral headaches, and to explore the cavernous sinus area with other techniques. This may promote our understanding of the relative significance of the cavernous sinus area on the one hand, and the neck on the other, in the cluster headache syndrome.

Thus what role do the local changes in the neck play in the entire picture? Is the neck only a relay station in a cascade of events, ultimately leading to the pain attack? There is some evidence to suggest that there are also 'central' regulation disturbances in CPH. During heating experiments, CPH patients take longer than controls to reach an arbitrary limit of forehead sweating (which we have set at $>75 \mathrm{~g} \mathrm{~m}^{-2} \mathrm{~h}^{-1}$). Furthermore, when the sweating starts in CPH, it may start abruptly, and it may be most irregular with high 'peaks' and deep 'valleys'. It, therefore, seems as though there is, at least occasionally, a deficient thermoregulation with decreased sensitivity for temperature increase and an 'over-sized' reaction when the mechanism signalling overheating is finally activated (Sjaastad *et al.*, 1986). When nocturnal attacks were studied, there proved to be a temporal link to the rapid eye movement sleep phase in the patient in whom attacks can be readily precipitated mechanically.

Several patients have, furthermore, experienced that anxiety may reduce the tendency to attacks, whereas looking forward to something might bring on attacks.

It will be understood that, despite the presented examples, there are so far no hard and fast pieces of evidence that point to a 'central' origin of CPH. My present view is that the cavernous sinus area is the locus of crucial pathology in both cluster headache and CPH. The relative independence of cervical factors seems to be much more marked in cluster headache than in CPH. Maybe cluster headache is absolutely independent of cervical influence. Mechanically precipitated attacks of CPH seem to be largely influenced by cervical factors. 'Ordinary' CPH (without mechanically precipitated attacks) may take an intermediate position, possibly having some connections with the neck, and possibly being more dependent on local abnormality in the cavernous sinus. This intermediate position cannot be defined accurately at the present time. The interplay between 'central' and cervical structures in the pathogenesis of these attacks is not fully understood at present. They may both be necessary factors for the generation of the attack.

References

Adams RD and Victor M (1985) *Principles of Neurology*, 3rd edn. New York: McGraw-Hill.

Ad Hoc Committee on Classification of Headache (1962) Classification of headache. *JAMA* **179**:717–718.

Adler CS, Adler SM and Graham JR (1987) Psychodynamics of cluster headache. In: Adler CS, Adler SM and Packard RW (Eds), *Psychiatric Aspects of Headache*, pp. 212–234. Baltimore: Williams & Wilkins.

Agnoli A and De Marinis M (1987) Trigeminal control of cranio-facial vasomotor response: its possible role in cluster headache. In: Sicuteri F, Vecchiet L and Fanciullacci M (Eds), *Trends in Cluster Headache*, pp. 283–381. Amsterdam: Excerpta Medica.

Ala-Hurula V, Myllylä VV, Arvela P, Kärki NT and Hokkanen E (1979) Systemic availability of ergotamine tartrate after three successive doses and during continuous medication. *Eur J Clin Pharmacol* **16**:355–360.

Alessi R, Nusynowitz M, Abildskob JA and Moe GK (1958) Non-uniform distribution of vagal effects on the atrial refractory period. *Am J Physiol* **194**:406–410.

Alford RI and Whitehouse FR (1945) Histamine cephalalgia with duodenal ulcer. *Ann Allergy* **3**:200–203.

Alvarez-Cermeno JC, Ferandez JM, O'Neill TA, Moral L and Saiz-Ruiz J. (1989) Lithium-induced headache. *Headache* **29**:246–247.

Andersson PG (1985) Migraine in patients with cluster headache. *Cephalalgia* **5**:11–16.

Andersson PG and Jespersen LT (1986) Dihydroergotamine nasal spray in the treatment of attacks of cluster headache: a double-blind trial versus placebo. *Cephalalgia* **6**:51–54.

Anselmi B, Baldi E, Cassacci F and Salmon S (1980) Endogenous opioids in cerebrospinal fluid and blood in idiopathic headache sufferers. *Headache* **20**:294–299.

Anthony M (1985) Arrest of attacks of cluster headache by local steroid injection of the occipital nerve. In: Rose FC (Ed), *Migraine*, pp. 169–173. Basel: Karger.

Anthony M and Lance JW (1971a) Histamine and serotonin in cluster headache. *Arch Neurol* **25**:225–231.

Anthony M and Lance JW (1971b) Whole blood histamine and plasma serotonin in cluster headache. *Aust Assoc Neurol* **8**:43–46.

Anthony M, Hinterberger H and Lance JW (1969) The possible relationship of serotonin to the migraine syndrome. *Res Clin Stud Headache* **21**:25–59.

Anthony M, Lord GDA and Lance JW (1978) Controlled trials of cimetidine in migraine and cluster headache. *Headache* **18**:261–264.

Antonaci F and Sjaastad O (1989) Chronic paroxysmal hemicrania (CPH): a review of clinical manifestations. *Headache* **29**:648–656.

Antonaci F, Sand T and Sjaastad O (1988) Sweating patterns in humans: I. Exercise- and pilocarpine-induced forehead sweating in healthy individuals. *Funct Neurol* **3**:89–94.

Antonaci F, Fredriksen TA, Sand T, Wysocka-Bakowska MM, Salvesen R, Bogucki A, Seim A and Sjaastad O (1989) Electronic pupillometry in healthy controls. Response to sympathicomimetics. *Funct Neurol* **4**:20–32.

Appenzeller O (1970) The autonomic nervous system. In: Vinken PJ and Bruyn GW (Eds), *Handbook of Clinical Neurology*, Vol. V, pp. 427–535. Amsterdam: North-Holland.

Appenzeller O, Becker W and Ragaz A (1978) Cluster headache. Ultra-structural aspects. *Neurology* **28**:371.

Appenzeller O, Becker WJ and Ragaz A (1981a) Cluster headache: Ultrastructural aspects and pathogenetic mechanisms. *Arch Neurol* **38**:302–306.

Appenzeller O, Atkinson RA and Standefer JC (1981b) Serum β-endorphin in cluster headache and common migraine. In: Clifford Rose F and Zilka E (Eds), *Progress in Migraine*, pp. 106–109. London: Pitman.

Ash ASF and Schild HO (1966) Receptor mediating some actions of histamine. *Br J Pharmacol* **27**:427–439.

Aubry M and Pialoux P (1968) Sluder's syndrome. In: Vinken PJ and Bruyn GW (Eds), *Handbook of Clinical Neurology*, Vol. V, pp. 326–332. Amsterdam: North-Holland.

Aver'ianov UN, Gordienko AF and Krotova IN (1983) Indomethacin-sensitive variant of migrainous neuralgia. *J Neuropath Psych* **12**:1796–1800.

Baldi E, Salmon S, Anselmi B, Spillantini MG, Copelli G, Brocchi A and Sicuteri F (1982) Intermittent hypoendorphinemia in migraine attack. *Cephalalgia* **2**:77–81.

Balla J and Walton JN (1964) Periodic migrainous neuralgia. *Br Med J* **1**:219–221.

Baringer JR and Swoveland P (1973) Recovery of herpes simplex virus from human trigeminal ganglion. *New Engl J Med* **288**:648–650.

Barré F (1982) Cocaine as an abortive agent in cluster headache. *Headache* **22**:69–73.

Barré F (1983) Thermography and tonometry in cluster headache. *International Headache Congress, Munich, September 1983, Book of Abstracts*, p. 103.

Barton JW and Margolis MT (1975) Rotational obstructions of the vertebral artery at the atlantoaxial joint. *Neuroradiology* **9**:117–120.

Beall G and Van Arsdel Jr PP (1960) Histamine metabolism in human disease. *J Clin Invest* **39**:676–683.

Bennett A, Magnæs B, Sandler M and Sjaastad O (1974) Prostaglandins and headache. In: *Background to Migraine. The Sixth Migraine Symposium*, pp. 12–13. London: The Migraine Trust.

Berde B, Cerletti A, Dengler HJ and Zoglio MA (1970) Studies of the interaction between ergot alkaloids and xanthine derivatives. In: Cochrane AL (Ed), *Background to Migraine*, pp. 80–102. London: W. Heinemann.

Bickerstaff ER (1959) The periodic migrainous neuralgia of Wilfred Harris. *Lancet* **i**:1069–1071.

Bickerstaff ER (1961) Basilar artery migraine. *Lancet*, **i**:15–17.

Bickerstaff ER (1968) Cluster headaches. In: Vinken PJ and Bruyn GW (Eds), *Handbook of Clinical Neurology*, Vol. V, pp. 111–118. Amsterdam: North-Holland.

Biemond A (1970) *Brain Diseases*. Amsterdam: Elsevier.

Bigo A, Delrieu F and Bousser MG (1989) Traitement des algies vasculaires de la face par injection de methylprednisolone dans la region du grand nerf occipital: 16 ca. *Rev Neurol (Paris)* **145**:160–162.

Bill A (1975) Blood circulation and fluid dynamics in the eye. *Physiol Rev* **55**:383–417.

Bill A, Stjernschantz J, Mandahl A, Brodin E and Nilsson G (1979) Substance-P: release on trigeminal nerve stimulation, effects in the eye. *Acta Physiol Scand* **106**:371–373.

Bill A, Mandahl A and Andersson S (1987) Role of tachykinins in the ocular response to noxious stimuli. In: Sicuteri F, Vecchiet L and Fanciullacci M (Eds), *Trends in Cluster Headache*, pp. 179–185. Amsterdam: Exerpta Medica.

Bille B (1981) Migraine in childhood and its prognosis. *Cephalalgia* **1**:71–75.

Bing R (1913) Lehrbuch der Nervenkrankheiten. Berlin, Ladischnikow.

Bing R (1930) Uber traumatische Erythromelalgie und Erythroprosopalgie. *Nervenarzt* **3**:506–512.

Bing R (1945) Lehrbuch der Nervenkrankheiten, 7th edn Basel: B. Schwabe & Co.

Bing R (1952) Histaminkopfschmerz oder Erythroprosopalgie. *J Nerv Ment Dis* **116**: 862–873.

Black JW, Duncan WAM, Durant GJ, Ganellin CR and Parsons EM (1972) Definition and antagonism of H_2-receptors. *Nature (London)* **236**:385–390.

Blau N (Ed) (1987) *Migraine*. London: Chapman and Hall.

Blumenthal LS (1950) Current histamine therapy. *Mod Med* **18**:51–53.

Blumhardt LD, Smith PEM and Owen L (1986) Electrocardiographic accompaniments of temporal lobe epileptic seizures. *Lancet* **i**:1051.

Boccuni M, Morace G, Pietrini U, Porciani MC, Fanciullacci M and Sicuteri F (1984) Co-existence of pupillary and heart sympathergic asymmetries in cluster headache. *Cephalalgia* **84**:9–15.

Bogduk N (1984) Headaches and the cervical spine. *Cephalalgia* **4**:7–8.

Bogduk N, Lambert GA and Duckworth JW (1981) The anatomy and physiology of the vertebral nerve in relation to cervical migraine. *Cephalalgia* **1**:11–24.

Bogucki A and Niewodniczy A (1984) Case report: chronic cluster headache with unusual high frequency of attacks. Differential diagnosis with CPH. *Headache* **24**:150–151.

Bogucki A and Kozubski W (1985) Indomethacin does not inhibit nitroglycerin-provoked cluster headache attack. In: Pfaffenrath V, Lundberg P-O and Sjaastad O (Eds), *Updating in Headache*, pp. 312–314. Berlin: Springer-Verlag.

Bogucki A and Kozubski W (1987) Cluster headache and chronic paroxysmal hemicrania: How to classify borderline cases? *J Neurol Neurosurg Psychiat* **50**:1698–1699.

Bogucki A and Prusinski A (1985) Cluster headache: histamine skin test in painful area. *Cephalalgia* **5**:91–94.

Bogucki A, Szymanska R and Braciak W (1984a) Chronic paroxysmal hemicrania: lack of pre-chronic stage. *Cephalalgia* **4**:187–189.

Bogucki A, Szymanska R and Braciak W (1984b) O nowoopisanej postaci samoistnych bolow glowni—ZW. przewleklej napadowej hamikranii (chronic paroxysmal hemicrania—zespól Sjaastada) *Neurol Neurochir Pol* **18**: 373–378.

Boiardi A, Bussone E, Martini A, di Giulio AM, Tansini E, Merati B and Panerai AE (1983) Endocrinological responses in cluster headache. *J Neurol Neurosurg Psychiat* **46**:956–958.

Boiardi A, Carenini L, Frediani F, Porta E, Sinatra MG and Bussone G (1986a) Visual evoked potentials in cluster headache; central structures involvement. *Headache* **26**:70–73.

Boiardi A, Gemma M, Porta E, Peccarisi C and Bussone G (1986b) Calcium entry blocker: treatment in acute pain in cluster headache patients. *Ital J Neurol Sci* **70**:531–534.

Boiardi A, Munari L, Milanesi I, Paggetta E, Lamperti E and Bussone G (1988a) Impaired cardiovascular reflexes in cluster headache and migraine patients: evidence for an autonomic dysfunction. *Headache* **28**:417–422.

Boiardi A, Frediani F, Leone M, Munari L and Bussone G (1988b) Cluster headache: lack of central modulation? *Funct Neurol* **3**:79–87.

Boniuk M and Schlezinger NS (1962) Ræder's paratrigeminal syndrome. *Am J Ophthalmol* **54**:1074–1084.

Bono G, Micieli G, Manzoni GC, Terzano MG, Covelli V, Sandrini G and Nappi G (1985) Chronobiological basis for the management of periodic headaches. In: Rose FC (Ed), *Migraine*, pp. 206–217. Basel: Karger.

Bordini C, Antonaci F, Stovner LJ, Schrader H and Sjaastad O (1991) Hemicrania continua. A clinical review. *Headache* **31**:20–26.

Boulant JA (1981) Hypothalamic mechanisms in thermoregulation. *Fed Proc* **40**:2843–2850.

Bourne PB, Smith SA and Smith SE (1979) Dynamics of the light reflex and the influence of age on the human pupil measured by television pupillometry. *J Physiol (London)* **293**:IP.

Bousser MG and Baron JC (1979) *Migraine et Algies Vasculaires de la Face*. Sandoz editions.

Brainin M and Eisenstädter A (1985) Lithium-triggered chronic cluster headache. *Headache* **25**:394–395.

Brickner RM and Riley HA (1935) Autonomic facio-cephalalgia. *Bull Neurol Inst New York* **4**:422–431.

Broch A, Hørven I, Nornes H, Sjaastad O and Tønjum A (1970) Studies of cerebral and ocular circulation in a patient with cluster headache. *Headache* **10**:1–8.

Brodal A (1969) Neurological anatomy in relation to clinical medicine, 2nd edn. London: Oxford University Press.

Bruyn GW (1984) Intracranial arteriovenous malformation and migraine. *Cephalalgia* **4**:191–207.

Bruyn GW Bootsma BK and Klawans HL (1976) Cluster headache and bradycardia. *Headache* **16**:11–15.

Bülow PM, Ibraeem JJ, Paalzow G and Tfelt-Hansen P (1986) Comparison of pharmacodynamic effects and plasma levels of oral and rectal ergotamine. *Cephalalgia* **6**:107–111.

Burn JH (1957) Acetylcholine and cardiac fibrillation. *Br Med Bull* **13**:181–184.

Bussone G, Giovannini P, Boiardi A and Boeri R (1977) A study of the activity of platelet monoamine oxidase in patients with migraine headaches or with 'cluster headaches'. *Eur Neurol* **15**:157–162.

Bussone G, Boiardi A, Merati B, Crenna P and Picco A (1979) Chronic cluster headache: response to lithium treatment. *J Neurol* **221**:181–185.

Bussone G, Sinatra MG, Boiardi A, Cocchini F, La Mantia L and Frediani F (1985) Auditory brainstem responses in headache. In: Clifford Rose F (Ed), *Migraine*, pp. 26–30. Basel: Karger.

Bussone G, Sinatra MG, Boiardi A, Frediani F, La Mantia L, Lamperti E and Peccarisi C (1986) Brainstem auditory evoked potential (BAEPs) in cluster headache (CH): new aspects for a central theory. *Headache* **26**:67–69.

Bussone G, Frediani F, Leone M, Grazzi L, Lamperti E and Boiardi A (1988) TRH test in cluster headache. *Headache* **28**:462–464.

Bussone G, Leone M, Vescovi A, Peccarisi C, Grazzi L and Parali EA (1989) Derangement of the hypothalamopituitary axis (HPa) in cluster headache: further considerations. *Cephalalgia* **9**: (Suppl. 10), 141–142.

Cala LA and Mastaglia FL (1976) Computerized axial tomography in patients with severe migraine. *Br Med J* **ii**:149–150.

Campbell AMG and Lloyd JK (1954) Atypical facial pain. *Lancet* **ii**:1034–1038.

Cannom DS, Graham AF and Harrison DC (1973) Electrophysiological studies in the denervated transplanted human heart: responses to atrial pacing and atropine. *Circ Res* **32**:268–278.

Cannon WB (1939) A law of denervation. *Am J Med Sci* **198**:737–750.

Caskey WH (1966) Cluster headache in a woman. Headache Rounds 12.1.1966. The Faulkner Hospital Boston, Mass. *Loc. cit.* Heyck.

Caviness VS and O'Brien P (1980) Cluster headache, response to chlorpromazine. *Headache* **20**:128–131.

Centonze V, Attolini E, Campanozzi F, Magrone D, Tesauro P, Vino M, Campanale G and Albano O (1987) Hemicrania continua: a new clinical entity or a further development from cluster headache? A case report. *Cephalalgia* **7**:167–168.

Charlin C (1931) Le syndrome du nerf nasal. *Ann Ocul* **168**:86–102.

Chazot G, Claustrat B, Brun J, Jordan D, Sassolas G and Schott B (1984) A chronobiological study of melatonin, cortisol, growth hormone and prolactin secretion in cluster headache. *Cephalalgia* **4**:213–220.

Chazot G, Claustrat B, Brun J and Zaidan R (1987) Effects on the patterns of melatonin and cortisol in cluster headache of a single administration of lithium at 7.00 a.m. daily over one week: a preliminary report. *Pharmacopsychiatry* **20**:222–223.

Chorobski J and Penfield W (1932) Cerebral vasodilator nerves and their pathway from the medulla oblongata, with observations on the pial and intracerebral vascular plexus. *Arch Neurol Psychiat* **28**:1257–1289.

Christoffersen B (1979) Kronisk paroxystisk hemicrani. *Ugeskr Læg* **141**:930–931.

Colle J, Duke-Elder PM and Duke-Elder WS (1931) Studies on the intraocular pressure. Part I. The action of drugs on the vascular and muscular factors controlling intraocular pressure. *J Physiol (Lond)* **71**:1–30.

Costen JB (1934) A syndrome of ear and sinus symptoms dependent upon disturbed function of the temporomandibular joint. *Ann Otol Rhinol Laryngol* **43**:1–15.

Costen JB (1951) The present status of mandibular joint syndrome in otolaryngology. *Trans Am Acad Ophthalmol Otolaryngol* 809–822.

Couch JR and Ziegler DK (1978) Prednisone therapy for cluster headache. *Headache* **18**:219–221.

Crawford N and Rudd BT (1962) A spectrophotofluorimetric method for the determination of serotonin (5-hydroxytryptamine) in plasma. *Clin Chim Acta* **7**:114–121.

Curless RG (1982) Cluster headache in childhood. *J Pediatrics* **101**:393–395.

Curran DA, Hinterberger H and Lance JW (1967) Methysergide. *Res Clin Stud Headache* **1**:74–122.

Cuypers J and Altenkirch H (1979) HLA antigens in cluster headache. *Headache* **19**:228–229.

Cuypers J, Altenkirch H and Bunge S (1979) Therapy of cluster headache with histamine H_1 and H_2 receptor antagonists. *Eur Neurol* **18**:345–347.

Cuypers J, Westphal K and Bunge S (1980) Mast cells in cluster headache. *Acta Neurol Scand* **61**:327–329.

Cuypers J, Altenkirch H and Bunge S (1981) Personality profiles in cluster headache and migraine. *Headache* **21**:21–24.

Dahl A, Russell D, Nyberg-Hansen R and Rootwelt H (1990) Cluster headache: transcranial Doppler ultrasound and rCBF studies. *Cephalalgia* **10**:87–94.

Dahl E (1973a) The fine structures of intracerebral vessels. *Z Zellforsch* **145**:577–586.

Dahl E (1973b) The innervation of the cerebral arteries. *J Anat* **115**:53–63.

Dahl E (1986) The ultrastructure of cerebral blood vessels. *Cephalalgia* **6** (Suppl. 4):45–48.

Dalessio DJ (1987) *Wolff's Headache and Other Head Pain*, 5th edn. New York: Oxford University Press.

Dalessio DJ, Waltz TH and Ott K (1983) Trigeminal cistern glycerol injections for facial pain. In: Pfaffenrath V, Lundberg P-O and Sjaastad O (Eds), *Abstracts of Papers Presented, 1st International Headache Congress*, Munich, p. 85.

D'Alessandro R, Gamberini G, Benassi G, Morganti G, Cortelli P and Lugaresi E (1986) Cluster headache in the Republic of San Marino. *Cephalalgia* **6**:159–162.

Dalsgaard-Nielsen T (1955) Migraine diagnostics with special reference to pharmacological tests. *Int Arch Allergy* **7**:312–322.

Dalsgaard-Nielsen T (1970) Some aspects of the epidemiology of migraine in Denmark. In: Klee A and Ulrich K (Eds), *Kliniske Aspekter i Migræneforskningen*, pp. 18–25. København: Norlundes Bogtrykkeri.

Damasio H and Lyon J (1980) Lithium carbonate in the treatment of cluster headache. *J Neurol* **224**:1–8.

D'Andrea G, Cananzi AR, Toldo M and Ferro-Milone F (1986) Platelet activity in cluster headache. *Cephalalgia* **6**:163–167.

Da Silva WF (1974) Consideracões sobre a enxaqueca e o sindrome de Horton. *Neurobiologia Recife* **37**:171–182.

Da Silva WF (1983) Cefaléia em salvas: quadro clinico e diagnostico differential. In: *32nd Encontro de Especialistas. III Curso de actualizacao em cefaleia*, pp. 10–15.

Day MD (1979) *Autonomic Pharmacology*. Edinburgh: Churchill Livingstone.

de Belleroche J, Cook GE, Das I, Joseph R, Tresidder J, Rouse S, Petty R and Rose FC (1984a) Erythrocyte choline concentrations and cluster headache. *Br Med J* **288**:268–270.

de Belleroche J, Cook GE, Das J, Joseph R, Tresider J, Petty R and Clifford Rose F (1984b) Choline levels in cluster headache. In: Corsini GU and Fanciullacci M (Eds), *Cefalea: Attuali Orientamenti Eziopathogenetici e Clinicoterapeutici*, pp. 65–67. Fidia Research Biomedical Information.

de Belleroche J, Kilfeather S, Das J and Rose FC (1986) Abnormal membrane composition and membrane-dependent transduction mechanisms in cluster headache. *Cephalalgia* **6**:147–153.

de Belleroche J, Morris R, Davies PTG and Clifford Rose F (1988) Differential changes in receptor-mediated transduction in migraine and cluster headache: studies on polymorphonuclear leucocytes. *Headache* **28**:409–413.

de Carolis R, Baldrati A, Agati R, de Capoa D, D'Alessandro R and Sacquena T (1987) Nimodipine in episodic cluster headache: results and methodological considerations. *Headache* **27**:397–399.

de Carolis P, de Capoa D, Agati R, Baldrati A and Sacquegna T (1988) Episodic cluster headache: short- and long-term results of prophylactic treatment. *Headache* **8**:475–476.

Del Bene E and Poggioni M (1987) Cluster headache in childhood: clinic and pharmacology. In: Sicuteri F, Vecchiet L and Fanciullacci M (Eds), *Trends in Cluster Headache*, pp. 313–322. Amsterdam: Excerpta Medica.

Del Bene E, Poggioni M and Sicuteri F (1985) The 'dysautonomic iris in cluster headache: a genetic marker of vegetative lateralization? In: Pfaffenrath V, Lundberg P-O and Sjaastad O (Eds), *Updating in Headache*, pp. 290–297. Berlin: Springer Verlag.

de Fine Olivarius B (1971) Hemicrania neuralgiformis chronica (Chronic migrainous neuralgia). *Proceedings of the Scandinav Migraine Society Annual Meeting, 1970*. Forskning och praktik. 1:8.

De Marinis M, Martucci N, Gagliardi FM, Feliciani M and Agnoli A (1984) Trigeminal control of cranio-facial vasomotor response: I. Histamine test in patients with unilateral gasserian ganglion lesions. *Cephalalgia* **4**:243–251.

de Souza Carvalho D, Salvesen R, Smith SE, Sand T and Sjaastad O (1988) Chronic paroxysmal hemicrania. XIII. The pupillometric pattern. *Cephalalgia* **8**:219–226.

Devoize J-L, Rigal F, Eschalier A and Tournilhac M (1986) Dexamethasone suppression test in cluster headache. *Headache* **26**:126–127.

Dexter JD (1974) Studies in nocturnal migraine. *Arch Neurobiol (Madr)* **37** (Suppl):281–300.

Dexter JD (1984) Sleep abnormalities in the chronic cluster headache patient. *Headache* **24**:171.

Dexter JD and Weitzman ED (1970) The relationship of nocturnal headaches to sleep stage patterns. *Neurology (Minneap)* **20**:513–518.

Dexter JD and Riley T (1975) Studies in nocturnal migraine. *Headache* **15**:51–62.

Diamond S (1982) Prolonged exertional headache: its clinical characteristics and response to indomethacin. *Headache* **23**:96–98.

Diamond S and Medina JL (1979a) Benign exertional headache, successful treatment with indomethacin. *Headache* **19**:249.

Diamond S, Mogabgab ER and Diamond M (1982) Cluster headache variant: spectrum of a new headache syndrome responsive to indomethacin. In: FC Rose (Ed) *Advances in Migraine Research and Therapy*, pp. 57–65. New York: Raven Press.

Dimitriadou V, Henry P, Mathiau P, Aubineau P and Brochet B (1989) Interrelations entre mastocytes et ners de l'adventice de l'artere temporale chez des sujets atteints de cluster headache. In: *Société Francaise d'Etudes des Migraines et Céphalées. Reunion 22 juin 1989, Paris, Book of Abstracts*, p.4.

Dinitz CR, Carvalho IF, Ryan J and Rocha e Silva M (1961) A micromethod for the determination of bradykininogen in blood plasma. *Nature (Lond.)* **192**:1194–1195.

Djupesland G (1975) Advanced reflex considerations. In: Jerger J (Ed) *Handbook of Clinical Impedance Audiometry*, pp. 85–126. New York: Dobbs Ferry/American Electromedics Corporation.

Døhlen H, Nornes H, Sjaastad O and Sjaastad ØV (1973) Histaminuria after parenteral L'histidine administration in man. *Acta Physiol Scand* **89**:51–60.

Drummond PD (1985) Thermographic and pupillary asymmetry in chronic paroxysmal hemicrania. A case study. *Cephalalgia* **5**:133–136.

Drummond PD (1988) Dysfunction of the sympathetic nervous system in cluster headache. *Cephalalgia* **8**:181–186.

Drummond PD (1988a) Autonomic disturbances in cluster headache. *Brain* **111**:1199–1209.

Drummond PD and Anthony M (1985) Extracranial vascular responses to sublingual nitroglycerin and oxygen inhalation in cluster headache patients. *Headache* **25**:70–74.

Drummond PD and Lance JW (1984) Thermographic changes in cluster headache. *Neurology (Minneap)* **34**:1292–1298.

Duke-Elder S (1963) *System of Ophthalmology*, Vol. III. London: Kingston.

Dunér H and Pernow B (1956) Urinary excretion of histamine in healthy human subjects. *Scand J Clin Lab Invest* **8**:296–303.

Dunér H and Pernow B (1958) Determination of histamine in blood and urine by absorption on Amberlite IRC-50. With special reference to the normal values for histamine in the blood and an analysis of the specificity of the method. *Scand J Clin Lab Invest* **10**:233–240.

Dutta AK (1984) Chronic paroxysmal hemicrania. *J Assoc Phys India* **32**:537.

Duvoisin RC, Parker GW and Kenoyer WL (1961) The cluster headache. *Arch Intern Med* **108**:711–716.

Eadie MJ and Sutherland JM (1966) Migrainous neuralgia. *Med J Aust* **1**:1053–1057.

Eagle WW (1942) Sphenopalatine ganglion neuralgia. *Arch Otolaryngol* **35**:66–84.

Earl CJ and McArdle MJ (1968) Chronic migrainous neuralgia. In: Locke S. (Ed), *Modern Neurology*, pp. 583–588. Boston: Little, Brown & Co.

Edvinsson L (1985) Functional role of perivascular peptides in the control of cerebral circulation. *Trends Neurol Sci* **8**:126–131.

Egeberg O (1970) Factor XII defect and hemorrhage. Evidence for a new type of hereditary hemostatic disorder. *Thrombos Diathes Hemorrh (Stuttg)* **23**:432–440.

Ekbom KA (1947) Ergotamine tartrate orally in Horton's histaminic cephalgia (also called Harris's 'ciliary neuralgia'): a new method of treatment. *Acta Psychiatr Scand* **46** (Suppl):106–113.

Ekbom K (1969) Prophylactic treatment of cluster headache with a new serotonin antagonist BC 105. *Acta Neurol Scand* **45**:601–610.

Ekbom K (1970) *Studies on Cluster Headache*. Stockholm: Solna Tryckeri.

Ekbom K (1974a) Abortive attacks in episodes of cluster headache. *Arch Neurobiol (Madr)* **37**:191–194.

Ekbom K (1974b) Clinical aspects of cluster headache. *Headache* **13**:176–180.

Ekbom K (1974c) Litium vid kroniska symptom av cluster headache. *Opusc Med* **19**:148–156.

Ekbom K (1975) Some observations on pain in cluster headache. *Headache* **14**:219–225.

Ekbom K (1977) Lithium in the treatment of chronic cluster headache. *Headache* **17**:39–40.

Ekbom K (1986) Chronic migrainous neuralgia. In: Vinken PJ, Bruyn GW, Klawans HL and Rose FC (Eds), *Handbook of Clinical Neurology*, Vol. 4, pp. 247–255. Amsterdam: Elsevier.

Ekbom K (1987) Pathogenesis of cluster headache. In: Blau N (Ed), *Migraine*, pp. 433–448. London: Chapman and Hall.

Ekbom K and Kudrow L (1979) Facial flush in cluster (Editorial). *Headache* **19**:47.

Ekbom K and Kugelberg E (1968) Upper and lower cluster headache (Horton's syndrome). In: *Brain and Mind Problems*, pp. 482–489. Rome: II Pensiero Scientifico.

Ekbom K and Lindahl J (1971) Remission of angina pectoris during periods of cluster headache. *Headache* **11**:57–62.

Ekbom K and Olivarius B de Fine (1971) Chronic migrainous neuralgia — diagnostic and therapeutic aspects. *Headache* **11**:97–101.

Ekbom K and Waldenlind E (1981) Cluster headache in women: evidence of hypofertility (?): headaches in relation to menstruation and pregnancy. *Cephalalgia* **1**:167–174.

Ekbom K and Waldenlind E (1982) Reply to Peatfield *et al. Cephalalgia* **2**:172.

Ekbom K, Ahlborg B and Schele R (1978) Prevalence of migraine and cluster headache in Swedish men of 18. *Headache* **18**:9–19.

Ekbom K, Paalzow L and Waldenlind E (1981) Low biological availability of ergotamine tartrate after oral dosing in cluster headache. *Cephalalgia* **1**:203–207.

Ekbom K, Krabbe AAE, Paalzow G, Paalzow L, Tfelt-Hansen P and Waldenlind E (1983) Optimal routes of administration of ergotamine tartrate in cluster headache patients. A pharmacokinetic study. *Cephalalgia* **3**:15–20.

Ekbom K, Lindgren L, Nilsson BY, Hardebo JE and Waldenlind E (1987) Retro-Gasserian glycerol injection in the treatment of chronic cluster headache. *Cephalalgia* **7**:21–27.

Eliassen KA (1969) Metabolism of ^{14}C-histamine in domestic animals. *Acta Physiol Scand* **76**:172–181.

Elliot FA (1971) Clinical Neurology, 2nd edn. London: W.B. Saunders.

Emblem L (1964) Vasculær hodepine. *Tidsskr Nor Lægeforen* **5**:416–423.

Espadaler JM (1986) *Diccionario Enciclopedico de Cefaleas*. Barcelona: Salvat.

Eszenyi-Halasy M (1949) Histamine headache. *Br Med J* **i**:1121–1123.

Eulenburg A (1878) *Lehrbuch der Nervenkrankheiten*, 2nd edn, Vol. 2, pp. 264–274. Berlin: Hirschwald.

Eulenburg A (1883) Subcutane injectionen von Ergotinin — (Tauret) = Ergotinum citricum solutum (Gehe). *Dtsch Med Wochenschr* **9**:637–639.

Facchinetti F, Nappi G, Cicoli C, Micieli G, Ruspa M, Bono G and Genazzani AR (1986) Reduced testosterone levels in cluster headache: a stress-related phenomenon? *Cephalalgia* **6**:29–34.

Facchinetti F, Martignoni E, Gallai V, Micieli G, Mercantini F, Nappi G and Genazzani AR (1987) Naloxone test in primary headache sufferers. *Cephalalgia* **7** (Suppl. 6), 39–42.

Facchinetti F, Martignoni E, Gallai V, Micieli G, Petralgia F, Nappi G and Genazzani AR (1988) Neuroendocrine evaluation of central opiate activity in primary headache disorders. *Pain* **34**:29–33.

Fagius J (1985) Muscle nerve sympathetic activity in migraine. Lack of abnormality. *Cephalalgia* **5**:197–203.

Fahlgren H (1986) Retropharyngeal tendinitis. *Cephalalgia* **6**:169–174.

Fanciullacci M (1979) Iris adrenergic impairment in idiopathic headache. *Headache* **19**:8–13.

Fanciullacci M, Pietrini U, Gatto G, Boccuni M and Sicuteri F (1982) Latent dysautonomic pupillary lateralization in cluster headache: a pupillometric study. *Cephalalgia* **2**:135–144.

Fanciullacci M, Pietrini U, Boccuni M, Gatto G and Gangi F (1983) Does lithium balance the neuronal bilateral asymmetries in cluster headache? *Cephalalgia* **3** (Suppl. 1):85–87.

Fanciullacci M, Murialdo G, Gatto G, Filippi U, De Palma D, Polleri A and Sicuteri F (1987) Further appraisal of sex hormones set up in cluster headache. *Cephalalgia* **7** (Suppl. 6):82–83.

Fanciullacci M, Pietrini U, Geppetti P, Nicolodi M, Curradi C and Sicuteri F (1988a) Substance-P in the human iris: possible involvement in echothiophate-induced miosis in cluster headache. *Cephalalgia* **8**:49–53.

Fanciullacci M, Pietrini U, Fusco BM, Alessandri M, Marabini S and Sicuteri F (1988b) Does anisocoria by clonidine reflect a central sympathetic dysfunction in cluster headache? *Clin Neuropharmacol* **11**:56–62.

Fanciullacci M, Fusco BM, Alessandri M, Campagnolo V and Sicuteri F (1989) Unilateral impairment of pupillary response to trigeminal nerve stimulation in cluster headache. *Pain* 36:185–191.

Fay T (1927) Atypical neuralgia. *Arch Neurol Psychiat* 18:309–313.

Fay T (1932) Atypical facial neuralgia, a syndrome of vascular pain. *Ann Otol Rhinol Laryngol* 41:1030–1062.

Ferrari E, Canepari C, Bossolo PA, Vailati A, Martignoni E, Micieli G and Nappi G (1983) Changes in biological rhythms in primary headache syndromes. *Cephalalgia* 3 (Suppl. 1):58–68.

Firenze C, Del Gatto F, Mazzotta G and Gallai V (1988) Somatosensory-evoked potential study in headache patients. *Cephalalgia* 8:157–162.

Firenze C, Gallai V, Del Gatto F, Galafi F and Bruni A (1989) Dysfunction of the autonomic nervous system in the cluster headache. *Cephalalgia* 9 (Suppl. 10):147.

Fisher CM (1968) Headache in cerebrovascular disease. In: Vinken PJ and Bruyn GW (Eds), *Handbook of Clinical Neurology*, Vol. 5, pp. 124–156. Amsterdam: North Holland.

Fisher CM (1982) The headache and pain of spontaneous carotid dissection. *Headache* 22:60–65.

Fogan L (1985) Treatment of cluster headache: a double-blind comparison of oxygen v. air inhalation. *Arch Neurol* 42:362–363.

Ford FR and Walsh FB (1958) Raeder's paratrigeminal syndrome. *John Hopkins Med J* 103:296–298.

Fragoso YD, Seim A, Stovner LJ, Mack M, Bjerve KS and Sjaastad O (1988) Arachidonic acid metabolism in polymorphnuclear cells in headaches. *Cephalalgia* 8:149–155.

Fragoso YD, Stovner LJ, Bjerve KS and Sjaastad O (1989a) Cluster headache: incorporation of (1-^{14}C) oleic acid into phosphatidyl-serine in polymorphonuclear cells. *Cephalalgia* 9:207–211.

Fragoso YD, Seim A, Stovner LJ, Mack M, Bjerve KS and Sjaastad O (1989b) Cluster headache: increased incorporation of (1-C^{14}) arachidonic acid into phosphaditylserine in polymorphonuclear cells. *Cephalalgia* 9:213–220.

Fragoso YD, Stovner LJ, Bjerve KS and Sjaastad O (1989c) Increased incorporation of L-(U-^{14}C) serine into phosphatidylserine in polymorphonuclear cells from cluster headache patients. *Cephalalgia* 9:221–225.

Frazier CH and Russell EC (1924) Neuralgia of the face: an analysis of 754 cases with relation to pain and other sensory phenomena before and after operation. *Arch Neurol Physchiat* 11:557–563.

Frediani F, Lamperti E, Leone M, Boiardi A, Grazzi L and Bussone G (1988) Cluster headache patients' responses to dexamethasone suppression test. *Headache* 28:130–132.

Fredriksen TA (1988) Cervicogenic headache: the forehead sweating pattern. *Cephalalgia* 8:203–209.

Fredriksen TA (1989) Studies on cervicogenic headache. Clinical manifestation and differentiation from other unilateral headache forms. Thesis. Trondheim: Tapir.

Fredriksen TA, Hovdal H and Sjaastad O (1987) 'Cervicogenic headache': clinical manifestation. *Cephalalgia* 7:147–160.

Fredriksen TA, Wysocka-Bakowska MM, Bogucki A and Antonaci F (1988) Cervicogenic headache. Pupillometric findings. *Cephalalgia* 8:93–103.

Friedenwald JS (1957) Tonometer calibration: An attempt to remove discrepancies found in the 1954 calibration scale for Schiøtz tonometers. *Trans Am Acad Ophthalmol Otolaryngol* 61:108–123.

Friedman AP (1969) Atypical facial pain. *Headache* 9:27–30.

Friedman AP and Elkind AH (1963) Appraisal of methysergide in treatment of vascular headache of migraine-type. *JAMA* 184:125–128.

Friedman AP and Mikropoulos HE (1958) Cluster headaches. *Neurology (Minneap)* 8:653–663.

Furlow LT (1942) Tic douloureux of the nervus intermedius. *JAMA* 119:255–259.

Gabai IJ and Spierings ELH (1989) Prophylactic treatment of cluster headache with verapamil. *Headache* 29:167–168.

Gardner WJ, Stowell A and Dutlinger R (1947) Resection of the greater superficial petrosal nerve in the treatment of unilateral headache. *J Neurosurg* 4:105–114.

Gawel MJ and Krajewski A (1988) Intracranial haemodynamics in cluster headache. *Headache* 28:484–487.

Gawel MJ, Willinsky RA and Krajewski A (1989) Reversal of cluster headache side following treatment of arteriovenous malformation. *Headache* 29:453–454.

Geaney DP (1983) Indomethacin-responsive episodic cluster headache. *J Neurol Neurosurg Psychiat* 46:860–861.

Geppetti P, Brocchi A, Caleri D, Marabini S, Raino L and Renzi D (1985) Somatostatin for cluster headache attack. In: Pfaffenrath V, Lundberg P-O and Sjaastad O (Eds), *Updating in Headache*, pp. 302–305. Berlin: Springer Verlag.

Giacovazzo M, Martelletti P, Romiti A, Gallo MF and Juvara E (1984) Relationship between HLA-system in cluster headache and clinical response to lithium therapy. *Headache* 24:162.

Giacovazzo M, Martelletti P, Romiti A and Gallo MF (1985) Cutaneous responsiveness to histamine in cluster headache. In: Pfaffenrath V, Lundberg P-O and Sjaastad O (Eds), *Updating in Headache*, pp. 298–301. Berlin: Springer Verlag.

Gilbert GJ (1965) Ménière's syndrome and cluster headache: recurrent paroxysmal focal vasodilatation. *JAMA* 191:691–694.

Gilbert GJ (1970) Cluster headache and cluster vertigo. *Headache* 9:195–200.

Glaser MA (1928) Atypical neuralgia, socalled: a critical analysis of 143 cases. *Arch Neurol Psychiat* 20:537–558.

Glaser MA (1940) Atypical facial neuralgia: diagnosis, cause and treatment *Arch Intern Med* 63:340–367.

Glaser MA and Beerman HM (1938) Atypical facial neuralgia: an analysis of 200 cases. *Arch Intern Med* 61:172–183.

Glover V, Peatfield R, ZammitPace RM, Littlewood J, Gawel M, Rose FC and Sandler M (1981) Platelet monoamine oxidase activity and headache. *J Neurol Neurosurg Psychiatry* 44:786–790.

Gonzales G, Onofrio BM and Kerr FWL (1975) Vasodilator system of the face. *J Neurosurg* 42:696–703.

Graham JG (1988) Cluster headache and pain in the face. In: Hopkins A (Ed) *Headache*, pp. 111–139. London: W.B. Saunders.

Graham JR (1960) Use of a new compound, UML-491 (1-methyl-D-lysergic acid butanolamide), in the prevention of various types of headache. A pilot study. *New Engl J Med* 263:1273–1277.

Graham JR (1963) Seven common headache profiles. *Neurology* 13:16–23.

Graham JR (1964) Methysergide for prevention of headache: experience in five hundred patients over three years. *N Engl J Med* 270:67–72.

Graham JR (1972) Cluster headache. *Headache* 11:175–185.

Graham JR (1974) Treatment of cluster headache (workshop). *Sixteenth Annual Meeting: Am Assoc Study Headache*, June 1974 (recorded on tape).

Graham JR (1975) Some clinical and theoretical aspects of cluster headache. In: Saxena PR (Ed), *Migraine and Related Headaches*, pp. 27–40. Rotterdam: Erasmus Universiteit.

Graham JR (1984) Personal communication to the author.

Graham JR, Suby HI, LeCompte PR and Sadowsky NL (1966) Fibrotic disorders associated with methysergide therapy for headache. *New Engl J Med* 274:359–368.

Graham JR, Suby HI, LeCompte PR and Sadowsky NL (1967) Inflammatory fibrosis associated with methysergide therapy. *Res Clin Stud Headache* 1:123–164.

Graham JR, Rogado AZ, Rahman M and Gramer IV (1970) Some physical, physiological and psychological characteristics of patients with cluster headache. In: Cochrane AL (Ed), *Background to Migraine*, pp. 38–51. London: Heinemann.

Grammeltvedt A, Hovig T and Sjaastad O (1975) Electronmicroscopy of blood platelets in migraine and cluster headache. *Headache* 14:226–230.

Granerus G (1968) Effects of oral histamine, histidine and diet on urinary excretion of histamine, methylhistamine and 1-methyl-4-imidazole acetic acid in man. *Scand J Clin Lab Invest* 104:49–58.

Granerus G and Magnusson R (1965) A method for semiquantitative determination of 1-methyl-4-imidazoleacetic acid in human urine. *Scand J Clin Lab Invest* 17:483–490.

Green M and Apfelbaum RI (1978) Cluster-tic syndrome. *Headache* 18:112.

Greve E and Mai J (1988) Cluster headache-like headaches: A symptomatic feature? A report of three patients with intracranial pathologic findings. *Cephalalgia* 8:79–82.

Grinker RR and Sahs AL (1966) *Neurology*, 6th edn Springfield, IL: Charles C. Thomas.

Grønbæk E (1982) *Traumatic Cervical Pain Generators*. Scientific exhibition. Scand Neurosurg Soc 34. Annual Meeting, Trondheim.

Grønbæk E (1985) Cervical anterolateral microsurgery for headache. In: Pfaffenrath V, Lundberg PO and Sjaastad O (Eds), *Updating in Headache*, pp. 17–23. Munich: Springer-Verlag.

Gruiloff RJ and Fruns M (1988) Limb pain in migraine and cluster headache. *J Neurol Neurosurg Psychiat* 51:1022–1031.

Guerra PR (1981) Hemicranea cronica paroxistica. *Rev Invest Clin (Mex)* 33:57–60.

Hanes WJ (1969) Histamine cephalalgia resembling tic douloureaux, differential diagnosis and treatment. *Headache* 8:162–166.

Håkanson S (1981) Trigeminal neuralgia treated by the injection of glycerol into the trigeminal cistern. *Neurosurgery* 9:638–646.

Hannerz J (1985) Pain characteristics of painful ophthalmoplegia (the Tolosa–Hunt syndrome). *Cephalgia* 5:103–106.

Hannerz J (1989) A case of parasellar meningioma mimicking cluster headache. *Cephalalgia* 9:265–269.

Hannerz J, Ericson K and Bergstrand G (1984) Orbital phlebography in patients with Tolosa–Hunt syndrome in comparison with normal subjects. *Acta Radiol (Diagn)* 25:457–463.

Hannerz J, Ericson K and Bergstrand G (1986) A new etiology for visual impairment and chronic headache. The Tolosa–Hunt syndrome may be only one manifestation of venous vasculitis. *Cephalalgia* 6:59–63.

Hannerz J, Ericson K and Bergstrand G (1987a) Orbital phlebography in patients with cluster headache. *Cephalalgia* 7:207–211.

Hannerz J, Ericson K and Bergstrand G (1987b) Chronic paroxysmal hemicrania: orbital phlebography and steroid treatment. A case report. *Cephalalgia* 7:189–192.

Hardebo JE (1984) The involvement of trigeminal substance-P neurons in cluster headache. An hypothesis. *Headache* 24:294–304.

Hardebo JE (1986) An association between cluster headache and herpes simplex. *N Engl J Med* 314:316.

Hardebo JE, Krabbe AA and Gjerris F (1980) Enhanced dilatory response to histamine in large extracranial vessels in chronic cluster headache. *Headache* 20:316–320.

Hardebo JE, Ekman R, Eriksson M, Holgersson S and Ryberg B (1985) CSF opioid levels in cluster headache. In: Clifford Rose F (Ed), *Migraine*, pp. 79–85. Basel: Karger.

Hardebo JE and Elner A (1987) Nerves and vessels in the pterygopalatine fossa and symptoms of cluster headache. *Headache* 27:528–532

Hardebo JE and Ryberg B (1988) CSF findings in cluster headache indicative of inflammatory disease or reaction. In: *Proceedings of the Scandinavian Migraine Society*, p. 26.

Hardebo JE, Ekman R and Eriksson M (1989) Low CSF met-encephalin levels in cluster headache are elevated by acupuncture. *Headache* 29:494.

Hardesty WH, Roberts B, Toole JF and Royster HP (1961) Studies on carotid artery flow. *Surgery* 49:251–256.

Hardman RA and Hopkins EJ (1966) A survey of migrainous neuralgia. *J Coll Gen Practit* 11:195–200.

Harris MC (1961) Prophylactic treatment of migraine headache and histamine cephalalgia with a serotonin antagonist (Methysergide), *Ann Allergy* 19:500–504.

Harris W (1926) *Neuritis and Neuralgia*. London: Oxford Med. Publ.

Harris W (1936) Ciliary (migrainous) neuralgia and its treatment. *Br Med J* i:457–460.

Harrison RH, Rogado A and Graham J (1975) The measurement of unconscious hostility in migraine and cluster headache patients and normal controls. In: Kunkel R, Sjaastad O and Stensrud P (Eds), *The Bergen Migraine Symposium*, Sandoz-informasjon (Suppl.), pp. 35–36.

Hasan Z, Sjaastad O and Lundervold A (1976) An electroencephalographical investigation of patients with cluster headache. *Clin Electroencephalography* 7:203–207.

Hauge T (1954) Catheter vertebral angiography. *Acta Radiol (Stockh)* (Suppl. 109).

Headache Classification Committee of the International Headache Society (1988) Classification and diagnostic criteria for headache disorders, cranial neuralgias and facial pain. 1 edn. *Cephalalgia* 8 (Suppl. 7), 1–96.

Heatley RV, Denburg JA, Bayer N and Bienenstock J (1982) Increased plasma histamine levels in migraine patients. *Clin Allergy* 12:145–149.

Hellem AJ (1971) Metabolic disorders of platelets. *Adv Intern Med Chicago: Year Book Publ.* 17:171–187.

Henry PY, Vernhiet J, Orgogozo JM and Caille JM (1978) Cerebral blood flow in migraine and cluster headache. *Res Clin Stud Headache* 6:81–88.

Hering R and Kuritzky A (1989) Sodium valproate in the treatment of cluster headache: an open trial. *Cephalalgia* **9**:195–198.

Herzberg L, Lenman JAR, Victoratos G and Fletcher F (1975) Cluster headaches associated with vascular malformations. *J Neurol Neurosurg Psychiatry* **38**:648–649.

Heyck H (1960) Serotoninantagonisten in der Behandlung der Migräne und der Erythroprosopalgie Bing's oder der Horton-syndromes. *Schweiz Med Wschr* **90**:203–209.

Heyck H (1975) *Der Kopfschmerz*. Stuttgart: Georg Thieme Verlag.

Heyck H (1976) 'Cluster'-Kopfschmerz (Bing-Horton-Syndrom?). *Fortschr Neurol Psychiatr* **44**:37–50.

Heyck H (1981) *Headache and Facial Pain*. Stuttgart: Thieme-Verlag.

Hildebrandt J and Jansen J (1984) Vascular compression of the C_2 and C_3 roots—yet another cause of chronic intermittent hemicrania? *Cephalalgia* **4**:167–170.

Hochman MS (1981) Chronic paroxysmal hemicrania: A new type of treatable headache. *Am J Med* **71**:169–170.

Hoes MJAJM, Bruyn GW and Vielvoye GJ (1981) The Tolosa–Hunt syndrome—literature review: seven new cases and a hypothesis. *Cephalalgia* **1**:181–194.

Holmsen H (1986) Platelets and prostaglandins. *Cephalalgia* **6** (Suppl. 4):33–42.

Hornabrook RW (1964) Migrainous neuralgia. *NZ Med J* **63**:774–779.

Horner F (1869) Über eine Form von Ptosis. *Klin Monatsbl Augenheilkd* **7**:193–198.

Horton BT (1941) The use of histamine in the treatment of specific types of headaches. *JAMA* **116**:377–383.

Horton BT (1944) Head and face pain. *Trans Am Acad Ophthalmol Otolaryngol* **49**:23–33.

Horton BT (1952) Histamine cephalgia. *Journal Lancet* **72**:92–98.

Horton BT (1956a) Histaminic cephalgia: differential diagnosis and treatment. *Mayo Clin Proc* **31**:325–333.

Horton BT (1956b) Histaminic cephalalgia. *JAMA* **160**:468–469.

Horton BT (1957) Histaminic cephalgia: provocative tests. *Triangle* **3**:66–71.

Horton BT (1961) Histaminic cephalgia (Horton's headache or syndrome). *Md State Med J* **10**:178–203.

Horton BT (1964) Histamine cephalgia linked with upper respiratory infections. *Headache* **4**:228–236.

Horton BT and Magath TB (1932) An undescribed form of arteritis of the temporal vessels. *Mayo Clin Proc* **7**:700–701.

Horton BT, MacLean AR and Craig WM (1939) A new syndrome of vascular headache: results of treatment with histamine: preliminary report. *Mayo Clin Proc* **14**:257–260.

Horton BT, Peters GA and Blumenthal LS (1945) A new product in the treatment of migraine: a preliminary report. *Mayo Clin Proc* **20**:241–248.

Horton BT, Ryan RE and Reynolds JT (1948) Clinical observations on the use E.C. 110, a new agent for the treatment of headache. *Mayo Clin Proc* **23**:105–108.

Hørven I (1968) Dynamic tonometry. I. The dynamic tonometer. *Acta Ophthalmol (Copenh)* **46**:1213–1221.

Hørven I (1970a) Dynamic tonometry. II. Methods of corneal indentation pulse registration. *Acta Ophthalmol (Copenh)* **48**:23–38.

Hørven I (1970b) Dynamic tonometry. III. The corneal indentation pulse in normal and glaucomatous eyes. *Acta Ophthalmol (Copenh)* **48**:39–58.

Hørven I (1975) Corneal temperature in normal subjects and arterial occlusive disease. *Acta Ophthalmol (Copenh)* **53**:863–874.

Hørven I and Gjønnæss H (1974) Corneal indentation pulse and intraocular pressure in pregnancy. *Arch Ophthalmol (Chic)* **91**:92–98.

Hørven I and Larsen CT (1975) Contact probe for corneal temperature measurements. *Acta Ophthalmol (Copenh)* **53**:856–862.

Hørven I and Sjaastad O (1977) Cluster headache syndrome and migraine: ophthalmological support for a two-entity theory. *Acta Ophthalmol (Copenh)* **55**:35–51.

Hørven I, Nornes H, Syrdalen P and Tønjum A (1971a) Dynamic tonometry in carotid occlusive disease. *Acta Opthalmol (Copenh)* **49**:913–920.

Hørven I, Nornes H and Sjaastad O (1971b) Dynamic tonometry in migraine and cluster headache. In: Dalessio DJ, Dalsgaard-Nielsen T and Diamond S (Eds), *Proceedings of the International Headache Symposium*, pp. 103–110. Elsinore, Denmark. Basle: Sandoz.

Hørven I, Nornes H and Sjaastad O (1972) Different corneal indentation pulse pattern in cluster headache and migraine. *Neurology (Minneap)* 22:92–98.

Hørven I, Russell D and Sjaastad O (1989) Ocular blood flow changes in cluster headache and chronic paroxysmal hemicrania. *Headache* 29:373–376.

Hovdal H, Syversen GB and Rosenthaler J (1982) Ergotamine in plasma and CSF after i.m. and rectal administration to humans. *Cephalalgia* 2:145–150.

Hungerford GD, Du Boulay GH and Zilkha KJ (1976) Computerized axial tomography in patients with severe migraine: a preliminary report. *J Neurol Neurosurg Psychiatry* 39:990–994.

Hunt WE, Meagher JN, LeFever HE and Zeman W (1961) Painful ophthalmoplegia. Its relation to indolent inflammation of the cavernous sinus. *Neurology (Minneap)* 11:56–62.

Hunter CR and Mayfield FH (1949) Role of the upper cervical roots in the production of pain in the head. *Am J Surg* 78:743–749.

Hyndman OR and Wolkin J (1941) The pilocarpine sweating test 1. A valid indicator in differentiation of preganglionic and postganglionic sympathectomy. *Arch Neurol Psychiatry (Chic)* 45:992–1006.

Igarashi H, Sakai F, Suzuki S and Tazaki Y (1987) Cerebrovascular sympathetic nervous activity during cluster headaches. *Cephalalgia* 7 (Suppl. 6):87–89.

Iordanidis T and Sjaastad O (1989) Hemicrania continua: a case report. *Cephalalgia* 8:301–303.

Isler H (1986) A hidden dimension in headache work: applied history of medicine. *Headache* 26:27–29.

Isler H (1987) Independent historical development of the concepts of cluster headache and trigeminal neuralgia. *Funct Neurol* 2:141–148.

Jacobsen LB (1969) Cluster headache: a rare cause of bradycardia. *Headache* 9:159–161.

Jaffe NS (1950) Localization of lesions causing Horner's syndrome. *Arch Ophthalmol* 44:710–728.

Jammes JL (1975) The treatment of cluster headaches with prednisone. *Dis Nerv Syst* 36:375–376.

Janowitz HD and Grossman MI (1950) The response of the sweat glands to some locally acting agents in human subjects. *J Invest Dermatol* 14:453–458.

Janowitz HD and Grossman MI (1951) An exception to Cannon's law. *Experientia* 7:275.

Jensen NB, Joensen P and Jensen PJ (1982) Chronic paroxysmal hemicrania: continued remission of symptoms after discontinuation of indomethacin. *Cephalalgia* 2:163–164.

Jose AD and Collison D (1970) The normal range and determinants of the intrinsic heart rate in man. *Cardiovasc Res* 4:160–167.

Joubert J (1988) Cluster headache in black patients. A report of 7 patients. *S Afr Med J* 73:552–554.

Joubert J, Powell D and Djikowski J (1987) Chronic paroxysmal hemicrania in a South African black. *Cephalalgia* 7:193–196.

Julou L, Guyonnet J-C, Ducrot R, Gariet G, Bardone MC, Maignan G and Pasquet J (1971) Etude des propriétés pharmacologiques d'un nouvel antiinflammatoire l'acide (benzoyl-3-phenyl)-2 proprionique (19583 R.P.). *J Pharmacol (Paris)* 2:259–286.

Kahlson G and Rosengren E (1971) *Biogenesis and Physiology of Histamine*. London: Arnold.

Kahn D and Rothman S (1942) Sweat response to acetylcholine. *J Invest Dermatol* 5:431–444.

Kayed K and Sjaastad O (1985) Nocturnal and early morning headaches. *Ann Clin Res* 17:243–246.

Kayed K, Godtlibsen OB and Sjaastad O (1978) Chronic paroxysmal hemicrania. IV. 'Remlocked' headache attacks. *Sleep* 1:91–95.

Kerr FWL (1964) A mechanism to account for frontal headache in cases of posterior fossa tumors. *J Neurosurg* 18:605–609.

Kerr FWL and Olafson RA (1961) Trigeminal and cervical volleys: convergence on single units in the spinal grey at C_1 and C_2. *Arch Neurol* 5:17–18.

Kettler HL and Martin DJ (1975) Arterial stationary wave phenomenon in Tolosa–Hunt syndrome. *Neurology (Minneap)* 25:765–770.

Kilpatrick CJ and King J (1982) Chronic paroxysmal hemicrania. *Med J Aust* 1:49–50.

Kirsch RE, Samet P, Kugel U and Axelrod S (1957) Electrocardiographic changes during ocular surgery and their prevention by retrobulbar injection. *Arch Ophthalmol* 58:348–356.

Kittrelle JP, Grouse DS and Seybold ME (1985) Cluster headache. Local anaesthetic abortive agents. *Arch Neurol* **42**:496–498.

Klimek A (1982a) Gastrin levels in patients with migraine and cluster headache. *Eur Neurol* **21**:305–308.

Klimek A (1982b) Plasma testosterone levels in patients with cluster headache. *Headache* **22**:162–164.

Klimek A (1985a) Growth hormone and prolactin levels in the course of metoclopramide test in headache patients. *Endocrynologia Polska* **36**:19–27.

Klimek A (1985b) Leczenie bolu glowy Hortona przy pomocy testosteronu. *Neurol Neurochir Pol* **19**:486–489.

Klimek A (1985c) Badania immunoglobulin i uk: ladu dope: lniacza w bolu glowy Hortona. *Neurol Neurochir Pol* **19**:295–301.

Klimek A (1987) Cluster-tic syndrome. *Cephalalgia* **7**:161–162.

Klimek A, Szulc-Kuberska J and Kawiorski S (1979) Lithium therapy in cluster headache. *Eur Neurol* **18**:267–268.

Kobayashi Y and Freeman H (1961) Histamine metabolism by schizophrenic and normal subjects. *J Neuropsychiat* **3**:112–117.

Krabbe AA (1986) Cluster headache: a review. *Acta Neurol Scand* **74**:1–9.

Krable AA (1989) Early clinical experience with subcutaneous GR 43 175 in acute cluster headache attacks. *Cephalalgia* **9** (Suppl. 10):406–407.

Krabbe AA (1989a) Limited efficacy of methysergide in cluster headache. A clinical experience. *Cephalalgia* **9** (Suppl. 10):404–405.

Krabbe AA and Olesen J (1980) Headache provocation by continuous intravenous infusion of histamine. Clinical results and receptor mechanisms. *Pain* **8**:253–259.

Krabbe AA and Rank F (1985) Histological examinations of the superficial temporal artery in patients suffering from cluster headache. *Cephalalgia* **5** (Suppl. 3):282–283.

Krabbe AA, Henriksen L and Olesen J (1984) Tomographic determination of cerebral blood flow during attacks of cluster headache. *Cephalalgia* **4**:17–23.

Kristiansen K and Krog J (1962) Electromagnetic studies on the blood flow through the carotid system in man. *Neurology (Minneap)* **12**:20.

Krog J (1964a) Autonomic nervous control of the cerebral blood flow in man. *J Oslo City Hosp* **14**:25–33.

Krog J (1964b) The effect of cervical sympathetic stimulation on cerebral blood flow in dogs. *J Oslo City Hosp* **14**:3–15.

Krüger H (1989) Different effects of bupidine for the prophylactic treatment of cluster headache, cluster migraine, and migraine. *Cephalalgia* **9** (Suppl. 10):408–409.

Krüger H, Kohlepp W, Reimann G and Przuntek H (1988) Prophylactic treatment of cluster headache with budipine. *Headache* **28**:344–346.

Kudrow L (1976a) Prevalence of migraine, peptic ulcer, coronary heart disease and hypertension in cluster headache. *Headache* **16**:66–69.

Kudrow L (1976b) Plasma testosterone levels in cluster headache: preliminary results. *Headache* **16**:28–31.

Kudrow L (1977) Lithium prophylaxis for chronic cluster headache. *Headache* **17**:15–18.

Kudrow L (1978) HLA-antigens in cluster headache and classical migraine. *Headache* **18**:167–168.

Kudrow L (1980) *Cluster Headache: Mechanisms and Management.* New York: Oxford University Press.

Kudrow L (1981) Response of cluster headache attacks to oxygen inhalation. *Headache* **21**:1–4.

Kudrow L (1983) A possible role of the carotid body in the pathogenesis of cluster headache. *Cephalalgia* **3**:241–247.

Kudrow L (1985) Treatment-resistant cluster headache. *Cephalalgia* **5** (Suppl. 3):270.

Kudrow L (1987) The cyclic relationship of natural illumination to cluster period frequency. *Cephalalgia* **7** (Suppl. 6):76–78.

Kudrow L (1987b) Subchronic cluster headache. *Headache* **27**:197–200.

Kudrow L (1989) An association of cluster headache onset and sustained oxygen desaturation. *Cephalalgia*, **9** (Suppl. 10):57–58.

Kudrow D and Kudrow L (1989) Successful aspirin prophylaxis in a child with chronic paroxysmal hemicrania. *Headache* **29**:280–281.

Kudrow L and Sutkus BJ (1979) MMPI pattern specificity in primary headache disorders. *Headache* **19**:18–24.

Kudrow L, McGinty DJ, Phillips ER and Stevenson M (1984) Sleep apnea in cluster headache. *Cephalalgia* **4**;33–38.

Kudrow L, Esperanza P and Vijayan N (1987) Episodic paroxysmal hemicrania? *Cephalalgia* **7**:197–201.

Kunkel RS (1981) Eleven clues to cluster headache—and tips on drug therapy. *Mod Med Aust* **Sep**:14–21.

Kunkel RS and Dohn DF (1974) Surgical treatment of chronic migrainous neuralgia. *Cleve Clin Q* **41**:189–192.

Kunkle EC (1959) Acetylcholine in the mechanism of headache of the migraine type. *Arch Neurol Psychiat* **84**:135–141.

Kunkle EC (1982) Clues in the tempos of cluster headache. *Headache* **22**:158–161.

Kunkle EC and Anderson WB (1960) Dual mechanisms of eye signs of headache in cluster pattern. *Trans Am Neurol Assoc* **85**:75–79.

Kunkle EC and Anderson WB (1961) Significance of minor eye signs in headache of migraine type. *Arch Ophthalmol* **65**:504–508.

Kunkle EC, Pfeiffer Jr JB, Wilhoit WM and Hamrick Jr LW (1952) Recurrent brief headaches in 'cluster' pattern. *Trans Am Neurol Assoc* **77**:240–243.

Kunkle EC, Pfeiffer JB, Wilhoit WM and Hamrick Jr LW (1954) Recurrent brief headaches in 'cluster' pattern. *NC Med J* **15**:510–512.

Kuritzky A (1984) Cluster headache-like pain caused by an upper cervical meningioma. *Cephalalgia* **4**:185–189.

Lance JW (1982) *Mechanisms and Management of Headache*, 4th edn. London: Butterworth.

Lance JW and Anthony M (1971a) Migrainous neuralgia or cluster headache? *J Neurol Sci* **13**:401–414.

Lance JW and Anthony M (1971b) Thermographic studies in vascular headache. *Med J Aust* **1**:240–243.

Lance JW, Fine RD and Curran DA (1963) An evaluation of methysergide in the prevention of migraine and other vascular headaches. *Med J Aust* **1**;814–818.

Leblanc B, Dordain G and Tournilhac M (1980) Indomethacin treatment of chronic paroxystic hemicrania. In: *Prostaglandin Synthetase Inhibitors: New Clinical Applications*, pp. 221–224. New York: A. R. Liss.

Ledermann RJ and Salanga V (1976) Fibromuscular dysplasia of the internal carotid artery—a cause of Raeder's paratrigeminal syndrome. *Neurology* **26**:353.

Lembeck F (1983) Sir Thomas Lewis's nocifensor system, histamine and substance-P-containing primary efferent neurons. *Trends Neurol Sci* **6**:106–108.

Lembeck F and Holzer P (1979) Substance-P mediator of antidromic vasodilation and neurogenic plasma extravasation. *Naunyn Schmiedebergs Arch Pharmacol* **310**:175–183.

Levy MN and Zieske H (1969) Autonomic control of cardiac pacemaker activity and atrioventricular transmission. *J Appl Physiol* **27**:465–470.

Levyman C, D'Agua Filho AdSP, Volpato MM, Settanni FAP and Lima WC (1991) Epidermoid tumour of the posterior fossa causing multiple facial pain—a case report. *Cephalalgia* **11**:33–36.

Liberski PP (1980) Zmiany ilosciowe komorektucznych skory okolicy skroniowej w bolu glowny Hortona. *Patol Pol* **31**:425–428.

Liberski PP and Prusinski A (1982) Further observations on the mast cells over the painful region in cluster headache patients. *Headache* **22**:115 117.

Liberski PP and Mirecka B (1984) Mast cells in cluster headache: ultrastructure, release pattern and possible pathogenetic significance. *Cephalalgia* **4**:101–106.

Lieder LE (1944) Histaminic cephalagia and migraine. *Ann Int Med* **20**:752–759.

Lindegaard K, Øvrelid L and Sjaastad O (1980) Naproxen in the prevention of migraine attacks. A double-blind placebo-controlled study. *Headache* **20**:96–98.

Lindell SE and Westling H (1966) Histamine metabolism in man. In: Eichler O and Farah A (Eds), *Handbook of Experimental Pharmacology*, Vol. 18, pp. 734–788. Berlin: Springer Verlag.

List CF and Peet MM (1938) Sweat secretion in man. I. Sweating responses in normal persons. *Arch Neurol Psychiatry* **39**:1128–1137.

Littlewood J, Glover V, Sandler M, Peatfield R, Petty R and Clifford Rose F (1984) Low platelet monoamine exidase activity in headache: no correlation with phenolsulphotransferase, succinate dehydrogenase, platelet preparation method or smoking. *J Neurol Neurosurg Psychiat* **47**:338–343.

Loewenfeld IE and Rosskothen HD (1974) Infrared pupil camera. A new method for mass screening and clinical use. *Am J Ophthalmol* **78**:304–313.

Loomis TA, Captain MC and Krop S (1955) Auricular fibrillation induced and maintained in animals by acetylcholine or vagus stimulation. *Circ Res* **3**:390–396.

Lovshin LL (1960) Vascular neck pain: a common syndrome seldom recognized, *Cleve Clin Q* **27**:5–13.

Lovshin LL (1961) Clinical caprices of histaminic cephalalgia. *Headache* **1**:3–6.

Lovshin LL (1963a) Use of methysergide in the treatment of extracranial vascular headache. *Headache* **3**:107–111.

Lovshin LL (1963b) Treatment of histaminic cephalalgia with methysergide (UML-491). *Dis Nerv Syst* **24**:3–7.

Lovshin LL (1977) Carotidynia. *Headache* **17**:192–195.

Macmillan JC and Nukuda H (1989) Chronic paroxysmal hemicrania. *NZ Med J* **102**:251–252.

Macmillan AL and Spalding JMK (1969) Human sweating response to electrophoresced acetylcholine: a test of postganglionic sympathetic function. *J Neurol Neurosurg Psychiatry* **32**:155–160.

Mainardi M, Maxwell V, Sturdevant RAL and Isenberg JI (1974) Metiamide, an H_2-receptor blocker, as inhibitor of basal and meal-stimulated gastric acid secretion in patients with duodenal ulcer. *New Engl J Med* **291**:373–376.

Malmros R (1973) Tractotomi ved migrænoid hovedpine. In: *Proceedings of the Meetings of the Scandinavian Migraine Society*. Copenhagen Meeting.

Maloney WF, Younge BR and Moyer NJ (1980) Evaluation of the causes and accuracy of pharmacologic localization in Horner's syndrome. *Am J Ophthalmol* **90**:394–402.

Mani S and Deeter J (1982) Arteriovenous malformation of the brain presenting as a cluster headache: a case report. *Headache* **22**:184–185.

Manzoni GC and Terzano MG (1979) Emicrania parossistica cronica: considerazioni a proposito di un caso. *Atti XXI Congresso Societa Italiana di Neurologica, Catania, 8–10 November*, p. 252.

Manzoni GC, Terzano MG and Moretti G (1981) A new case of 'chronic paroxysmal hemicrania'. *Ital J Neurol Sci* **2**:411–414.

Manzoni GC, Bono G, Lanfrachi M, Micieli G, Tezano MG and Nappi G (1983a) Lithium carbonate in cluster headache: assessment of its short- and long-term therapeutic efficacy. *Cephalalgia* **3**:109–114.

Manzoni GC, Terzano MG, Bono G, Micieli G, Martucci N and Nappi G (1983b) Cluster headache — clinical findings in 180 patients. *Cephalalgia* **3**:21–30.

Manzoni GC, Michieli G, Granella F, Martignoni E, Farina S and Nappi G (1988) Cluster headache in women: clinical findings and relationship with reproductive life. *Cephalalgia* **8**:37–44.

Mapstone R (1968) Determinations of corneal temperature. *Br J Ophthalmol* **52**:729–741.

Marchesi C, De Ferri A, Petrolini N, Govi A, Manzoni GC, Coiro V and Derisio C (1989) Prevalence of migraine and muscle tension headache in depressive disorders. *J Affective Disord* **16**:33–36.

Markowitz S, Saito K and Moskowitz MA (1988) Neurologically mediated plasma extravasation in dura mater: effect of ergot alkaloids. A possible mechanism of action in vascular headache. *Cephalalgia* **8**:83–91.

Martin RC (1942) Atypical facial neuralgia. *Arch Otolaryngol* **35**:735–739.

Masland WS, Friedman AP and Buchsbaum HW (1978) Computerized axial tomography of migraine. *Res Clin Stud Headache* **6**:136–140.

Mathew NT (1978) Clinical subtypes of cluster headache and response to lithium therapy. *Headache* **18**:26–30.

Mathew NT (1981) Indomethacin responsive headache syndromes. *Headache* **21**:147–150.

Mathew NT and Frost JD (1984) Sleep apnea and other abnormalities in primary headache disorders. *Headache* **24**:171.

Mathew NT and Hurt W (1988) Percutaneous radiofrequency trigeminal gangliorhizolysis in intractable cluster headache. *Headache* **28**:328–331.

Mathew NT, Meyer JS, Welch KMA and Neblatt CR (1977) Abnormal CT-scans in migraine. *Headache* **16**:272–279.

Maxwell RE (1982) Surgical control of chronic migrainous neuralgia by trigeminal ganglio-rhizolysis. *J Neurosurg* **57**:459–466.

McArdle MJ (1969) Variants of migraine. In: Smith R (Ed), *Background to Migraine*, pp. 1–9. London: Heinemann.

McElin TW and Horton BT (1945) Clinical observations on the use of benodryl: a new antihistaminic substance. *Mayo Clin Proc* **20**:417–429.

McElin TW and Horton BT (1947) Atypical face pain; a statistical consideration of 66 cases. *Ann Intern Med* **27**:749–768.

McGovern JP and Haywood TJ (1963) Histaminic cephalalgia. *Headache* **3**:39–40.

McKinney AS (1983) Cluster headache developing following ipsilateral orbital exenteration. *Headache* **23**;305–306.

Medina JL and Diamond S (1977) The clinical link between migraine and cluster headache. *Arch Neurol* **34**:470–472.

Medina JL and Diamond S (1981) Cluster headache variant. Spectrum of a new headache syndrome. *Arch Neurol* **38**:705–709.

Medina JL, Diamond S and Fareed J (1979) The nature of cluster headache. *Headache* **19**:309–322.

Merskey H (1979) *The Analysis of Hysteria*. London: Bailliére Tindall.

Merskey H (1981) Headache and hysteria. *Cephalalgia* **1**:109–119.

Merskey H (1983) Development of a universal language of pain syndromes. In: Bonica JJ (Ed), *Advances in Pain Research and Therapy*, pp. 37–52. New York: Raven Press.

Merskey H, Bond MR, Bonica JJ, Boyd DB, Carmon A, Deathe AB, Dehen H, Lindblom U, Mumford JM, Noordenbos W, Sjaastad O, Sternbach RA and Sunderland S (1986) Classification of chronic pain. Description of chronic pain syndromes and definitions of pain terms. *Pain* (Suppl. 3):1–226.

Meyer JS and Hardenberg J (1983) Clinical effectiveness of calcium entry blockers in prophylactic treatment of migraine and cluster headache. *Headache* **23**:266–277.

Meyer JS, Binns PM, Ericsson AP and Vulpe M (1970) Sphenopalatine ganglionectomy for cluster headache. *Arch Otolaryngol* **92**:475–484.

Meyer JS, Nance M, Walker M, Zetusky WJ and Dowell Jr RE (1985) Migraine and cluster headache treatment with calcium antagonist supports a vascular pathogenesis. *Headache* **25**:358–367.

Meyer JS, Hata T and Imai A (1987) Evidence supporting a vascular pathogenesis of migraine and cluster headache. In: Blau JN (Ed), *Migraine*, pp. 265–302. London: Chapman and Hall.

Micieli G, Facchinetti F, Martignoni E, Manzoni GC, Cleva M and Nappi G (1987) Disordered pulsatile LH release in cluster headache. *Cephalalgia* **7** (Suppl. 6): 79–81.

Micieli G, Magri M, Sandrini G, Tassorelli C and Nappi G (1988) Pupil responsiveness in cluster headache: a dynamic TV pupillometric evaluation. *Cephalalgia* **8**:193–201.

Micieli G, Cavallini A, Facchinetti F, Sances G and Nappi G (1989) Chronic paroxysmal hemicrania: a chronobiological study (case report). *Cephalalgia* **9**:281–286.

Milstein BA and Morretin LB (1971) Report of a case of sphenoid fissure syndrome studied by orbital venography. *Am J Ophthalmol* **72**:600–603.

Milton-Thompson GJ, Williams JG, Jenkins DJA and Miseiwicz JJ (1974) Inhibition of nocturnal acid secretion in duodenal ulcer by one oral dose of metiamide. *Lancet* **i**:693–694.

Minton LR and Bounds Jr GW (1964) Ræder's paratrigeminal syndrome. *Am J Ophthalmol* **58**:271–275.

Mokri B (1982) Ræder's paratrigreminal syndrome. *Arch Neurol* **39**:395–399.

Mokri B, Sundt Jr TM and Houser OW (1979) Spontaneous internal carotid dissection, hemicrania, and Horner's syndrome. *Arch Neurol* **36**:677–680.

Möllendorff V (1867) Uber Hemikranie. *Virchows Arch (Pathol Anat)* **41**:385–395.

Moore S (1955) *Hyperostosis Cranii*. Springfield, IL: Thomas.

Moskowitz MA (1984) The neurobiology of vascular head pain. *Ann Neurol* **16**:157–168.

Moskowitz MA (1988) Cluster headache: evidence for a pathophysiologic focus in the superior pericarotid cavernous sinus plexus. *Headache* **28**:584–586.

Moskowitz MA, Reinhard JF, Romero J, Melamed E and Pettibone DJ (1979) Neurotransmitters and the fifth cranial nerve: is there a relation to the headache phase of migraine? *Lancet* **ii**:883–885.

Moskowitz MA, Henrikson BM and Markowitz S (1986) Experimental studies on the sensory innervation of the cerebral blood vessels. *Cephalalgia* **6** (Suppl. 4):63–66.

Muhletaler CA and Gerlock AJ (1979) Orbital venography in painful ophthalmoplegia (Tolosa–Hunt syndrome). *Am J Roentgenol* **133**:31–34.

Murialdo G, Masturzo P, Filippi U, de Palma D, Balbi D, Fanciullacci M, Gatto G, Sicuteri F and Polleri A (1987) Integrative neuroendocrine approach to gonadotropine function in cluster headache. In: Sicuteri F, Vecchiet L and Fanciullacci M (Eds), *Trends in Cluster Headache*, pp. 361–370. Amsterdam: Excerpta Medica.

Murialdo G, Fanciullacci M, Nicolodi M, Filippi U, De Palma D, Sicuteri F and Polleri A (1989) Cluster headache in the male: sex steroid pattern and gonadotropic response to luteinizing hormone releasing hormone. *Cephalalgia* **9**:91–98.

Nappi G and Savoldi F (1983) *Le céfalée*. Milano: Workshop Italiana.

Nappi G, Ferrari E, Polleri A, Savoldi F and Vailati A (1981) Chronobiological study in cluster headache. *Chronobiologia* **2**:140.

Nappi G, Micieli G, Sandrini G, Martignoni E, Lottici P and Bono G (1983) Headache temporal patterns: towards a chronobiological model. *Cephalalgia* **3** (Suppl. 1):21–30.

Nappi G, Facchinetti F, Bono G, Petraglia F, Micieli G, Volpe A and Genazzani AR (1985a) Lack of β-endorphin and β-lipotropin circadian rhythmicity in episodic cluster headache: a model for chronopathology. In: Pfaffenrath V, Lundberg P-O and Sjaastad O (Eds), *Updating in Headache*, pp. 269–275. Berlin: Springer-Verlag.

Nappi G, Facchinetti F, Martignoni E, Petralgia F, Bono G, Micieli G, Rosachino G, Manzoni GC and Genazzani AR (1985b) Plasma and CSF endorphin levels in primary and symptomatic headaches. *Headache* **25**:141–144.

Nappi G, Facchinetti F, Martignoni E, Petralgia F, Manzoni GC, Sances G, Sandrini G and Genazzani AR (1985c) Endorphin patterns within the headache spectrum disorders. *Cephalalgia* **5** (Suppl. 2):201–210.

Nappi G, Micieli G, Facchinetti F, Sandrini G and Martignoni E (1987) Changes in rhythmic temporal structure in cluster headache. In: Sicuteri F, Vecchiet L and Fanciullacci M (Eds), *Trends in Cluster Headache*, pp. 351–359. Amsterdam: Excerpta Medica.

Nappi G, Sjaastad O, Raffaelli Jr E, Leston JA, Micieli G, Manzoni GC, Bussone G, Helde G, Dacua ASE, Martins OJ, Figuerola M and Bruera O (1989) Weather interference on cluster headache temporal pattern. A cooperative international long-term study. *Cephalalgia* **9** (Suppl. 10):195–196.

Nattero G and Savi L (in press) Cluster headache and hypertension: case report. *Cephalalgia*.

Nattero G, Savi L, Piantino P, Priolo C and Corno M (1985) Serum gastrin levels in cluster headache and migraine attacks. In: Pfaffenrath V, Lundberg P-O and Sjaastad O (Eds), *Updating in Headache*, pp. 306–311. Berlin: Springer-Verlag.

Nattero G, Savi L and Piantino P (1987a) Gastrin in cluster headache. In: Sicuteri F, Vecchiet L and Fanciullacci M (Eds), *Trends in Cluster Headache*, pp. 371–376. Amsterdam: Excerpta Medica.

Nattero G, Allais G, Biale L and De Lorenzo C (1987b) Cluster headache: a clinical model of 'lateralization of pain'? *Cephalalgia* **7** (Suppl. 6):341–342.

Nebudova J (1987) Chronic paroxysmal hemicrania. *Cez Neurol Neurochir* **50**:69–72.

Nelson RF (1970) Cluster migraine—an unrecognized common entity. *Can Med Assoc J* **103**.1026–1030.

Nelson RF (1978) Testosterone levels in cluster and non-cluster migrainous headache patients. *Headache* **18**:265–267.

Nelson RF, du Boulay GH, Marshall J, Ross Russell RW, Symon L and Zilkha E (1980) Cerebral blood flow studies in patients with cluster headache. *Headache* **20**:184–189.

Netsky MG (1948) Studies on sweat secretion in man 1. Innervation of the sweat glands of the upper extremity, newer methods of studying sweating. *Arch Neurol Psychiatry (Chic)* **60**:279–287.

Newsome DA and Loewenfeld IE (1974) Pilocarpine re-examined an old puzzle. *Surv Ophthalmol* **19**:399–424.

Nieman EA and Hurwitz LJ (1961) Ocular sympathetic palsy in periodic migrainous neuralgia. *J Neurol Neurosurg Psychiatry* **24**:369–373.

Nilsson GE (1977) On the measurement of evaporative water loss, Dissertation (No. 48), Linköping University, Linköping, Sweden.

Nilsson K, Lindell SE, Schayer RW and Westling H (1959) Metabolism of ^{14}C-labelled histamine in pregnant and nonpregnant women. *Clin Sci* **18**:313–319.

Nornes H, Hørven I and Tønjum A (1971a) Simultaneous recording of corneal indentation pulse and internal carotid blood flow. *Acta Neurol Scand* **47**:291–306.

Nornes H, Hørven I, Tönjum AM and Syrdalen P (1971b) Corneal indentation pulse in carotid occlusion disease. *Acta Neurol Scand* **47**:525–540.

Norris JW, Hachinski VC and Cooper PW (1976) Cerebral blood flow changes in cluster headache. *Acta Neurol Scand* **54**:371–374.

Ofstad E (1970) Formation and destruction of plasma kinins during experimental acute hemorrhagic pancreatitis in dogs. *Scand J Gastroenterol* **5** (Suppl. 5):1–44.

Okayasu H, Meyer JS, Mathew N, Amano T and Hardenberg J (1984) Lithium carbonate has no measurable effect on cerebral hemodynamics in cluster headache. *Headache* **24**:1–4.

Onofrio BM and Campbell JK (1986) Surgical treatment of chronic cluster headache. *Mayo Clin Proc* **61**:537–544.

Oppermann ICU (1747) *Dissertatio medica inauguralis de hemicrania horologica*. Halle.

Othmer E, Hayden MP and Sgelbaum R (1969) Encephalic cycles during sleep and wakefulness in humans: a 24-hour pattern. *Science* **64**:447–449.

Owman C and Hardebo JE (1986) Multiple transmitter amines and peptides in cerebrovascular nerves: possible links in migraine pathophysiology. *Cephalalgia* **6** (Suppl. 4):49–62.

Pavesi G, Granella F, Brambilla S, Medici D, Mancia D and Manzoni GC (1987) Blink reflex in cluster headache: evidence of a trigeminal system dysfunction. *Cephalalgia* **7** (Suppl. 6):100–102.

Pearce JMS (1980) Chronic migrainous neuralgia: a variant of cluster headache. *Brain* **103**:149–159.

Peatfield RC and Rose FC (1981) Exacerbation of migraine by treatment with lithium. *Headache* **21**:140–142.

Peatfield RC, Petty RG and Rose FC (1982) Cluster headache in women. *Cephalalgia* **2**:171.

Pelz M and Merskey H (1982) A case of pre-chronic paroxysmal hemicrania. *Cephalalgia* **2**:47–50.

Penman J (1968) Trigeminal neuralgia. In: Vinken PJ and Bruyn GW (Eds), Handbook of clinical neurology, Volume V, Amsterdam: North-Holland Publ. Co, pp. 296–322.

Peters GA (1953) Migraine: diagnosis and treatment with emphasis on the migraine tension headache, provocative tests and use of rectal suppositories. *Mayo Clin Proc* **28**:673–686.

Petty RG and Rose FC (1983) Chronic paroxysmal hemicrania: first reported British case. *Br Med J* **286**:438.

Pfaffenrath V, Mayer ET, Pöllmann W, Kufner GM and Auberger T (1984a) The cervicogenic headache: correlation of the symptomatology with results of a computer-aided evaluation of the cervical spine with special attention to the atlantoaxial articulations. *Migraine Trust Symposium. Book of Abstracts*, pp. 21–22.

Pfaffenrath V, Kufner G and Pöllmann W (1984b) Die chronisch paroxysmale Hemicranie (CPH). *Nervenarzt* **55**:402–406.

Pfaffenrath V, Pöllmann W, Rüther E, Lund R and Hajak G (1986) Onset of nocturnal attacks of chronic cluster headache in relation to sleep stages. *Acta Neurol Scand* **73**:403–407.

Pfaffenrath V, Dandekar R, Mayer E, Hermann G and Pöllmann W (1988) Cervicogenic headache: results of computer-based measurements of cervical spine mobility in 15 patients. *Cephalalgia* **8**:45–48.

Pickering GW (1933) Observations on the mechanism of headache produced by histamine. *Clin Sci* **1**:77–101.

Polich J, Aung M and Dalessio DJ (1987) Pattern-shift visual evoked responses in cluster headache. *Headache* **27**:446–451.

Polleri A, Nappi G, Murialdo G, Bono G, Martignoni E and Savoldi F (1982) Changes in the 24-hour prolactin pattern in cluster headache. *Cephalalgia* **2**:1–7.

Polleri A, Nappi G, Murialdo G, Sances G, Masturzo P and Savoldi F (1983) Neuro-endocrinological signs of central neurotransmission disorders. *Cephalalgia* **3** (Suppl. 1):122–128.

Polleri A, Bono G, Murialdo G, Martignoni E, Manzoni GC, Bonura ML and Nappi G (1983b) Gonadotropic function in cluster headache. In: Myllylä V and Tokola RA (Eds), *Twelfth Meeting of the Scandinavian Migraine Society, Helsinki*, pp. 58–59.

Porter M and Jankovic J (1981) Benign coital cephalalgia. Differential diagnosis and treatment. *Arch Neurol* **38**:710–712.

Pradalier A and Dry J (1984) Hémicranie paroxystique chronique. *Therapie* **39**:185–188.

Price RW and Posner JB (1978) Chronic paroxysmal hemicrania: a disabling headache syndrome responding to indomethacin. *Ann Neurol* **3**:183–184.

Procacci P, Zoppi M, Maresca M, Zamponi A, Fanciullacci M and Sicuteri F (1989) Lateralisation of pain in cluster headache. *Pain* **38**:275–278.

Prusinski A (1976) *Migrena*. Warszawa: Panstwowy Zaklad Wydawnictw Lekarskich.

Prusinski A and Liberski PP (1979) Is the cluster headache local mastocytic diathesis? *Headache* **19**:102.

Prusinski A, Liberski PR and Szulc-Kuberska J (1985) Cluster headache in a patient without an ipsilateral eye. *Headache* **25**:134–135.

Pöllmann W and Pfaffenrath V (1986) Chronic paroxysmal hemicrania: the first possible bilateral case. *Cephalalgia* **6**:55–57.

Ræder JG (1924) "Paratrigeminal" paralysis of oculo-pupillary sympathetic. *Brain* **47**:149–158.

Raffaelli Jr E (1979) Cefaléias chronicas e enxaqueca. Diagnostico e terapeutica. *Rev Terapeut Med* **11**:5–46.

Raffaelli Jr E (1984) Nomenclatura em cefaleia. *4th Encontro de Especialistas*, pp. 61–64.

Raffaelli Jr E (1986) Personal communication to the author.

Raffaelli Jr E, Martins OJ and D'Aqua Filho SP (1983) Lisuride in cluster headache. *Headache* **23**:117–121.

Raffaelli Jr E, Martins OJ and D'Aqua Filho SP (1985) Electronystagmography in chronic headache. *Cephalalgia* **5** (Suppl. 3):498.

Rapoport AM, Sheftell FD and Baskin SM (1981) Chronic paroxysmal hemicrania—case report of the second known definite occurrence in a male. *Cephalalgia* **1**:67–69.

Raskin NH (1987) Is the brain pain-insensitive? *Cephalalgia* **7** (Suppl. 6):23–25.

Raskin NH (1989) Cluster headache: localization. *Headache* **29**:579–580.

Raskin NH and Prusiner S (1977) Carotidynia. *Neurology (Minneap)* **27**:43–46.

Raskin NH and Schwartz RK (1980) Icepick-like pain. *Neurology (Minneap)* **30**:203–205.

Ray BS, Wolff HG (1940) Experimental studies on headache. Pain sensitive structures of the head and their significance in headache. *Arch Surg* **41**:813–856.

Rechschaffen A and Kales A (1968) A manual of standardized terminology, technique and scoring of sleep stages of human subjects. In: *Public health Publications No. 204*. Washington, DC: Government Printing Office.

Reik Jr L (1987) Cluster headache after head injury. *Headache* **27**:509–510.

Riley C and Moyer NJ (1971) Oculosympathetic paresis associated with cluster headache. *Am J Ophthalmol* **72**:763–768.

Robinson BW (1958) Histamine cephalalgia. *Medicine (Baltimore)* **37**:161–180.

Rogado AZ and Graham JR (1979) Through a glass darkly. *Headache* **19**:58–62.

Romberg MH (1840) *Lehrbuch der Nervenkrankheiten des Menschen*, Bd I, pp. 58–60. Berlin: Dunker.

Romiti A, Martelletti P, Gallo MF and Giacovazzo M (1983) Low plasma testosterone levels in cluster headache. *Cephalalgia* **3**:41–44.

Rooke ED (1968) Benign exertional headache. *Med Clin North Am* **52**:801–808.

Rooke ED, Rushton JG and Peters GA (1962) Vasodilating headache: a suggested classification and results of prophylactic treatment with UML 491 (methysergide). *Mayo Clin Proc* **37**:433–443.

Roseman DM (1967) Carotidynia. A distinct syndrome. *Arch Otolaryngol* **85**:81–84.

Roseman DM (1968) Carotidynia. In: Vinken PJ and Bruyn GW (Eds), *Handbook of Clinical Neurology*, Vol. V, pp. 375–377. Amsterdam: North Holland.

Roszkowski AP, Rooks WH, Tomolonis AJ and Miller LM (1971) Antiinflammatory and analgesic properties of d-2-(6-methoxy-2-naphthyl) proprionic acid (Naproxen). *J Pharm Exp Ther* **179**:114–123.

Rozniecki JJ, Kuzminska B and Prusinski A (1989) The possible mechanism of nitroglycerin induced cluster headache attack—a proposal explanation. *Cephalalgia* **9** (Suppl. 10):80–81.

Rugstad HE (1966) Kininase production by some microbes. *Brit J Pharmacol* **28**:315–323.

Russell D (1978a) Cluster headache. Histamine H_1 and H_2 antagonist treatment. *Acta Neurol Scand* **57** (Suppl. 67):264–265.

Russell D (1978b) Measurement of the pain-threshold and pain-tolerance in a cluster headache population. In: *Proceedings of the Meetings of the Scandinavian Migraine Society*, p. 27.

Russell D (1981) Cluster headache: severity and temporal profiles of attacks and patient activity prior to and during attacks. *Cephalalgia* **1**:209–216.

Russell D (1984) Chronic paroxysmal hemicrania: severity, duration and time of occurrences of attacks. *Cephalalgia* **4**:53–56.

Russell D (1985) Studies of autonomic functions in cluster headache syndrome, Thesis. Oslo.

Russell D and Lindegaard F (1985) Cluster headache: Doppler examination of the extracranial arteries. *Cephalalgia* **5** (Suppl. 3):276–277.

Russell D and Sjaastad O (1985) Chronic paroxysmal hemicrania: diagnosis and treatment. In: Pfaffenrath V, Lundberg P-O and Sjaastad O (Eds), *Updating in Headache*, pp. 1–6. Berlin: Springer-Verlag.

Russell D and Storstein L (1983) Cluster headache: a computerized analysis of 24 h Holter ECG recordings and description of ECG rhythm disturbances. *Cephalalgia* **3**:83–107.

Russell D and Storstein L (1984) Chronic paroxysmal hemicrania: Heart rate changes and EEG rhythm disturbances. A computerized analysis of 24 h ambulatory EEG recordings. *Cephalalgia* **4**:135–144.

Russell D and von der Lippe A (1982) Cluster headache: heart rate and blood pressure changes during spontaneous attacks. *Cephalalgia* **2**:61–70.

Russell D, Veger T and Sjaastad O (1977) Trial of a histamine H_2 receptor antagonist, cimetidine, in the treatment of cluster headache. In: Sicuteri F (Ed), *Headache: New Vistas*, pp. 191–199. Florence: Biomedical Press.

Russell D, Nakstad P and Sjaastad O (1978) Cluster headache—pneumoencephalographic and cerebral computerized axial tomography findings. *Headache* **18**:272–273.

Ryan RE (1950) Cafergone for relief of headache. A further study. *J Missouri Med Assoc* **47**:107–108.

Ryan RE (1951) A new agent for the treatment of migraine and histaminic cephalalgia. *J Missouri Med Assoc* **48**:963–965.

Ryan RE (1963) Modern concepts of the management of histaminic cephalalgia. *South Med J* **56**:1384–1387.

Ryan Sr RE and Ryan Jr RE (1978) *Headache and Head Pain*. St Louis: Mosby Comp.

Sachs Jr E (1968) The role of the nervus intermedius in facial neuralgia. Report of four cases with observations on the pathways for taste, lacrimation, and pain in the face. *J Neurosurg* **28**:54–60.

Sacquegna T, Cortelli P, Amici R, Pich EM, de Carolis P, Baldrati A, Cirignotta F, D'Alessandro R and Lugaresi E (1955) Cardiovascular changes in cluster headache. *Headache* **25**:75–78.

Sacquegna T, de Carolis P, Agati R, de Capoa D, Baldrati A and Cortelli P (1987) The natural history of episodic cluster headache. *Headache* **27**:370–371.

Sadjadpour K. Studies on cluster headaches role of cigarette smoking and incidence of oculosympathic palsy. In: Kunkel R, Sjaastad O and Stensrud P (Eds), *The Bergen Migraine Symposium. Sandoz-informasjon* (Suppl.):66.

Safer LA (1962) Cluster headache. Case report of a variant type. *Ohio State Med J* **58**:917.

Sakai F and Meyer JS (1978) Regional cerebral hemodynamics during migraine and cluster headache measured by the 133 Xe inhalation method. *Headache* **18**:122–132.

Sakai F and Meyer JS (1979) Abnormal cerebrovascular reactivity in patients with migraine and cluster headache. *Headache* **19**:257–266.

Salvesen R and Sjaastad O (1987) Cluster headache pathogenesis: a pupillometric study. *Cephalalgia* **7** (Suppl. 6):94–96.

Salvesen R, Fredriksen T, Bogucki A and Sjaastad O (1986) Sweating and pupillary responsiveness in Horner's syndrome. *Ups J Med Sci* (Suppl. 43):56.

Salvesen R, Fredriksen T, Bogucki A and Sjaastad O (1987a) Sweat gland and pupillary responsiveness in Horner's syndrome. *Cephalalgia* **7**:135–146.

Salvesen R, Bogucki A, Wysocka-Bakowska MM, Antonaci F, Fredriksen TA and Sjaastad O (1987b) Cluster headache pathogenesis: a pupillometric study. *Cephalalgia* **7**:273–284.

Salvesen R, de Souza Carvalho D, Sand T and Sjaastad O (1988) Cluster headache: forehead sweating pattern during heating and pilocarpine tests. Variation as a function of time. *Cephalalgia* 8:245–253.

Salvesen R, Sand T and Sjaastad O (1988a) Cluster headache: combined assessment with pupillometry and evaporimetry. *Cephalalgia* 8:211–218.

Salvesen R, de Souza Carvalho D and Sjaastad O (1989) Horner's syndrome. Sweat gland and pupillary responsiveness in two cases with a probable 3rd neuron dysfunction. *Cephalalgia* 9:63–70.

Salvesen R, Sand T, Zhao J-M and Sjaastad O (1989a) Cluster headache: pupillometric patterns as a function of the degree of anisocoria. *Cephalalgia* 9:131–138.

Sandler M (1972) Migraine: a pulmonary disease? *Lancet* ii:618–619.

Sandrini G, Micieli G, Magri M, Bono G and Nappi G (1984) Reattivita pupillare a stimoli esterocettivi nella cefalea a grappolo e nell'emicrania. In: Corsini GU and Fanciullacci M (Eds), *Cefalea: Attuali Orientamenti Eziopatogenetici e Clinicoterapeutici*, pp. 217–223. Italia: Fidia Research.

Sandrini G, Micieli G, Martignoni E, Bono G, Savoldi F and Nappi G (1985) Unilateral impairment of pupillary responsiveness to noxious stimulation of sural nerve in episodic cluster headache. In: Pfaffenrath V, Lundberg P-O and Sjaastad O (Eds), *Updating in Headache*, pp. 283–289. Berlin: Springer-Verlag.

Saunte C (1983) Quantification of salivation, nasal secretion and tearing in man. *Cephalalgia* 3:159–173.

Saunte C (1984a) Autonomic disorders in cluster headache, with special reference to salivation, nasal secretion and tearing. *Cephalalgia* 4:57–64.

Saunte C (1984b) *Cluster Headache Syndrome: Studies on Autonomic Dysfunctions*. Trondheim: Tapir.

Saunte C (1984c) Chronic paroxysmal hemicrania: salivation, tearing and nasal secretion. *Cephalalgia* 4:25–32.

Saunte C, Russell D and Sjaastad O (1983a) Chronic paroxysmal hemicrania. IX. On the mechanism of attack-related sweating. *Cephalalgia* 3:191–199.

Saunte C, Russell D and Sjaastad O (1983b) Cluster headache: on the mechanism behind attack-related sweating. *Cephalalgia* 3:175–185.

Saxena PR (1975) Two types of histamine receptors in a vascular bed of relevance to migrainous headaches. In: Diamond S, Dalessio DJ, Graham JR and Medina JC (Eds), *Vasoactive Substances Relevant to Migraine*, pp. 34–44. Springfield, IL: Thomas.

Schayer RW (1962) Evidence that induced histamine is an intrinsic regulator of the microcirculatory system. *Am J Physiol* 202:66–72.

Schayer RW and Cooper JAD (1956) Metabolism of ^{14}C-histamine in man. *J Appl Physiol* 9:481–483.

Schiffter R and Pohle P (1972) Zum Verlauf der absteigenden zentralen Sympathicusbahn. *Arch Psychiatr Nervenkr* 216:379–392.

Schirmer O (1909) Über den Einfluss des Sympathicus auf die Funktion der Tränendrüse. *Pfluegers Arch* 126:351–370.

Schlake H-P, Hofferberth B, Grotemeyer K-H and Husstedt IW (1989) Electronystagmographic investigations in migraine and cluster headache during the pain-free interval. *Cephalalgia* 9:271–275.

Schliack H (1962) Zum Problem der Schweissdrüseninnervation. *Nervenarzt* 33:421–423.

Schliack II and Simon J (1974) Über Sympathicusläsionen. *Aktuelle Neurol* 1:18–26.

Schroth G, Gerber WD and Langohr HD (1983) Ultrasonic doppler flow in migraine and cluster headache. *Headache* 23:284–288.

Scuk-Kuberska J and Klimek A (1979) Lithium treatment of chronic Horton's headache. *Neurol Neurochir Pol* 12:409–411.

Sejersen P (1971) *Measurement of Cutaneous Blood Flow by Freely Diffusible Radioactive Isotopes*. Copenhagen: Costers bogtrykkeri.

Selby G (1983) *Migraine and its Variants*. Sydney: ADIS Health Science Press.

Selmaj K and Pruszcynski M (1984) Nasal smears in cluster headache patients. *Headache* 24:120.

Selmaj K, de Belleroche J, Das I and Clifford Rose F (1986) Leukotriene B$_4$ generation of polymorphonuclear leucocytes: possible involvement in the pathogenesis of headache. *Headache* 26:460–464.

Selye H (1956) *The Stress of Life*. New York: McGraw Hill.

Shafar, J (1966) The syndromes of the third neurone of the cervical sympathetic system. *Am J Med* **40**:97–109.

Shore PA, Burkhalter A and Cohn VH (1959) A method for the fluorimetric assay of histamine in tissues. *J Pharmacol Exp Therap* **127**;182–186.

Sicuteri F (1959) Prophylactic and therapeutic properties of 1-methyl-D-lysergic acid butanolamide in migraine. *Int Arch Allergy* **15**:300–307.

Sicuteri F (1965) Termination of migraine headache by a new antiinflammatory vasoconstrictor agent. *Clin Pharmacol Ther* **6**:336–344.

Sicuteri F (1985) Symptomatologic interdependence or interindependence as a key alternative in migraine and cluster headache mechanisms. *Cephalalgia* **5** (Suppl. 2):233–235.

Sicuteri F (1988) Antiandrogenic medication of cluster headache. *Int J Clin Pharmacol Res* **8**:21–24.

Sicuteri D, Raino L and Geppetti P (1983) Substance-P and endogeneous opioids: how and where they could play a role in cluster headache. *Cephalalgia* **3** (Suppl. 1):143–145.

Sicuteri F, Geppetti P, Marabini S and Lembeck F (1984) Pain relief by somatostatin in attacks of cluster headache. *Pain* **18**;359–365.

Sicuteri F, Fanciullacci M, Geppetti P, Renzi D, Caleri D and Spillantini MG (1985) Substance-P mechanism in cluster headache: evaluation in plasma and cerebrospinal fluid. *Cephalalgia* **5**;143–149.

Sinforiani E, Farina S, Mancuso A, Manzoni GC, Bono G and Mazzucchi A (1987) Analysis of higher nervous functions in migraine and cluster headache. *Funct Neurol* **2**:69–77.

Sjaastad O (1966a) Urinary excretion of free and conjugated histamine in healthy individuals. *Scand J Clin Lab Invest* **18**:617–628.

Sjaastad O (1966b) Fate of histamine and N-acetylhistamine administered to the gut of man. *Acta Pharmacol Toxicol (Kbh.)* **24**:189–202.

Sjaastad O (1966c) Histamine formation after oral L-histidine in health and dystrophia myotonica. *Acta Med Scand* **180**:581–588.

Sjaastad O (1970) Kinin- and histamine-investigations in vascular headache. In: Klee A and Ullrich K (Eds), *Kliniske Aspekter i Migræneforskningen*, pp. 61–69. København: Norlundes Bogtrykkeri.

Sjaastad O (1975a) Is histamine of significance in the pathogenesis of vascular headache? In: Diamond S, Dalessio DJ, Graham JR and Medina JI (Eds), *Vasoactive Substances Relevant to Migraine*, pp. 45–66. Springfield, IL: Thomas.

Sjaastad O (1975b) Vascular and biochemical changes in migraine. In: Saxena PR (Ed), *Migraine and Related Headaches*, pp. 55–69. Rotterdam: Erasmus Universiteit.

Sjaastad O (1976) So-called 'vascular headache of the migraine type': one or more nosological entities? *Acta Neurol Scand* **54**:125–139.

Sjaastad O (1978) Pathogenesis of the cluster headache syndrome. *Res Clin Stud Headache* **6**:53–64.

Sjaastad O (1979) Chronic paroxysmal hemicrania (CPH). The clinical picture. In: Kärrlander G and Lundberg P-O (Eds), *Proceedings of the Scandinavian Migraine Society, 10th Annual Meeting*, Uppsala, 21–22 September 1979, p. 10.

Sjaastad O (1981) Evaporimetry in the cluster headache syndrome. In: Sjaastad O and Russell D (Eds), *Proceedings of the Scandinavian Migraine Society Meetings. Sandoz-informasjon 1981 (Suppl. 1)*, 41–42.

Sjaastad O (1982a) Cluster headache syndromet. *Sandoz-informasjon 1982a* **2**:1–11.

Sjaastad O (1982b) Chronic paroxysmal hemicrania (CPH)—a treatable headache entity. In: Gänshirt H and Soyka D (Eds), *Migräne. Ursachen-Therapie*, pp. 154–159. Stuttgart: Enke Verlag.

Sjaastad O (1983) Cluster headache: unilaterality as demonstrated by ictal forehead sweating. *Cephalalgia* **3** (Suppl. 1):88–90.

Sjaastad O (1985a) The so-called 'partial Horner syndrome' in cluster headache. *Cephalalgia* **3**:59–61.

Sjaastad O (1985b) Migraine and therapy. *Cephalalgia* **5**:121–123.

Sjaastad O (1986a) On the classification of cluster headache. *Cephalalgia* **6**:65–68.

Sjaastad O (1986b) Chronic paroxysmal hemicrania (CPH). In: Vinken PJ, Bruyn GW, Klawans HL and Rose FC (Eds), *Handbook of Clinical Neurology*, Vol. 4, pp. 257–266. Amsterdam: Elsevier.

Sjaastad O (1986c) Cluster headache. In: Vinken PJ, Bruyn GW, Klawans HL and Rose FC (Eds), *Handbook of Clinical Neurology*, Vol. 4, pp. 217–246. Amsterdam: Elsevier.

Sjaastad O (1986d) 'Cervicogenic headache'. *Sandoz-informasjon* **2**:13–16.

Sjaastad O (1987a) Headache and the influence of stress. A personal view. *Ann Clin Res* **19**:122–128.

Sjaastad O (1987b) Chronic paroxysmal hemicrania: recent developments. *Cephalalgia* **7**:179–188.

Sjaastad O (1987c) Chronic paroxysmal hemicrania (CPH) and similar headaches. In: Dalessio DJ (Ed), *Wolff's Headache and Other Head Pain*, 5th edn, pp. 131–135. New York: Oxford University Press.

Sjaastad O (1987d) 'Hemicrania continua'—new developments. *Cephalalgia* **7**:163–166.

Sjaastad O (1987e) Chronic paroxysmal hemicrania: clinical aspects and controversies, In: Blau N (Ed), *Migraine*, pp. 135–152. London: Chapman and Hall.

Sjaastad O (1988a) Cluster headache: on the inadequacy of existing hypotheses concerning the origin of the autonomic phenomena. *Cephalalgia* **8**:133–137.

Sjaastad O (1988b) Cluster headache: the possible significance of midline structures. *Cephalalgia* **8**:229–236.

Sjaastad O (1988c) Cluster headache and its variants. *Headache* **28**:667–668.

Sjaastad O (1989) Chronic paroxysmal hemicrania (CPH): nomenclature as far as the various stages are concerned. *Cephalalgia* **9**:1–2.

Sjaastad O and Antonaci F (1987) Chronic paroxysmal hemicrania: a case report. Longlasting remission in the chronic stage. *Cephalalgia* **7**:203–205.

Sjaastad O and Bjerve K (Eds) (1986) Prostaglandins and migraine. *Cephalalgia* **6** (Suppl. 4):1–110.

Sjaastad O and Dale I (1974) Evidence for a new (?) treatable headache entity. *Headache* **14**:105–108.

Sjaastad O and Dale I (1976) A new (?) clinical headache entity: 'chronic paroxymal hemicrania' 2. *Acta Neurol Scand* **54**:140–159.

Sjaastad O and Fredriksen TA (1986) Cluster headache syndrome: interrelationship of autonomic phenomena and pain. *Cephalalgia* **6**:3–5.

Sjaastad O and Haggag K (1987) Cluster headache: symptomatology and pathophysiology. In: Ferrari MD, Bruyn GW, Padberg G and Zitman FG (Eds), *Migraine and Other Headaches*, pp. 61–75. Leiden: Boerhaave.

Sjaastad O and Hørven I (1982) Indomethacin and headache. *Headache* **22**:90–92.

Sjaastad O and Salvesen R (1986) Cluster headache: are we only seeing the tip of the iceberg? *Cephalalgia* **6**:127–129.

Sjaastad O and Saunte C (1982) Sweating in cluster headache: patterns and possible underlying mechanisms. In: Rose FC (Ed), *Advances in Migraine Research and Therapy*, pp. 67–78. New York: Raven Press.

Sjaastad O and Saunte C (1983) Unilaterality of headache: Hauge's studies revisited. Cephalalgia **3**:201–205.

Sjaastad O and Saunte C (1984) Cluster headache: on the significance of the sweating abnormality—an editorial. *Cephalalgia* **4**:145–148.

Sjaastad O and Saunte C (1985) Unilaterality of headache. In: Pfaffenrath V, Lundberg P-O, and Sjaastad O (Eds), *Updating in Headache*, pp. 41–46. Berlin: Springer-Verlag.

Sjaastad O and Sjaastad ØV (1964) Urinary excertion of histamine in patients with headache. *Nord Med* **71**:526–527.

Sjaastad O and Sjaastad ØV (1970) The histaminuria in vascular headache. *Acta Neurol Scand* **46**:331–342.

Sjaastad O and Sjaastad ØV (1974) Catabolism of orally administered ^{14}C-histamine in man. *Acta Pharmacol (Copenh)* **34**;33–45.

Sjaastad O and Sjaastad ØV (1977a) Histamine metabolism in cluster headache and migraine: catabolism of ^{14}C histamine. *J Neurol* **216**:105–117.

Sjaastad O and Sjaastad ØV (1977b) Urinary histamine excretion in migraine and cluster headache. *J Neurol* **216**:91–104.

Sjaastad O and Spierings ELH (1984) 'Hemicrania continua': another headache absolutely responsive to indomethacin. *Cephalalgia* **4**:65–70.

Sjaastad O and Stensrud P (1969) Appraisal of BC-105 in migraine prophylaxis. *Acta Neurol Scand* **45**:594–600.

Sjaastad O and Tjørstad K (1987) 'Hemicrania continua': a third Norwegian case. *Cephalalgia* **7**:175–177.

Sjaastad O, Rootwelt K and Hørven I (1974) Cutaneous blood flow in cluster headache. *Headache* **13**:173–175.

Sjaastad O, Hørven I and Vennerød A-M (1976) A new headache syndrome? Headache resembling cluster headache (Horton's headache), with recurring bouts of homolateral retrobulbar neuritis, partial factor XII deficiency, bleeding tendency and a heterolateral convulsive episode. *Headache* **16**:4–10.

Sjaastad O, Djupesland G, Hørven I, Kayed K, Rootwelt K, Schrader H, Sundby A and Veger T (1977) Chronic paroxysmal hemicrania. A cluster headache variant. 3. Some new observations. In: Sicuteri F (Ed), *Headache: New Vistas*, pp. 123–137. Florence: Biomedical Press.

Sjaastad O, Russell D, Hørven I and Bunæs U (1978) Multiple neuralgiform, unilateral headache attacks associated with conjunctival injection appearing in clusters. A nosological problem. *Proceedings of the Scandinavian Migraine Society*, p. 31.

Sjaastad O, Egge K, Hørven I, Kayed K, Lund-Roland L, Russell D and Slørdahl Conradi I (1979) Chronic paroxysmal hemicrania. V. Mechanical precipitation of attacks. *Headache* **19**:31–36.

Sjaastad O, Apfelbaum R, Caskey W, Christoffersen B, Diamond S, Graham J, Green M, Hørven I, Lund-Roland L, Medina J, Rogado AZ and Stein H (1980) Chronic paroxysmal hemicrania (CPH): the clinical manifestations. A review. *Ups J Med Sci* **31**:27–35.

Sjaastad O, Saunte C, Russell D, Hestnes A and Mårvik R (1981) Cluster headache: the sweating pattern during spontaneous attacks. *Cephalalgia* **1**:233–244.

Sjaastad O, Russell D, Saunte C and Hørven I (1982) Chronic paroxysmal hemicrania. VI. Precipitation of attacks. Further studies on the precipitation mechanism. *Cephalalgia* **2**:211–214.

Sjaastad O, Russell D and Saunte C (1983a) Chronic paroxysmal hemicrania. VIII. The sweating pattern. *Cephalalgia* **3**:45–52.

Sjaastad O, Saunte C, Aasly J and Breivik H (1983b) Chronic paroxysmal hemicrania (CPH). Autonomic disturbances and mechanism of pain. In: Meyer JS, Lechner H, Reivich M and Ott EO (Eds), *Cerebral Vascular Disease*, pp. 268–269. Amsterdam: Excerpta Medica.

Sjaastad O, Saunte C, Hovdahl H, Breivik H and Grønbæk E (1983c) 'Cervicogenic' headache. An hypothesis. *Cephalalgia* **3**:249–256.

Sjaastad O, Saunte C and Russell D (1983d) Chronic paroxysmal hemicrania (CPH)—a treatable headache entity with a partly known pathogenesis. *Neuropsych Clin* **2**:79–85.

Sjaastad O, Saunte C and Breivik H (1984) Chronisch-paroxysmale Hemikranie. Eine Sonderform des zervicogenen (vertebragenen) Kopfschmerzes. In: Pfaffenrath V, Schrader H and Neu IS (Eds), *Primäre Kopfschmerzen*, pp. 9–16. München: MMV Medizin Verlag.

Sjaastad O, Saunte C and Graham JR (1984a) Chronic paroxysmal hemicrania VII. Mechanical precipitation of attacks: new cases and localization of trigger points. *Cephalalgia* **4**:113–118.

Sjaastad O, Saunte C and Russell D (1984b) Migraine and cluster headache. A continuum or separate nosological entities? *Neuropsych Clin* **3**:7–14.

Sjaastad O, Spierings ELH, Saunte C, Wysocka-Bakowska MM, Sulg I and Fredriksen TA (1984c) 'Hemicrania continua': and indomethacin-responsive headache. II. Autonomic function studies. *Cephalalgia* **4**:265–273.

Sjaastad O, Saunte C and Fredriksen TA (1985) Bilaterality of cluster headache. An hypothesis. *Cephalalgia* **5**:55–58.

Sjaastad O, Aasly J, Fredriksen T and Wysocka-Bakowska MM (1986) Chronic paroxysmal hemicrania. X. On the autonomic involvement. *Cephalalgia* **6**:113–124.

Sjaastad O, Salvesen R and Antonaci F (1987a) Headache research strategy. *Cephalalgia* **7**:1–6.

Sjaastad O, Salvesen R and Antonaci F (1987b) The sweating anomaly in cluster headache. Further observations on the underlying mechanism. *Cephalalgia* **7**:77–81.

Sjaastad O, de Souza Carvalho D and Fragoso YD (1988a) The cluster phenomenon: an unspecific feature? *Cephalalgia* **8**:61–65.

Sjaastad O, Saunte C, Fredriksen TA, de Souza Carvalho D, Fragoso YD, Dale LG and Hørven I (1988b) Cluster headache-like headache, Hageman trait deficiency, retrobulbar neuritis and giant aneurysm. Autonomic function studies. *Cephalalgia* **8**:111–120.

Sjaastad O, de Souza Carvalho D and Zhao Jing-Ming (1988c) 'Mild' cluster headache. *Cephalalgia* **8**:121–126.

Sjaastad O, Antonaci F and Fragoso YD (1988d) Cluster headache. Further observations on the dissociation of pain and autonomic findings. *Cephalalgia* **8**:127–132.

Sjaastad O, de Souza Carvalho D and Zhao Jing-Ming (1988e) On the significance of the so-called minibouts. *Cephalalgia* **8**:285–291.

Sjaastad O, Fredriksen TA and Antonaci F (1989a) Unilaterality of headache in classic migraine. *Cephalalgia* **9**:71–77.

Sjaastad O, Saunte C, Salvesen R, Fredriksen TA, Seim A, Røe OD, Fostad K, Løbben O-P and Zhao Jing-Ming (1989b) Shortlasting, unilateral neuralgiform headache attacks with conjunctival injection, tearing, sweating, and rhinorrhea. *Cephalalgia* **9**:147–156.

Sjaastad ØV (1967) Determination and occurrence of histamine in the rumen liquor of sheep. *Acta Vet Scand* **8**:50–70.

Sjaastad ØV and Sjaastad O (1965) Salicylates and urinary excretion of histamine. *Acta Pharmacol (Copenh)* **23**:303–311.

Sjaastad ØV and Sjaastad O (1971) Rupture of the imidazole ring of histamine and *N*-acetylhistamine by human intestinal contents. *Acta Pharmacol Toxicol (Copenh)* **30**:366–371.

Sluder G (1908) Role of the sphenopalatine (Meckel's) ganglion in nasal headache. *NY State J Med* **87**:989–990.

Sluder G (1910) The syndrome of sphenopalatine ganglion neurosis. *Am J Med Sci* **140**:868–878.

Sluder G (1913) Etiology, diagnosis, prognosis and treatment of sphenopalatine ganglion neuralgia. *JAMA* **61**;1201–1206.

Sluder G (1915) Hyperplastic sphenoiditis and its clinical relation to the second, third, fourth, fifth, sixth and vidian nerves and nasal ganglion. *Trans Am Laryngol Assoc* 215–242.

Sluder G (1918) *Concerning some Headaches and Eye Disorders of Nasal Origin.* St. Louis: CV Mosby.

Smith SA and Smith SE (1983) Reduced pupillary light reflexes in diabetic autonomic neuropathy. *Diabetologia* **24**:330–332.

Smith SA, Ellis CJK and Smith SE (1979) Inequality of the direct and consensual light reflexes in normal subjects. *Br J Ophthalmol* **63**:523–527.

Snyder SH, Baldessarini RJ and Axelrod J (1966) A sensitive and specific enzymatic isotopic assay for tissue histamine. *J Pharmacol Exp Therap* **153**:544–549.

Solomon S (1986) Cluster headache and the nervus intermedius. *Headache* **26**:3–8.

Solomon S and Apfelbaum RJ (1986) Surgical decompression of the facial nerve in the treatment of chronic cluster headache. *Arch Neurol* **43**:479–482.

Solomon S and Cappa KG (1986) The time relationships of migraine and cluster headache when occurring in the same patient. *Headache* **26**:500–502.

Solomon S and Guglielmo KM (1985) Symptoms of salivary secretion accompanying cluster headache. In: Rose FC (Ed), *Migraine,* pp. 151–155. Basel: Karger.

Solomon S, Apfelbaum RJ and Guglielmo KM (1985) The cluster-tic syndrome and its surgical therapy. *Cephalalgia* **5**:83–89.

Solomon S, Lipton RB and Newman L (1989) Nuchal features of cluster headache. *Cephalalgia* **9** (Suppl. 10):201–202.

Spierings ELH (1980) The involvement of the autonomic nervous system in cluster headache. *Headache* **20**:218–219.

Spierings ELH, Sjaastad O, Saunte C, Wysocka-Bakowska MM and Fredriksen T (1985) Two cases of chronic continuous unilateral headache absolutely responsive to indomethacin—hemicrania continua. In: Rose FC (Ed), *Migraine,* pp. 236–246. Basle: Karger.

Split W, Szmidt M, Prusinski A and Rosniecki J (1983) Ketotifen (Zaditen) as a new drug in cluster headache treatment. Presented at the Vth Symposium 'Migraine and related headaches', *Lodz* 6–7 June 1983.

Stein HJ and Rogado AZ (1980) Chronic paroxysmal hemicrania—two new patients. *Headache* **20**:72–76.

Steinhilber RM, Pearson JS and Rushton JG (1960) Some psychologic considerations of histaminic cephalalgia. *Mayo Clin Proc* **35**:691–699.

Stern FH (1969) Histamine cephalalgia: an often overlooked cause of headache. *Psychosomatics* **10**:53–56.

Stinson EB, Griepp RB, Schroeder JS, Dong Jr E and Shumway NE (1972) Haemodynamic observations one and two years after cardiac transplantation in man. *Circulation* **45**:1183–1194.

Stowell A (1970) Physiologic mechanisms and treatment of histaminic or petrosal neuralgia. *Headache* **9**:187–194.

Sulg IA and Sjaastad O (1983) Multivariable monitoring in the cluster headache syndrome. I. *International Headache Congress, Munich 1983, Book of Abstracts,* p. 33.

Sutherland JM and Eadie MJ (1972) Cluster headache, *Res Clin Stud Headache* **3**:92–125.

Sveinsdottir E, Thorlöf P, Risberg J, Ingvar DH and Lassen N (1971) Calculation of regional cerebral blood flow (rCBF): Initial-slope-index compared height-over-total-area values. In: *Brain and Blood Flow*, pp. 85–93. Bath: The Pitman Press.

Sweet WH (1988) Surgical treatment of chronic cluster headache. *Headache* **28**:669–670.

Sweet WH, Poletti CE and Macon JB (1981) Treatment of trigeminal neuralgia and other facial pains by retro-gasserian injection of glycerol. *Neurosurgery* **9**:647–653.

Symonds C (1952) Migrainous variants. *Trans Med Soc Lond* **67**:237–250.

Symonds C (1956) A particular variety of headache. *Brain* **79**:217–232.

Tabor H and Mosettig E (1949) Isolation of actylhistamine from urine following oral administration of histamine. *J Biol Chem* **180**:703–706.

Tervo T and Tervo K (1987) Distribution of neuropeptides in the anterior segment of the eye: A minireview. In: Sicuteri F, Vecchiet L and Fanciullacci M (Eds), *Trends in Cluster Headache*, pp. 167–178. Amsterdam: Excerpta Medica.

Terzano MG, Manzoni GC and Maione R (1981) Cluster headache in a one year old infant? *Headache* **21**:255–256.

Testa D, Frediani F and Bussone G (1988) Cluster headache-like syndrome due to arteriovenous malformation. *Headache* **28**:36–38.

Tfelt-Hansen, P. (1986) The effect of ergotamine on the arterial system in man, Thesis, Copenhagen.

Tfelt-Hansen P, Paulson OB and Krabbe A (1982) Invasive adenoma of the pituitary gland and chronic migrainous neuralgia: a rare coincidence or a causal relationship? *Cephalalgia* **2**:25–28.

Tham R (1965) Identification of 1-methylimidazole-4 acetic acid—a histamine metabolite—by gas chromatography. *Life Sci* **4**:293–296.

Thevenet JP, Delestrain MC and Dordain G (1983) Hemicranie paroxystique chronique sensible a l'indomethacine. *Presse Med* **12**:2855–2858.

Thomas AL (1975) Periodic migrainous neuralgia associated with an arteriovenous malformation. *Postgrad Med J* **51**:460–462.

Thompson HS (1987) The pupil. In: Moses RA and Hart Jr WM (Eds), *Adler's Physiology of the Eye*, 8th edn. St. Louis: CV Mosby.

Thompson HS and Mensher JH (1971) Adrenergic mydriasis in Horner's syndrome. *Am J Ophthalmol* **72**:472–480.

Tolosa E (1954) Periarteritic lesions of the carotid siphon with the clinical features of a carotid infraclinoidal aneurysm. *J Neurol Neurosurg Psychiat* **17**:300–302.

Toshuiwal P (1986) Anterior ischaemic optic neuropathy secondary to cluster headache. *Acta Neurol Scand* **73**:213–218.

Toussaint D (1968) Raeder's syndrome. In: Vinken PJ and Bruyn GW (Eds), *Handbook of Clinical Neurology*, Vol. V, pp. 333–336. Amsterdam: North Holland.

Tucker WI and O'Neill PB (1952) Benadryl in histamine headache. *Lahey Clin Bull* **7**:218–221.

Turner P (1969) The human eye as a target to analyse the mechanism of action of substances. *Triangle (Eng)* **9**:91–97.

Turner P (1975) The human pupil as a model for clinical pharmacological investigations. *J R Coll Phys (Lond)* **9**:165–172.

Turner P (1980) Tests of autonomic function in assessing centrally-acting drugs. *Br J Clin Pharmacol* **10**:93–99.

Turner P and Sneddon JM (1968) Alpha receptor blockade by thymoxamine in the human eye. *Clin Pharmacol Ther* **9**:45–49.

Unger WG, Stamford IF and Bennett A (1971) Extraction of prostaglandins from human blood. *Nature* **233**:336–337.

Urbach KF (1949) Nature and probable origin of conjugated histamine excreted after ingestion of histamine. *Proc Soc Exp Biol Med* **70**:146–152.

Vail HH (1932) Vidian neuralgia. *Ann Otol Rhinol Laryngol* **41**:837–856.

Vaisrub S (1975) Brain and heart—the autonomic connection. *JAMA* **234**:959.

Vallery-Radot P and Blamoutier P (1925) Syndrome de vasodilatation hémicéphalique d'origine sympathique (hémicraine, hémihydrorrée nasale, hémilarmoiement). *Bull Soc Med Hôp, Paris* **49**:1488–1493.

Vallery-Radot P, Wolfromm R and Barbizet J (1951) Syndrome de vasodilatation hémicéphalique ou céphalée histaminique. *Presse Méd* **59**:589–590.

Vecchiet L, Geppetti P, Marchionini A, Frille S, Spillantini MG, Fanciullacci M and Sicuteri F (1987) Cerebrospinal fluid (Methionin⁵)-, enkephalin-, substance-P- and somastatin-like immunoreactivities in painful and painless human diseases. In: Sicuteri F, Vecchiet L and Fanciullacci M (Eds), *Trends in Cluster Headache*, pp. 135–143. Amsterdam: Excerpta Medica.

Veger T, Russell D and Sjaastad O (1976) Histamine H_2 antagonists and cluster headache. *Br Med J* **ii**:585.

Vijayan N and Dreyfus PM (1975) Posttraumatic dysautonomic cephalalgia. *Arch Neurol* **32**:649–652.

Vijayan N and Watson C (1978) Pericarotid syndrome. *Headache* **18**:244–254.

Vijayan N and Watson CE (1982) Evaluation of oculocephalic sympathetic function in vascular headache syndromes. Part II. Oculocephalic sympathetic function in cluster headache. *Headache* **22**:200–202.

Vijayan N and Watson C (1984) Corneal sensitivity in cluster headache. *Headache* **24**:162.

Vijayan N and Watson C (1989) The pericarotid region and cluster headache. *Headache* **29**:189.

Vincent MB (1988) Hemicrania paroxistica cronica (CPH). Centro de Ciencias Biologicas e de Medicina Pontifica Universidade Catolica do Rio de Janeiro, Brazil, Thesis.

Vistinini D, Trabattoni G, Manzoni GC, Lechi A, Bortone L and Behan PO (1986) Immunological studies in cluster headache and migraine. *Headache* **26**:398–402.

Waldenlind E (1987) Cluster headache: Studies on monoaminergic platelet functions and endocrine rhythms. Stockholm: Repro Print A/S.

Waldenlind E and Gustafsson SA (1987) Prolactin in cluster headache: Diurnal secretion, response to thyrotropin-releasing hormone, and relation to sex steroids and gonadotropins. *Cephalalgia* **7**:43–54.

Waldenlind E, Ekbom K, Friberg Y, Sääf J and Wetterberg L (1984a) Decreased nocturnal serum melatonin levels during active cluster headache periods. *Opusc Med* **29**:109–112.

Waldenlind E, Saar J, Ekbom K, Ross S, Wahlund L-O and Wetterberg L (1984b) Kinetics and thermolability of platelet monoamine oxidase in cluster headache and migraine. *Cephalalgia* **4**:125–134.

Waldenlind E, Ross SB, Sääf J, Ekbom K and Wetterberg L (1985) Concentration and uptake of 5-hydroxytryptamine in platelets from cluster headache and migraine patients. *Cephalalgia* **5**:45–54.

Waltz TA, Dalessio D and Ott KH (1985) Trigeminal cistern glycerol injections for facial pain. In: Pfaffenrath V, Lundberg P-O and Sjaastad O (Eds), *Updating in Headache*, pp. 35–40. Berlin: Springer-Verlag.

Waters WE and O'Connor PJ (1970) The clinical validation of a headache questionnaire. In: Cochrane AL (Ed), *Background to Migraine*, pp. 1–10. London: Heinemann.

Watson CP, Morley TP, Richardson JC, Schutz H and Tasker RR (1983) The surgical treatment of chronic cluster headache. *Headache* **23**:289–295.

Weiss LD, Ramasastry SS and Eidelman BH (1989) Treatment of a cluster headache patient in a hyperbaric chamber. *Headache* **29**:109–110.

Welch KM (1986) Naproxen sodium in the treatment of migraine. *Cephalalgia* **6** (Suppl. 4):85–92.

West TE, Davies RJ and Kelly RE (1976) Horner's syndrome and headache due to carotid artery disease. *Br Med J*, **i**:818–820.

Wetterqvist H and White T (1970) Bioassay of histamine in human urine. An improved method for purification of samples. *Scand J Clin Lab Invest* **25**:325–328.

Wilkinson M (1982) *Migraine and Headaches*. London: Martin Dunitz.

Williams RL, Karacan I and Hursh CJ (1974) *EEG of Human Sleep*. New York: Wiley.

Wilson WC (1936) Observations relating to the innervation of the sweat glands of the face. *Clin Sci* **2**:273–286.

Wolff HG (1972) In: Dalessio D (Ed), *Headache and Other Head Pain*, 3rd edn. New York: Oxford University Press.

Wood EH and Friedman AP (1974) Thermography in cluster headache. *Arch Neurobiol (Madr)* **37**:85–94.

World Federation of Neurology's Research Group on Migraine and Headache (1970) Definition of migraine. In: Cochrane AL (Ed), *Background to Migraine*, pp. 181–182. London: Heinemann.

Yamamoto M and Meyer JS (1980) Hemicranial disorder of vasomotor adrenoceptors in migraine and cluster headache. *Headache* **20**:321–335.
Ziegler DK and Ellis DJ (1985) Naproxen sodium in prophylaxis of migraine. In: Pfaffenrath V, Lundberg P-O and Sjaastad O (Eds), *Updating in Headache*, pp. 192–196. Berlin: Springer Verlag.

Index

abortive attacks   55–7
acetylcholine   210, 246, 388
  assay   180
acetylsalicylic acid   377
acupuncture   384
adenosine diphosphate (ADP)   170–1
adenosine triphosphate (ATP)   170
adenylate cyclase   174
adrenaline   171, 246
adrenocorticotrophic hormone (ACTH)   165
alcohol consumption   26, 80, 242, 176–7
angina pectoris   243
anhidrosis, facial   212, 215
anorexia   69
anterior cerebral artery stimulation   264
anterior communicating artery aneurysm   262
arteriovenous malformations   110–11
antihistamines   384
ataxia, mild   70
atrial fibrillation   188, 190 (fig.)
atrioventricular block   188
atropine   386, 388
atypical cluster headache (cluster headache variant)   104–6, 194–6
  corneal temperature   198
atypical facial neuralgia   2, 102–4
atypical facial pain   103
auriculotemporal nerve resection   282
autonomic faciocephalalgia   2, 15
autonomic nervous system (episodic cluster headache)   48, 49 (fig.), 235, 247–57, 260
  blockade of autonomic impulses   237–8
  cardiac disturbances   188–9
  fibres to forehead   213
  first-neuron dysfunction   214, 220–1
  parameters   205 (table)
  second-neuron dysfunction   214, 220–1
  third-neuron dysfunction   48, 214–15, 216, 220–1, 224, 256

autonomic nervous system (episodic cluster headache) (cont.)
  variables   49–50
  see also parasympathetic system; sympathetic system

benadryl   132
benign exertional headache   371 (table)
bilateral headache   48–51, 98–107, 260–1
  atypical cluster headache (cluster headache variant)   104–6, 194–6
  atypical facial neuralgia   102–4
  cluster migraine   99–100
  migraine see migraine
  psychogenic headache   106–7
  sinusitis   98
  Sluder's sphenopalatine ganglion headache   100–2
  vidian neuralgia   102
biological rhythms (circannual rhythms)   240, 265
Bing's description   13
β-blocking agents   94, 128
blood pressure   189, 244
blurred vision   63, 64
bradycardia   70, 235, 249
brufen   378, 384
budipine   128–9, 384
butazolidine   137, 378

calcium blocking agents   118 (table), 124, 279–80
cardiovascular reflexes   189
carotid artery
  occlusive disease   200
  spontaneous dissecting aneurysm   87–8
  see also external carotid artery; internal carotid artery
carotid body   257–9